Waste Management and Environmental Health

Waste Management and Environmental Health

Editor: Victor Bonn

Callisto Reference
www.callistoreference.com

Callisto Reference,
118-35 Queens Blvd., Suite 400,
Forest Hills, NY 11375, USA

Visit us on the World Wide Web at:
www.callistoreference.com

ISBN: 978-1-63239-886-4 (Hardback)

The publisher's policy is to use permanent paper from mills that operate a sustainable forestry policy. Furthermore, the publisher ensures that the text paper and cover boards used have met acceptable environmental accreditation standards.

Printed in China.

Cataloging-in-Publication Data

Waste management and environmental health / edited by Victor Bonn.
p. cm.
Includes bibliographical references and index.
ISBN 978-1-63239-886-4
1. Refuse and refuse disposal. 2. Environmental health. 3. Salvage (Waste, etc.).
4. Factory and trade waste. 5. Sewage--Environmental aspects. I. Bonn, Victor.

TD791 .W37 2017
628.4--dc23

Table of Contents

Preface

Every book is initially just a concept; it takes months of research and hard work to give it the final shape in which the readers receive it. In its early stages, this book also went through rigorous reviewing. The notable contributions made by experts from across the globe were first molded into patterned chapters and then arranged in a sensibly sequential manner to bring out the best results.

Waste management refers to the processes, methods and tools that are used in the handling and management of waste. This book on waste management deals with the challenges of waste accumulation and its increasing adverse impact on environmental health. Waste management techniques seek to convert potentially hazardous material into usable substances while reducing the overall negative impacts. Contents in this book highlight the various methods and technologies that are used in turning hazardous waste into biodegradable substances and promoting the health and sustainability of the environment. This book attempts to assist those with a goal of delving into the fields of waste management and ecotoxicology. It is a collective contribution of a renowned group of international experts. This book is a resource guide for experts as well as students.

It has been my immense pleasure to be a part of this project and to contribute my years of learning in such a meaningful form. I would like to take this opportunity to thank all the people who have been associated with the completion of this book at any step.

Editor

1

Bio-ethanol production by a novel autochthonous thermo-tolerant yeast isolated from wastewater

Azadeh Tofighi[1*], Mahnaz Mazaheri Assadi[2], Mohammad Hosein Arash Asadirad[3] and Shohreh Zare Karizi[1]

Abstract

Background: It has been known for years that ethanol is a bio-fuel to replace fossil fuels. The ethanol industry requires the utilization of micro-organisms capable production with stresses. The purpose of present study was to isolate and characterize ethanologenic yeast with high potential application at high temperature to produce bio-ethanol.

Methods: To isolate ethanologenic yeasts, wastewater samples from a starch producer plant in Varamin, Iran were used. The isolates were identified by molecular characterization. Characteristics of the isolated strains were determined at 30, 35, 40 and 45°C for 48 hours.

Results: 50 yeast strains capable of growing well in agar plates in a temperature range of 30–45°C were isolated. Out of the isolated strains, only three strains were screened for their ability to grow at 45°C. Selected yeast, designated as AT-3 strain which showed efficient flocculation capabilities with higher ethanol production and grew faster as compared to the rest of strains in media with 180 g/L glucose at 35°C. The selected yeast was identified as a new strain of *Saccharomyces cerevisiae* and submitted to the Gene-Bank database. Its' optimum growth temperature was between 35 and 40°C. The results showed that during the bio-ethanol production 2.5×10^{10} and 8.5×10^{9} (CFU/mL) were a good indication of strain capability in heat tolerance. Also, ethanol produced at a raise of 6.9% and 6.85% (w/v) at 35 and 40°C, respectively, whereas glucose-to-ethanol conversion yield was about 75% of the theoretical value.

Conclusions: Results emphasized that the isolated strain identified as *Saccharomyces cerevisiae*. This specific strain has thermo-tolerant, osmo-tolerant, flocculating capabilities with potential for application in developing a low cost ethanol industry.

Keywords: Ethanol, Isolation, Stress, Thermo stability, Wastewater, Yeast

Background

Ethanol is an important liquid product with potential as a bio-fuel to replace fossil fuels [1]. To be able to substitute bio-ethanol for gasoline, one must overcome many obstacles including low cost bio-ethanol production [2]. The ability of microbes for adaptation can be used for decreasing ethanol prices [3]. Industrial ethanol production depends on microbial activity, particularly that of yeasts. In industrial ethanol production, there are many important factors which should be considered. Temperature is one of the most important environmental factors affecting microbial activity [4]. Two of the problems associated with fermentation of sugar are the high temperatures (35-45°C) and high ethanol concentration (over 20%) [5]. Like all microorganisms, yeasts exhibit specific characteristics when growing at different growth temperatures [6]. Thermo-tolerant yeast refers to the yeasts possess optimum temperatures values above 40°C, as well as, the maximum temperature values range from 35°C up to 40–41°C for *Saccharomyces cerevisiae* strains [7,8]. Using thermo-tolerant yeasts for bio-ethanol production have several benefits: (i) Rapid metabolic activity, high fermentation rate and output. (ii) Reduction of gas solubility. (iii) Decreasing the viscosity of the media along with increasing temperature. (iv) Reduction of energy requirement. (v) Minimizing the chance of contamination [2,3,5,6,9].

* Correspondence: a_assadirad@yahoo.com
[1]Department of Biology, Varamin-Pishva Branch, Islamic Azad University, Pishva, Iran
Full list of author information is available at the end of the article

The ability of micro-organisms to adapt to different temperature environments has attracted considerable attention. Ethanol production in the world is sustained by fermentation with ethanologenic yeast. The growth of yeasts varies according to temperature [4,8]. In many countries, summer temperatures frequently reach over 35°C. Cooling costs during the process of ethanol production are expensive. Therefore, thermo-tolerant ethanologenic yeast strains would be useful for reducing the production cost [2,3]. Tolerance to high temperatures and ethanol concentrations are important factors of microorganisms for increasing efficiency on the industrial scale [1,5].

Therefore using the micro-organism with tolerance toward the inhibitors like high temperature, can increase the yield of ethanol production [5,10] and decrease the price of production [2]. The aim of this study was to isolate and screen indigenous thermo-tolerant yeasts producing ethanol at high temperature from wastewater in the city of Varamin in Iran during summer season.

Materials and methods

Media

The media and chemicals were purchased from Merck (Germany). The main sources of all the chemicals concentrations for culture medium were chosen based on the literature [11]. Rose Bengal Chloramphenicol Agar was used for yeast isolation, which consisted of 10 g glucose; 5 g papaic digest of soybean meal, 1 g KH_2PO_4, 0.5 g $MgSO_4$, 7 H_2O and 15 g agar in 1 litre distilled water. 0.05 g/L Rose Bengal and 0.5 g/L Chloramphenicol were also added for the inhibition of fast growing fungi and bacterial growth [11]. Potato Dextrose Agar (PDA) medium containing 300 g potato, 20 g Dextrose and 20 g agar in 1 litre distilled water was used for preparing inoculums. Two other media were used for screening process. These two media were designated as pre-culture and fermentation media. Pre-culture medium, consisted of 30 g glucose, 10 g yeast extract, 0.6 g ammonium phosphate and 1.2 g ammonium sulphate, per litre. A synthetic medium used for fermentation which consisted, per litre, 180 g glucose, 10 g yeast extract, 0.6 g ammonium phosphate and 1.2 g ammonium sulphate. These screening media were adjusted to pH 5.5 with 1 N HCl. All the media were autoclaved at 121°C and 15 Lb pressure for 15 minutes. For each purpose, experiments were performed in triplicates. The medium was prepared as reported by Tofighi et al. [11].

Sampling

To isolate ethanol producing yeasts, wastewater samples (200 mL) were collected from ten different sites of same sampling station in a starch producing plant in Varamin (Iran) on Jul. 2010, in to sterilized Erlenmeyer flasks, which were loosely covered and transported on ice to the laboratory within 1 h of collection. At the time of sampling some physicochemical parameters of effluents such as, temperature (°C), pH, BOD and COD were checked [12].

Yeast isolation and maintenance

For balancing the buffering capacity, 90 mL phosphate buffer (pH: 7.0) was added to the samples and shaken vigorously for 1 h. After that, 100 μL of the supernatants were spread on sterilized Rose Bengal Chloramphenicol Agar plates. The cultivated media were incubated aerobically at 30, 35, 40 and 45°C for 3 days. Representative colonies were selected randomly on the basis of colony color and distinct morphological appearance, purified and observed under microscope. In this order, the classical methods described by Barnnet et al. were used [13]. Subsequently, they were stored in 20% glycerol at −75°C for further analysis [14] and deposited at PTCC (Persian Type Culture Collection).

Molecular identification procedures

Total genomic DNA from the isolates was extracted [15]. Primarily, the selected yeast isolates were identified based on 18S rRNA gene (partial), ITS1, 5.8S rRNA gene, ITS2 and 26S rRNA (partial) gene. 18S rRNA gene was amplified by primers NS-1 (5′-GTAGTCATATGCTTGTCTC) as forward and NS-8 (5'-TCCGCAGGTTCACCTAC GGA) as reverse primer. It was sequenced using D1/D2 domain of the 26S rRNA gene sequencing. 26S rRNA gene was amplified with NL-1 (5′-GCATATCAATAAGCG GAGGAAAAG) as a forward primer and NL-4 (5′-GG TCCGTGTTTCAAGACGG) as a reverse primer to specific differentiation ITS region of *S. cerevisiae* [16]. PCR was performed in a final volume of 50 μL containing 1× Buffer, 2.5 mM MgCl2, 250 μM (each) dNTP Mix, 1U Taq Polymerase, 0.2 μM of each primers and 20 ng of the extracted DNA. Amplifications were performed for 36 PCR cycles with denaturing at 94°C for 1 min, annealing at 52°C for 1 min, and extension at 72°C for 2 min, with the final extension for 10 min [17]. Polymerase chain reaction products were separated by 1.5% (w/v) agarose gel electrophoresis in 0.5× TBE buffer with ethidium bromide (05 μg/mL) [15]. Purification and sequencing were performed by the Iranian Biological Resource Center (IBRC). Research for DNA similarity was performed with the National Centre of Biotechnology Information Gene-Bank.

Screening the thermo-tolerant, osmo-tolerant and ethanologenic yeasts

To prepare inoculums, pure isolated strains were streaked on sterilized PDA plates and incubated at 30°C. After 48 h incubation time, one loop-full of cells was transferred to 250 mL sterilized conical flask containing 50 mL pre-culture medium. The pre-culture media were incubated on rotary shaker at 30°C, 150 rev/min for 20 h. Then, the ability of the selected strains to produce ethanol was determined by transferring 6.16×10^7 CFU/mL cells from pre- culture to fermentation media. Since the yeast cells should grow in aerobic conditions for the first 8 hours, the flasks were placed on a shaker-incubator at 30°C, 150 rev/min. After this period, the cultures were aseptically transferred to a 100 mL sterilized Erlenmeyer flask, equipped with rubber stoppers and sterile syringe needles. Subsequently, to complete the fermentation process and screen the thermo-tolerant yeasts, the fermentation medium was incubated at 30, 35, 40 and 45°C for a further 40 hours under anaerobic conditions [10]. All experiments were performed in triplicates.

Analytical method

The sugar consumption during cultivation were quantified using an enzymatic method (Kit Glucose (GOD – PAP), Pars Azmun, Iran). Samples were aseptically taken to determine the optical density at 600 nm [18]. Ethanol concentrations were determined using gas chromatography on 14A Shimadzu as described previously by Tofighi et al. [11]. The bio-ethanol concentration in each sample was determined using a standard curve of ethanol.

Results and discussion

Isolation of yeast strains

During industrial bio-ethanol production, microorganisms are exposed to numerous environmental stresses such as high temperature and high sugar concentrations. Cellular micro molecules are seriously damaged under stress conditions, which leading to inhibition of cell growth and fermentation. To avoid lethal damage, bio-ethanol industry requires the utilization of microorganisms capable of working with stresses. Stress-tolerant microorganisms are thought to naturally occur; primarily in contaminated area. Studies suggested that physicochemical parameters of contaminated area, such as Hydrogen ion concentration (pH), can contribute to survive and tolerance of microorganisms against stresses. General effect of pH on cells is related to the rates of enzymatic reactions [19]. The measurement of Biological Oxygen Demand (BOD) and Chemical Oxygen Demand (COD) of the wastewater samples exhibited the rate of effluent pollution [20]. In the present study, the pH values of wastewater samples was about 4 and revealed no significant differences at all locations. Also, BOD and COD measurements was about 33 mg/L and 179 mg/L, respectively; which, indicated the wastewater samples were belonged to weakly contaminant wastewater [20]. Survival of microorganisms in the unfavorable conditions depends on their tolerance mechanisms. So, in this research, efforts were made to isolate and screen thermo-tolerant yeasts from wastewater. 50 colonies were isolated from studied industrial effluents.

Selection and identification of the thermo-tolerant and osmo-tolerant yeast strains

Out of the 50 yeast isolated colonies, three strains showed high growth rate at 40 and 45°C on the solid medium. The selected colonies were designated as AT-3, AT-7 and AT-16. Among the isolated, AT-3 was capable of producing floccules whereas AT-7 and AT-16 did not flocculate in fermentation media.

Molecular identification of the isolates according to the 5.8S-ITS rRNA sequence analysis showed that the AT-7 and AT-16 strains belonged to the species *Candida tropicalis* and the strain AT-3 belonged to the species *Saccharomyces cerevisiae* which exhibited 95% homology with *Saccharomyces cerevisiae* with accession number of *GU080045.1*. Then, to achieve a certain identification of the yeasts D1/D2 region of 26S rRNA was sequenced and compared with those available in the EMBL nucleotide sequence database. Gene analysis of AT-3 strain based on 26S rRNA (partial) showed 98% phylogenetic relationships among strain AT-3 and *Saccharomyces cerevisiae* with accession number of *GQ376089.1*. The species-specific partial D1/D2 domain and 5.8S ITS region sequences were submitted to the Gene-Bank database as *Saccharomyces cerevisiae* AT-1350 under accession number: KF725624.

Phylogenetic tree of AT-3 strain was constructed using the neighbour-joining method and illustrated in Figure 1.

Effect of high temperatures on growth

The cell mass of the yeast strains after 48 hours of incubation was measured by optical density at 600 nm. Moreover, at this time, pH values of the fermentation media was determined between 3.8-4.3. The influence of different temperatures (30, 35, 40 and 45°C) on growth of the isolated strains in the media with 180 g/L glucose, during the 48 h batch cultivation is displayed in Figure 2. As showed, the highest cell mass productivity was obtained at 30°C for AT-16 and at 35, 40 and 45°C for AT-3 strain. The results indicated that, the AT-3 strain is able to survive at higher temperatures. The highest cell mass productivity in anaerobic conditions was obtained at 35 and 40°C for AT-3. The cell mass in the first 8 hours (aerobic condition) and in the second part (40 h, anaerobic condition) was determined at the temperature studied. As presented in Figure 2, the cell mass productivity is affected with increasing the temperatures. These results agree with Ali Shah et al. [6] and Torija et al. [4] reported that yeast's viability decreases and the fermentation process is inhibited as the temperature increases. This may be related to the passage of time (48 hours), reduction of

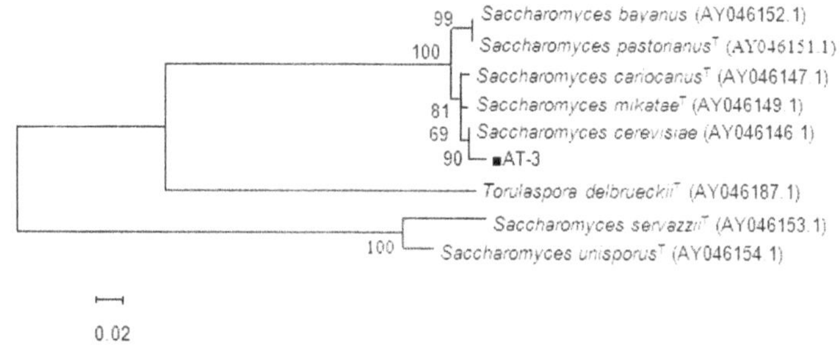

Figure 1 Neighbour-joining tree of the AT-3 isolate and type strains of related genera. Neighbour-joining tree based on 18S rRNA gene (partial), ITS1, 5.8S rRNA gene, ITS2 and 26S rRNA (partial) gene sequence showing the phylogenetic relationships among Strain AT-3 and type strains of related genera. Numbers at branch nodes are bootstrap values (percentages of 1000 replicates). Bar 2 substitutions per 100 nucleotide positions.

pH [19], the differences between the regulatory elements of stress responses in aerobic and anaerobic conditions as well as their sensitivity to ethanol toxicity [21-23].

Effect of high temperatures on ethanol productivity

The effect of elevated temperature on ethanol productivity (w/v)% in isolated yeasts was investigated (Figure 3). As illustrated, the ethanol productivity within 48 hours was determined to be about 5.32, 3.3 and 3.2 (w/v)% for the AT-3, AT-7 and AT-16 strains at 30°C; 6.9, 2.69 and 2.65 (w/v)% at 35°C; 6.85, 1.4 and 1.02 (w/v)% at 40°C as well as 2.8, 0.62 and 0.2(w/v)% at 45°C, respectively. As shown, the AT-3 strain could also tolerate and produce ethanol at higher temperatures. Our results indicated that the optimum temperature of the AT-3 strain was between 30–40°C and showed a tolerance against high temperature. Also, the highest ethanol productivity within 48 hours was obtained for the AT-3 strain at 30°C. It rose up to 150% at 35°C and decreased sharply over this temperature. At the same time the AT-3 ethanol concentration rate (Figure 3) increased about 130% at 35°C and was maintained at 40°C, further decreased occurred slowly at 45°C. Yeast growth and ethanol production decreased at 45°C too. The cells remained active but not progressive at temperatures above that. Cimpeanu et al. [9] also isolated thermo-tolerant yeast belonged to *Saccharomyces cerevisiae.* They confirmed that, thermo-tolerant yeast could promote high yield of ethanol at high temperatures [9].

Effect of high temperatures on glucose consumption

Media containing 180 g/L glucose was used in batch fermentations at the temperature range of 30–45°C for 48 h (Figure 4). As shown, glucose metabolism of AT-3 strain was stimulated from 17.14 -17.88 g/L, with increasing temperature from 30–35°C. When fermentation continued at temperatures over 35°C, production decreased rapidly. Glucose consumption of AT-7 and AT-16 strains was about 12.5 g/L at 30°C which decreased with increasing the temperature. In this work, we have shown that increasing the temperature up to 40°C did not have any negative effects on the AT-3 strain. Also, inhibition effects of the high glucose concentration were shown for the AT-7 and AT-16 strains. The highest metabolized glucose rate for AT-3 was obtained at 40°C and then at 35 and 30°C. This is may be because of the cells effort to survive at undesired conditions [24-26].

The data showed that the AT-3 strain could remain active at high temperatures to continue the fermentation process. Glucose-to-ethanol conversion yield of AT-3 was about 75% of the theoretical value at 35 and 40°C.

On the other hand, the AT-7 and AT-16 strains showed a good activity regarding the fermentation process using the media with high concentration of glucose at the range of 30–45°C.

The results indicated that the growth rate and ethanol productivity of the isolated yeasts were significantly affected by the temperature studied. The results showed that, in comparison with AT-7 and AT-16, AT-3 strain exhibited a good advantage at the highest temperature in the osmotic pressure, and we considered them osmo-tolerant and flocculating. These results were consistent with Kiran Sree et al. [10], and Nahvi et al. [27] studies which reported that flocculation ability could help the yeast strains to withstand the environmental pressures. The optimum temperature for the growth of AT-3 in aerobic conditions was between 35 and 40°C, for AT-7 and AT-16 was about 30°C.

The ability of microorganisms to adapt to different temperatures has attracted considerable attention, but the mechanism underlying this phenomenon is not well understood. Yeast cells exhibit a rapid molecular response when exposed to elevated temperatures [28]. Thermo-tolerance appears to involve a range of complex

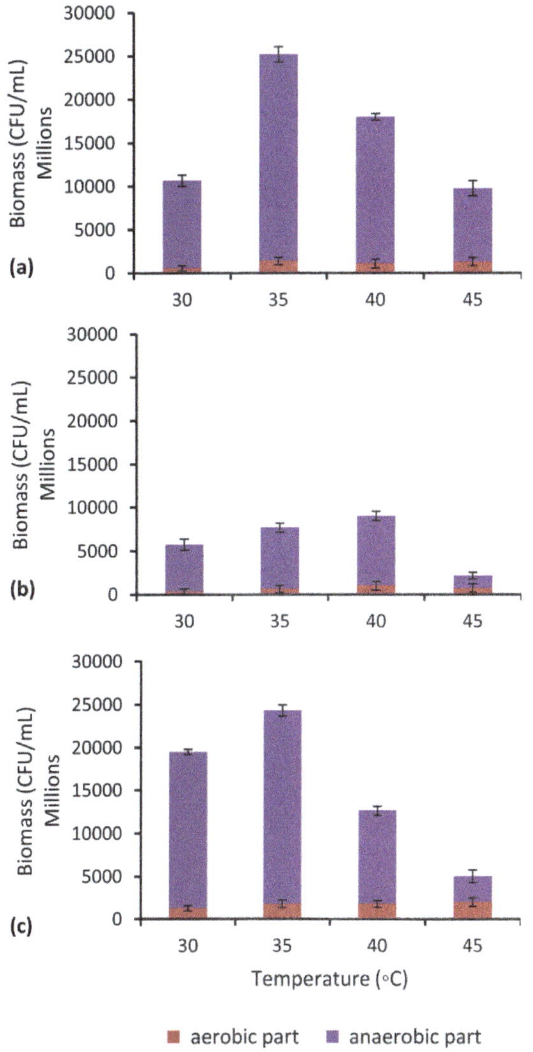

Figure 2 Effect of temperature on growth of selected strains. The growth of selected strains in different temperatures during the batch cultivation. Fermentation process was separated in aerobic (8 h) and anaerobic (40 h) parts. Error bars represent standard deviation of three replicates. **(a)**: AT-3; **(b)**: AT-7 and **(c)**: AT-17.

mechanisms [5,23,28,29]. Several mechanisms have been reported to be associated with stress responses, based on the ability to produce flocculated cells [10,27,30] and/or cause changes in gene expression [31,32], to affect membrane or cellular composition [23,29], and induce heat shock proteins such as Hsp90 [33]. Markedly, the heat shock response in yeast is one of the best molecularly characterized responses of eukaryotic cells and has been widely reviewed [34]. Some researchers have demonstrated that in some yeasts, the heat shock elements (HSE) are unresponsive to other stress (osmotic, oxidative, DNA damage, glucose repression, etc.) [23]. Moreover, the stress

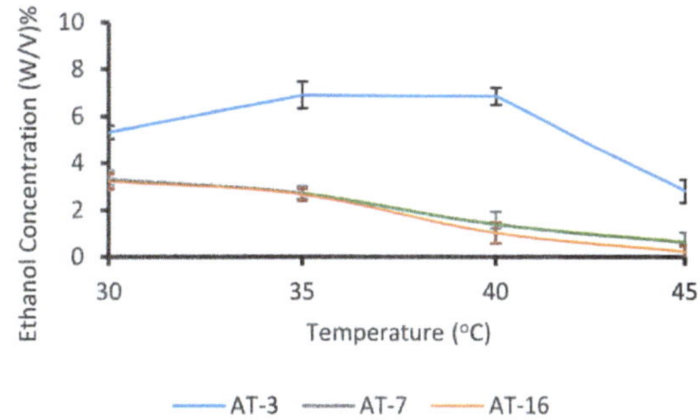

Figure 3 Effect of temperature on ethanol productivity of the selected strains. Ethanol concentrations of the selected strains in different temperatures during the batch cultivation after 48 hours. Error bars represent standard deviation of three replicates.

of environmental changes and selective pressures can actually influence the evolutionary processes [33,35]. Also, Kiran Sree et al. [10], and Cimpeanu et al. [9] indicated that, high concentration of glucose in the medium inhibited the growth of yeast cells and the production of ethanol, and the inhibitory effect is attributed to high osmotic pressure.

Conclusions

In this study, the AT-3 strain was found as autochthonous yeast with tolerance against high glucose concentrations. It is a flocculent strain that belongs to *Saccharomyces cerevisiae* with the optimum temperature over 35°C. The growth rate and ethanol productivity are stable at high temperatures (between 35–45°C). The glucose-to-ethanol conversion yields are about 75% of the theoretical value at 35 and 40°C. According to the data, we would like to highlight the AT-3 strain as a novel, highly desirable thermo-tolerant, osmo-tolerant, and flocculent *Saccharomyces* for

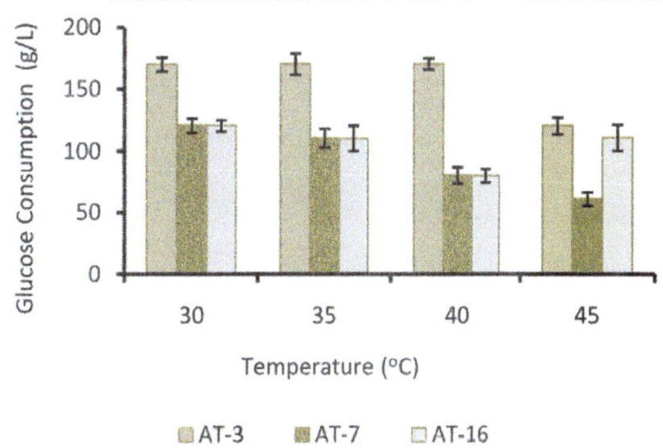

Figure 4 Effect of temperature on glucose consumption of the selected strains in the fermentation media. Glucose consumption of the selected strains in the media with 180 g/L glucose, in different temperatures during the batch cultivation after 48 hours. Error bars represent standard deviation of three replicates.

the low cost alcohol production industry especially in hot areas.

Competing interests

The authors declare that they have no competing interests.

Authors' contributions

AT and MHAA participated in the design and carried out the experimental studies. AT and SZK carried out the molecular genetic studies. AT, MMA, MHAA and SZK participated in draft the manuscript. All authors read and approved the final manuscript.

Acknowledgements

We would like to thank Deputy of Research of Varamin-Pishva Branch, Islamic Azad University for financial support of the project. The help rendered by Dr. Geoffrey Lin-Cereghino, Dr. Amir M. Assadi-Rad and Ms. Tarlan Tofighi are highly appreciated.

Author details

[1]Department of Biology, Varamin-Pishva Branch, Islamic Azad University, Pishva, Iran. [2]Departments of Biotechnology, Iranian Research Organization for Science and Technology, Tehran, Iran. [3]Departments of Microbiology, Zanjan Branch, Islamic Azad University, Zanjan, Iran.

References

1. Basso LC, Amorim HV, Oliveira AJ, Lopes ML: **Yeast selection for fuel ethanol production in Brazil.** *FEMS Yeast Res* 2008, **8**:1155–1163.
2. Rosenberger A, Kaul HP, Senn T, Aufhammer W: **Costs of bioethanol production from winter cereals: the effect of growing conditions and crop production intensity levels.** *Ind Crop Prod* 2002, **15**:91–102.
3. Abdel-Banat BM, Hoshida H, Ano A, Nonklang S, Akada R: **High-temperature fermentation: how can processes for ethanol production at high temperatures become superior to the traditional process using mesophilic yeast?** *Appl Microbiol Biotechnol* 2010, **85**(4):861–867.
4. Torija MJ, Rozes N, Poblet M, Guillamon JM, Mas A: **Effects of fermentation temperature on the strain population of *Saccharomyces cerevisiae*.** *Int J Food Microbiol* 2003, **80**:47–53.
5. Banat IM, Nigam P, Singh D, Marchant R, McHale AP: **Review: ethanol production at elevated temperatures and alcohol concentrations: part I- yeasts in general.** *World J Microbiol Biotechnol* 1998, **14**:809–821.
6. Ali Shah F, Aziz S, Memon HR, Rajoka MI: **Ethanol production kinetics by a thermo-tolerant mutant of *Saccharomyces cerevisiae* from starch industry waste (Hydrol).** *Pak J Anal Environ Chem* 2010, **11**(1):16–21.
7. Koedrith P, Dubois E, Scherens B, Jacobs E, Boonchird C, Messenguy F: **Identification and characterization of a thermotolerant yeast strain isolated from banana leaves.** *ScienceAsia* 2008, **34**:147–152.
8. Van Uden N: **Temperature profiles of yeasts.** *Adv Microb Physiol* 1984, **25**:195–251.
9. Cimpeanu C, Campeanu G, Begea M, Vladescu M, Cornea CP: **Bioethanol production by new thermotolerant Romanian yeast strains.** *Rom Biotechnol Lett* 2010, **15**(3):5310–5316.
10. Kiran Sree N, Sridhar M, Suresh K, Banat IM, Venkateswar RL: **Isolation of thermotolerant, osmotolerant, flocculating *Saccharomyces cerevisiae* for ethanol production.** *Bioresour Technol* 2000, **72**:43–46.
11. Tofighi A, Azin M, Mazaheri Assadi M, Assadi-rad MHA, Nejadsattari T, Fallahian MR: **Inhibitory effect of high concentrations of furfural on industrial strain of *Saccharomyces cerevisiae*.** *Int J Environ Res* 2010, **4**(1):137–142.
12. Health Association APHA - A: *Standard Methods for the Examination for Water and Wastewater.* 20th edition. Washington: AWWA, WPCF; 1998.
13. Barnnet JA, Payne RW, Yarow P: *A guide to identifying and classifying yeasts.* London: Cambridge University Press; 1978.
14. Ayogu TE: **Evaluation of the performance of yeast isolate from Nigerian palm wine in wine production from pineapple fruits.** *Bioresour Technol* 1999, **69**:189–190.
15. Kurtzman CP, Robnett CJ: **Identification and phylogeny of ascomycetous yeasts from analysis of nuclear large subunit (26S) ribosomal DNA partial sequences.** *Antonie Van Leeuwenhoek* 1998, **73**:331–371.
16. Kurtzman CP, Robnett CJ: **Phylogenetic relationships among yeasts of the 'Saccharomyces complex' determined from multigene sequence analyses.** *FEMS Yeast Res* 2003, **3**:417–432.
17. Kurtzman CP: **Recognition of yeast species from gene sequence comparisons.** *Open Appl Inf J* 2011, **5**(Suppl M4):S20–S29.
18. Wikandari R, Millati R, Lennartsson PR, Harmayani E, Taherzadeh MJ: **Isolation and characterization of zygomycetes fungi from tempe for ethanol production and biomass applications.** *Appl Biochem Biotechnol* 2012, **167**(6):1501–1512.
19. Cheng KK, Zhang JA, Ling HZ, Ping WX, Huang W, Ge JP, Xu JM: **Optimization of pH and acetic acid concentration for bioconversion of hemicellulose from corncobs to xylitol by *Candida tropicalis*.** *Biochem Eng J* 2009, **43**:203–207.
20. Samudro G, Mangkoedihardjo S: **Review on BOD, COD and BOD/COD ratio: a triangle zone for toxic, biodegradable and stable levels.** *Int J Academic Res* 2010, **2**(4):235–239.
21. Edgardo A, Carolina P, Manuel R, Juanita F, Baeza J: **Selection of thermotolerant yeast strains *Saccharomyces cerevisiae* for bioethanol production.** *Enzyme Microb Tech* 2008, **43**(2):120–123.
22. Pinilla L, Torres R, Ortiz C: **Bioethanol production in batch mode by a native strain of Zymomonas *mobilis*.** *World J Microbiol Biotechnol* 2011, **27**:2521–2528.
23. Stanley D, Bandara A, Fraser S, Chambers PJ, Stanley GA: **The ethanol stress response and ethanol tolerance of *Saccharomyces cerevisiae*.** *J Appl Microbiol* 2010, **109**(1):13–24.
24. Balakumar S, Arasaratnam V, Balasubramaniam K: **Isolation and improvement of a thermotolerant *Saccharomyces cerevisiae*s train.** *World J Microbiol Biotechnol* 2001, **17**:739–746.
25. Endo A, Nakamura T, Shima J: **Involvement of ergosterol in tolerance to vanillin, a potential inhibitor of bioethanol fermentation, in *Saccharomyces cerevisiae*.** *FEMS Microbiol Lett* 2009, **299**:95–99.
26. Garay-Arroyo A, Covarrubias AA, Clark I, Nino I, Gosset G, Martinez A: **Response to different environmental stress conditions of industrial and laboratory *Saccharomyces cerevisiae* strains.** *Appl Microbiol Biotechnol* 2004, **63**:734–741.
27. Nahvi I, Emtiazi G, Alkabi L: **Isolation of a flocculating *Saccharomyces cerevisiae* and investigation of its performance in the fermentation of beet molasses to ethanol.** *Biomass Bioenergy* 2002, **23**:481–486.
28. Ma M, Liu ZL: **Mechanisms of ethanol tolerance in *Saccharomyces cerevisiae*.** *Appl Microbiol Biotechnol* 2010, **87**(3):829–845.
29. Levin DE: **Cell wall integrity signaling in *Saccharomyces cerevisiae*.** *Microbiol Mol Biol Rev* 2005, **69**(2):262–291.
30. Silva CLC, Vianna CR, Cadete RM, Santos RO, Gomes FCO, Oliveira ES, Rosa CA: **Selection, growth, and chemo-sensory evaluation of flocculent starter culture strains of *Saccharomyces cerevisiae* in the large-scale production of traditional Brazilian cachaça.** *Int J Food Microbiol* 2009, **131**:203–210.
31. Hirasawa T, Yamada K, Nagahisa K, Dinh TN, Furusawa C, Katakura Y, Shioya S, Shimizu H: **Proteomic analysis of responses to osmotic stress in laboratory and sake-brewing strains of *Saccharomyces cerevisiae*.** *Process Biochem* 2009, **44**:647–653.
32. Kim HS, Kim NR, Yang J, Choi W: **Identification of novel genes responsible for ethanol and/or thermotolerance by transposon mutagenesis in *Saccharomyces cerevisiae*.** *Appl Microbiol Biotechnol* 2011, **91**(4):1159–1172.
33. Jarosz DF, Lindquist S: **Hsp90 and environmental stress transform the adaptive value of natural genetic variation.** *Science* 2010, **330**(6012):1820–1824.
34. Verghese J, Abrams J, Wang Y, Morano KA: **Biology of the heat shock responces: building yeast (*Saccharomyces cerevisiae*) as a model system.** *Microbiol Mol Biol Rev* 2012, **76**(2):115–158.
35. Zhao XQ, Bai FW: **Mechanisms of yeast stress tolerance and its manipulation for efficient fuel ethanol production.** *J Biotechnol* 2009, **144**(1):23–30.

2

Application of molecular imprinted polymer nanoparticles as a selective solid phase extraction for preconcentration and trace determination of 2,4-dichlorophenoxyacetic acid in the human urine and different water samples

Fariborz Omidi[1], Mohammad Behbahani[2], Hamid Sadeghi Abandansari[2], Alireza Sedighi[3] and Seyed Jamaleddin Shahtaheri[4*]

Abstract

A molecular-imprinted polymer nanoparticles (MIP-NP) for the selective preconcentration of 2,4-dichlorophenoxyacetic acid (2,4-D) is described. It was obtained by precipitation polymerization from methacrylic acid (the functional monomer), ethylene glycol dimethacrylate (the cross-linker), 2,2′-azobisisobutyronitrile (the initiator) and 2,4-D (the template molecule) in acetonitrile solution. The MIP-NPs were characterized by thermogravimetric analysis, and by scanning electron microscopy. Imprinted 2,4-D molecules were removed from the polymeric structure using acetic acid in methanol (15:85 v/v %) as the eluting solvent. The sorption and desorption process occur within 10 min and 15 min, respectively. The maximum sorbent capacity of the molecular imprinted polymer is 89.2 mg g^{-1}. The relative standard deviation and limit of detection for water samples by introduced selective solid phase extraction were 4.2% and 1.25 µg L^{-1}, and these data for urine samples were 4.7% and 1.80 µg L^{-1}, respectively. The method was applied to the determination of 2,4-D in the urine and different water samples.

Keywords: Molecular imprinted polymer nanoparticles, 2,4-dichlorophenoxyacetic acid, Selective preconcentration, Urine and water samples

Introduction

In recent years, the hazards of using pesticides have been accentuated by the sharp rise in their use in agriculture and industry. Phenoxy herbicides compounds are currently among the most frequently used pesticides worldwide [1]. They have been used on a large scale in agriculture to control the growth of broad-leaved weeds on rice, maize, wheat, and in post-emergence applications in most developing countries [2,3]. Among them, 2,4-dichlorophenoxyacetic acid (2,4-D) is a common important phenoxy herbicide that is selective, systemic auxin-type herbicide extensively used throughout the world for the past 50 years [4]. Exposures to 2,4-D occurs not only in general population groups through trace residues in the diet, from drinking water and direct contact with lawns recently treated with 2,4-D [5] but also persons who occupationally handle (mix, load or apply) it. 2,4-D is rapidly absorbed into the body following ingestion, inhalation and/or dermal contact and is rapidly excreted, predominantly in the urine unchanged [6,7]. Some recent well-documented studies show an association between the agricultural use of the 2,4-dichlorophenoxyacetic acid (2,4-D) and the risk of non- Hodgkin's lymphoma [8]. It has been classified as possibly carcinogenic to humans (IARC, group 2B) [4]. Furthermore, continuous use of 2,4-D may cause soil percolation and groundwater contamination [9]. Due to the presence of the carboxylate group in its structure, this compound can react with metal ions to form complexes which are

* Correspondence: shahtaheri@tums.ac.ir
[4]Department of Occupational Health Engineering, School of Public Health and Institute for Environmental Research, Tehran University of Medical Sciences, Tehran, Iran
Full list of author information is available at the end of the article

sparingly soluble in water. The World Health Organization (WHO), U.S. Environmental Protection Agency (EPA), and national governments such as New Zealand and United State of America (USA) regulation set the maximum contaminant level (MCL) of chlorophenoxy acid herbicides in drinking water in the range of 10-70 ng mL^{-1} [10,11]. Because of its adverse effect on humans, sensitive determination of 2,4-D in environmental and biological samples is necessary.

In the literature, several methods have been developed for determining 2,4-D in different environmental samples, including solid phase microextraction gas chromatography-mass spectrometry (SPME-GC-MS) [12], solid phase extraction high-performance liquid chromatographic with UV detector (SPE-HPLC-UV) [13] and liquid - liquid extraction gas chromatography-mass spectrometry (LLE-GC-MASS) [14] methods. The mentioned methods have major drawbacks as they are very time consuming procedure, requiring expensive instrumentation, affected by matrix effects and have low selectivity and recoveries. According to the complexity of matrix and low content of 2,4-D in real samples, an efficient sample treatment technique with high clean-up and high enrichment factor are required prior to analysis. Thus, development of a rapid and selective extraction technique for determination of 2,4-D from environmental and biological matrices is of great importance.

In recent years, molecularly imprinted polymers (MIPs) and ion imprinted polymers (IIPs) have been extensively used (e.g. SPE sorbent) for preconcentration and high efficient separation of different trace analytes in complex matrices [15-28], based on their unique imprinting and recognition properties. MIPs demonstrate high potential for sample clean-up of very complicated matrix [29], solid-phase extraction [30-34], and solid-phase micro extraction fibers [35]. The most widely employed preparation method for synthesis of MIPs is bulk polymerization. The prepared polymer with this method is then ground and sieved, and particles of usually about 25 mm are collected for subsequent studies.

Although the bulk MIP prepared by conventional methods exhibits high selectivity [36,37], some disadvantages were suffered, such as the heterogeneous distribution of the binding sites, embedding of most binding sites, and poor site accessibility for template molecule [38]. Consequently, the consideration of researchers has moved toward achieving highly uniform spherical imprinted particles, particularly on the nanoscale [39]. In contrast to monoliths, MIPs possess cavities designed for a target analyte, providing a retention mechanism based on molecular recognition; by this, imprinted cavities are more easily available to templates and the binding kinetic is increased [40]. Different methods are used to obtain MIPs Nano particles, namely suspension, multistep swelling and precipitation polymerization. The different methods of preparation have been well documented in a recent review by Haginaka [41]. Among them, the precipitation technique is the most convenient one, because it is a homogeneous, one-step synthesis and does not require the use of a surfactant or stabilizer that can remain adsorbed to the surface of the polymer, interfering with the selective binding of the target to the imprinted materials. The first prepared MIPs, using precipitation polymerization technique, were reported by Ye et al. [42]. The polymer particles were obtained according to this procedure, have more uniform particles size and require no crushing and sieving steps in comparison tothe polymers obtained by bulk polymerization.

The aim of the present study was the preparation of 2,4-D imprinting polymer via non-covalent precipitation polymerization as well as its application in selective sample preparation in order to eliminate the matrix effects. HPLC-UV was used for determination of 2,4-D after preconcentration by MIP-NPs in urine and different water samples.

Experimental

Reagents and chemicals

2,4-D was purchased from Fluka (Buchs, Switzerland). Azobisisobutyronitrile (AIBN) as the initiator was obtained from Acros Organic (NJ, USA). Methacrylic acid (MAA), ethylene glycol dimethacrylare (EGDMA), acetic acid (HOAC), sodium hydroxide (NaOH), acetonitrile (ACN) and methanol (MeOH) were purchased from Merck (Darmstadt, Germany, www.merck.de). All the reagents used were of analytical grade. Ultrapure water was prepared using a Milli-Q® system (Millipore, Milford, MA, USA). Stock standard solution of 2,4-D (1000 mg L^{-1}) was prepared in methanol and stored at refrigerator.

Instrumentation

All measurements were performed by a reversed-phase HPLC system from the Knauer Company (Germany), consisting of a K-1001 series high-pressure pump, a K-2006 photo diode-array detector and a VS injection valve, equipped with a 20-μL loop. The analytes were separated on a Chromolith performance RR-C_{18} 100 mm × 4.6 mm i.d. (MerchKGa A, Germany) and column guards (Chromolith Guard Cartridge Kit RP- C_{18} and 5 cm × 4.6 mm i.d., 5 μm). The mobile phase composition was 79.5% acetonitrile, 19.5% purified water and 1% acetic acid The flow-rate was set at 1 mL min^{-1} in isocratic mode with the detector's wavelength set at 280 nm. A digital pH meter, WTW Metrohm 827 Ion analyzer (Herisau, Switzerland), equipped with a combined glass calomel electrode was used for the pH adjustments at 25 ± 1°C temperature. Scanning electron microscopy (SEM) was carried out by gently distributing the powder sample on the stainless steel stubs, using SEM (Philips, XL-30, Almelo, the Netherlands) instrument. BAHR-Thermoanalyse GmbH (Germany) was used to determine the thermal properties of synthesized polymers with employing, heating and cooling rates of 10°C min^{-1} and using a condenser as the coolant. The samples were weighed as a thin film and carefully packed into a clean aluminum pan (11.5-12.5 mg), and sealed by crimping an aluminum lid on the pan (Shimadzu universal crimper). An Al_2O_3 empty pan sealed with a cover pan was used as a reference sample. A scanning range of 10 to 800°C was used for samples at 10°C min^{-1} in nitrogen gas.

Synthesis of molecular imprinted and non imprinted polymer nanoparticles

Precipitation polymerization technique was used for preparation of MIP-NPsaccording to following procedure (Figure 1): 1 mmol of 2,4-D (template) 4 mmol of MAA (functional monomer)which were dissolved in 40 mL of acetonitrile (progen solvent)in a 100 mL glass flask. The solution was mixed by ultrasonic wave for 10 min and then 1 mmol of AIBN (initiator) and 25 mmol of EGDMA (cross-linker agent) were added to the solution. The polymerization mixture was purged with a gentle flow of nitrogen gas for 6 min and the flask was sealed under nitrogen then; polymerization was performed in an oil bath at 60°C for 24 h in the presence of nitrogen under magnetic stirring at 400 rpm. The polymer nanoparticles were collected by centrifugation and washed with acetone and methanol, respectively for removing additional reagents and solvent. The template was removed from the cavity of MIP-NP using soxhlet extraction (acetic acid-methanol (85:15 v/v)), This step was confirmed through analysis of the eluted template molecules by HPLC analysis. Afterwards, the polymer was washed with deionized water until neutralization

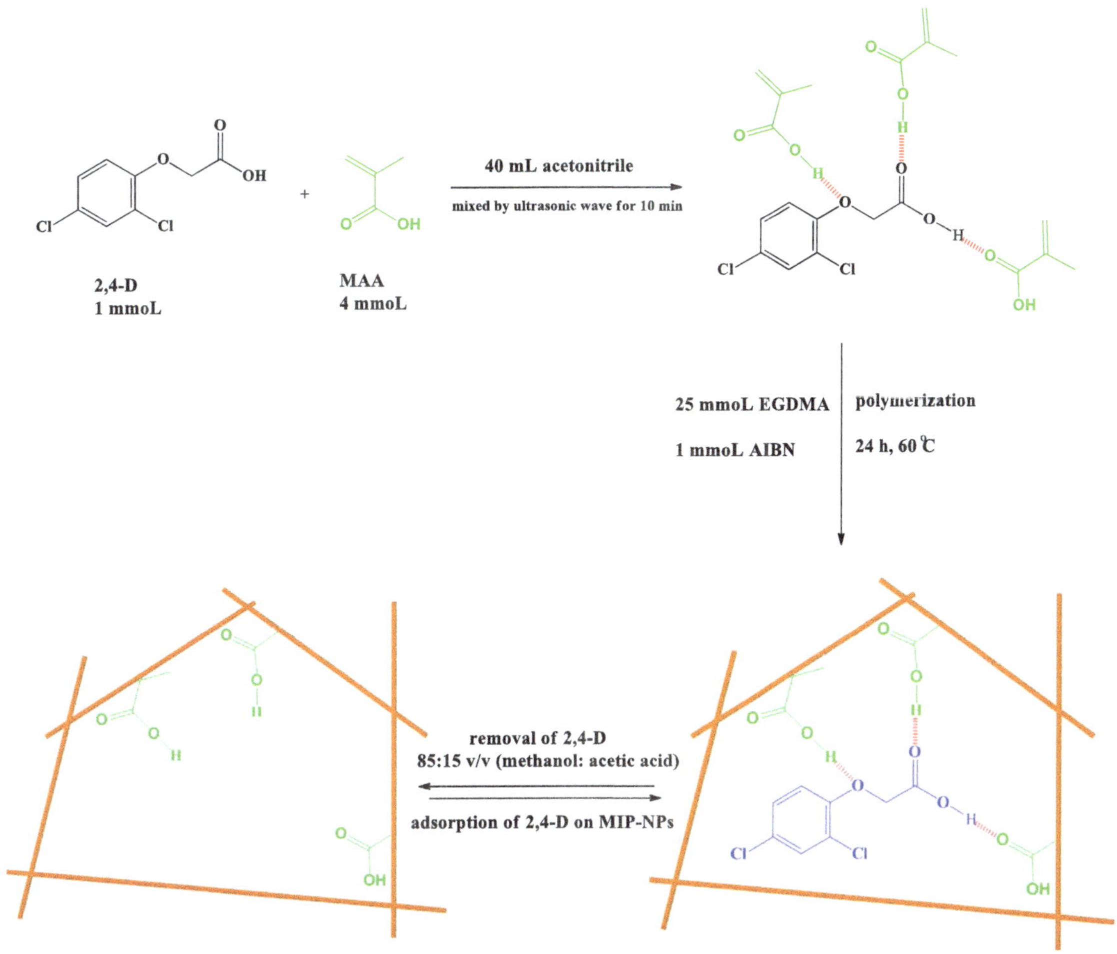

Figure 1 A scheme for the synthesis of 2,4-D imprinted polymer nanoparticles.

was obtained. Furthermore, non-imprinted polymers (NIP), as a reference, was prepared using the same process without the addition of the template molecule.

Preparation of standard solutions and real samples

Stock standard solution of the 2,4-D was prepared at concentration level of 1000 mg L^{-1} in methanol. The stock solution was protected from light and stored at 4°C and brought to ambient temperature just prior to use. The required working solutions were prepared daily in double-distilled water prior to use. For analysis of urine sample, 2 mL of spiked urine was diluted to 7.0 mL with ultrapure water. The water samples, including distilled water, tap water (Tehran, Iran), river waters obtained from Siahrood river and Derka river (Ghaemshahr, Iran) and sea water (Caspian Sea, Sari, Iran) were collected in cleaned polyethylene bottles and filtered through a 0.45 mm pore size nylon filter (Millipore) immediately after sampling. The amounts of 2,4-D was successfully determined by the present method.

Extraction procedure

All factors affecting sorption and desorption steps were investigated using batch method. Extraction of 2,4-D molecules from modeling solutions and real samples is followed by two steps: sorption and desorption. In the sorption step, the pH of sample solution was adjusted to 4.0 by drop wise addition of 2 mol L^{-1} sodium hydroxide or hydrochloric acid solutions. Then, 50 mg of dried polymer was suspended in aqueous solution (10 mL) containing 0.02 mg L^{-1} concentration of 2,4-D and stirred for 10 min with a magnetic stirrer, after that the polymer nanoparticles were separated from the solution by centrifugation. In washing step, in order to remove the potential interfering compounds and loosely retained molecules, the MIP-NPs were washed several times with double distilled water, then in desorption step, the elution of 2,4-D from MIP-NPs was performed by 1.5 mL of HOAC in methanol (15:85 v/v %) for 15 min. The eluate (separated by centrifuge) evaporated to almost dry under a gentle stream of nitrogen and the residue was dissolved in 0.3 mL mobile phase under sonication. Finally, 20 μL of the separated phase was drawn out by a Hamilton syringe and directly injected into the HPLC-Uv for analysis. Figure 2 provides a scheme for illustration of the mentioned extraction procedure.

Extraction percent of 2,4-D was calculated by the following equation:

$$\text{Adsorption efficiency}\% = C_A - C_B / C_A \times 100$$

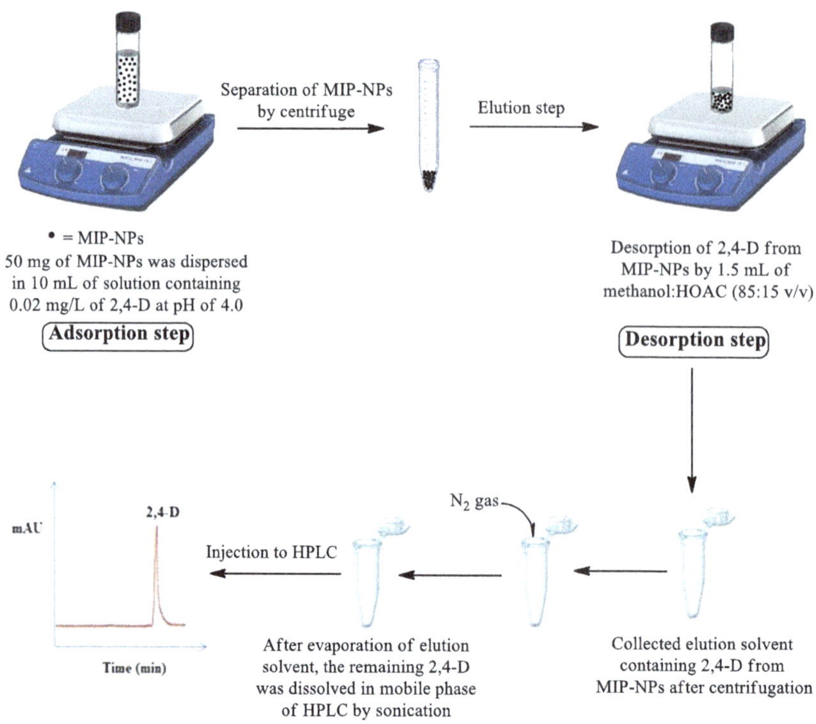

Figure 2 A schematic illustration of extraction procedure.

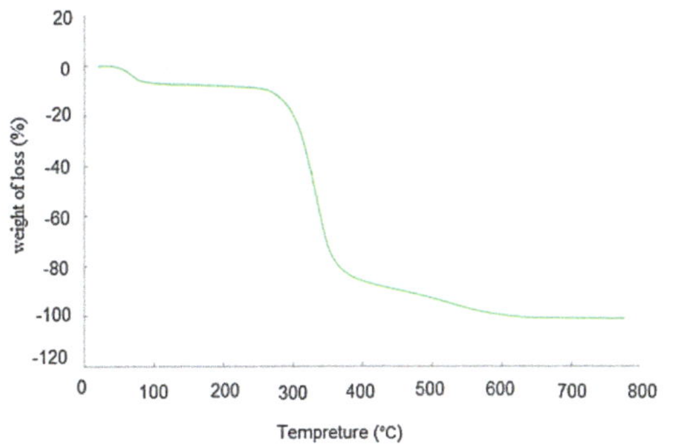

Figure 3 **The thermogram of synthesized molecular imprinted polymer nanoparticles.**

C_A and C_B are the concentrations of 2,4-D before and after extraction in the solution, respectively.

Results and discussion

Characterization of the synthesized molecular imprinted polymer nanoparticles

The resulting nanosized imprinted polymers were characterized by scanning electron microscopy (SEM), and thermogravimetric analysis (TGA). Thermal stability of the synthesized imprinted polymer nanoparticles was evaluated by TGA. Figure 3 shows TGA plot for the imprinted polymer. TGA plot for MIP-NPs can prove the thermal stability of the synthesized polymer. The morphology of the MIP-NPs was assessed by scanning electron microscopy, and the SEM micrograph is shown in Figure 4. As you can see in the Figure 4, the particle size of synthesized imprinted polymer was in range of 25-37 nm. These observation indicate that the formation 2,4-D imprinted nano particles was performed successfully and it can be used as a nano-size selective solid phase for very fast extraction of ultra-trace amounts of 2,4-D. The prepared MIP in the nanosize particles have many advantages such as: fast extraction of analyte from the real samples, high adsorption capacity of the prepared nanosized MIP toward conventional MIP according to the simple diffusion of target molecules to formed cavity due to high surface area of nanosized MIP.

Removal step

Effect of solution's pH

To evaluate the effect of pH on the extraction efficiency, the pH of 10 mL of sample solutions containing 0.02 mg L^{-1} of 2,4-D was adjusted in the range of 2-9. The pH of the suspensions was adjusted to desired values by adding sodium hydroxide or hydrochloric acid. Figure 5 illustrates the effect of solution's pH on percent of Adsorption efficiency. As it shows, the adsorption of 2,4-D by MIP-NPs was approximately constant from pH 2.0 to 4.0 but decreased from pH 5.0 to 9.0. Therefore, the pH of 4.0 was chosen as optimized pH, for quantitative adsorption of 2,4-D on the synthesized MIP-NPs in the subsequent experiments.

Equilibrium sorption time

In a typical uptake kinetics test, 50 mg of the sorbent was added to 10 mL of 0.02 mg L^{-1} 2,4-D aqueous solution at pH 4.0. The resulting suspension was stirred in different times (i.e., from 5 to 20 min) under magnetic stirring (Figure 6a). Consequently, an optimum equilibration

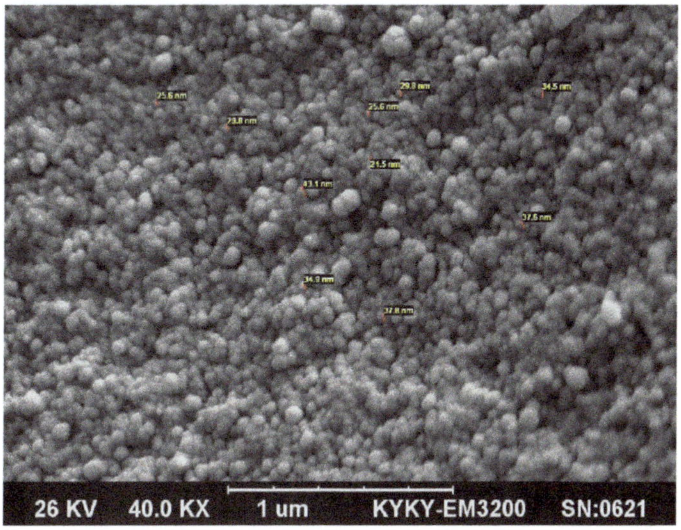

Figure 4 **The SEM micrograph of synthesized molecular imprinted polymer nanoparticles.**

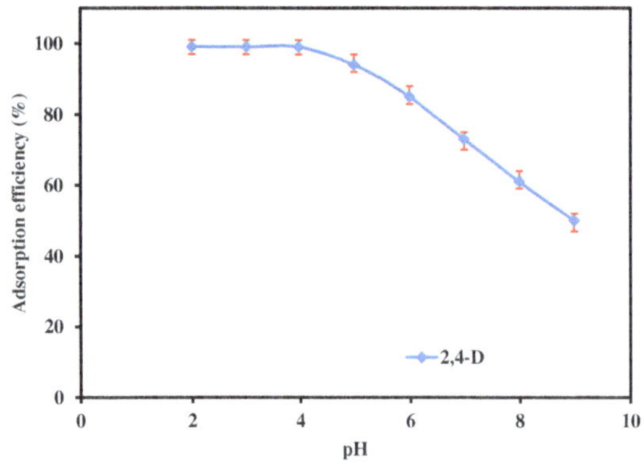

Figure 5 The effect of solution's pH on the adsorption efficiency of 2,4-D on MIP-NPs. (Conditions: 2,4-D concentration: 0.02 mgL^{-1}, Sample volume: 10 mL, Adsorption time: 10 min).

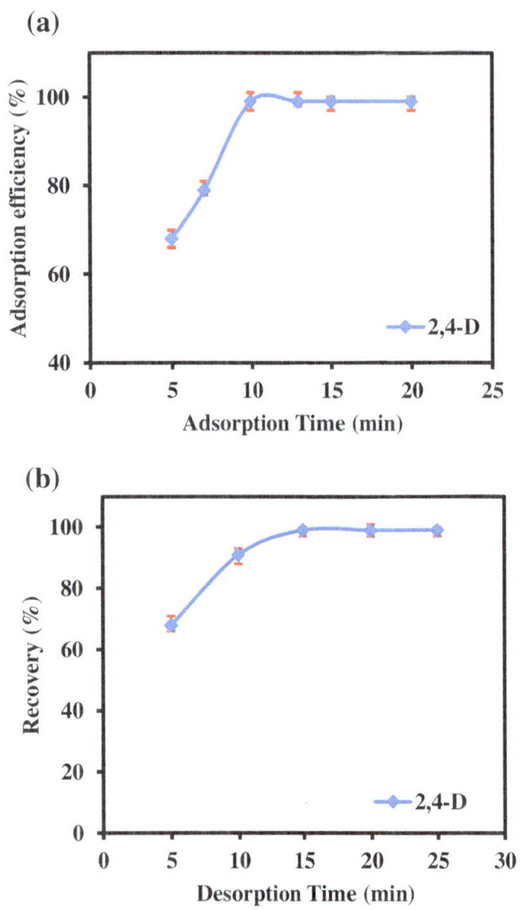

Figure 6 The effect of adsorption time (a) and desorption time (b) on the adsorption efficiency and recovery of 2,4-D from MIP-NPs.

Table 1 The effect of elution solvent type (The volume for each elution solvent was 5 mL) on the recovery of the target molecule from MIP-NPs (The obtained results are the mean of three measurements)

Elution solvent	Concentration (V/V (%))	$R^a \pm S^b$
Methanol	100	70.0 ± 1.4
Water	100	52.0 ± 1.6
Methanol: Acetic acid	95:5	82.0 ± 1.0
Water: Acetic acid	95:5	66.0 ± 1.2
Methanol: Acetic acid	90:10	90.0 ± 1.7
Methanol: Acetic acid	85:15	99.0 ± 1.0
Methanol: Acetic acid	80:20	97.0 ± 0.8
Methanol: Acetic acid	75:25	89.0 ± 1.0

[a]Recovery (%) [b]Standard deviation.

time of 10 minutes was obtained for quantitative removal of 2,4-D from solution into the solid phase.

Desorption step

Choice of eluent and desorption time

Complete removal of template from synthesized polymer isa very crucial step to guarantee the absence of memory effect. In this step, several solvents were examined; whose results are provided in Table 1. It is obvious that HOAC in methanol (15:85 v/v %) shows better recovery compared with the other solvents. Acetic acid can affect the hydrogen bonding between template and functional monomer, so that the removal of the template would be easier. In subsequent experiments (Table 2), 1.5 mL of HOAC in methanol (15:85 v/v %) was used as optimum eluent.

In order to investigate the optimum desorption time, various times were examined in the range of 5 to 25 min, while other parameters were kept in optimum conditions. According to measurements, extraction recovery was increased up to 15 min and it was constant in longer times. Therefore, 15 minutes can be considered to be the best quantitative time for the elution of 2,4-D from the imprinted polymer (Figure 6b).

Table 2 The effect of elution solvent volume on the recovery of the target molecule from MIP-NPs (The obtained results are the mean of three measurements)

Elution solvent (V/V (%))	Volume (mL)	$R^a \pm S^b$
Methanol: Acetic acid (85:15)	5	99.0 ± 0.8
Methanol: Acetic acid (85:15)	4	99.0 ± 1.0
Methanol: Acetic acid (85:15)	3	99.0 ± 0.9
Methanol: Acetic acid (85:15)	2	99.0 ± 1.0
Methanol: Acetic acid (85:15)	1.5	99.0 ± 1.0
Methanol: Acetic acid (85:15)	1.0	74.0 ± 1.2

[a]Recovery (%) [b]Standard deviation.

Table 3 The comparison between extraction recovery and adsorption capacity of MIP and NIP

Sorbent	$R^a \pm S^b$	Adsorption capacity (mg g^{-1})
Molecular imprinted polymer (MIP)	99.0 ± 1.0	89.2
Non imprinted polymer (NIP)	34.0 ± 1.3	12.1

[a]Recovery (%) [b]Standard deviation.

The effect of centrifugation time

The final parameter which evaluated and optimized was centrifugation time. If the centrifugation time is not enough, the MIP nanoparticles cannot be completely collected on bottom of the vial. A series of extraction with varying centrifugation times from 1 to 5 min at a rate of 3000 rpm were performed. The extraction recovery for the analytes was lower when the centrifugation time was shorter than 3 min. However; longer centrifugation has not significant effect on the extraction efficiency of the target molecule. Therefore, 3 min was selected as the optimum centrifuging time.

Investigation of the selectivity of the synthesized molecular imprinted polymer for 2,4-D

The effect of interfering agents on extraction recovery of 2,4-D were investigated in the presence of methylbenzene, aniline and 2-(4-chloro-2-methylphenoxy) propanoic acid with hundred fold concentration as interfering agents separately, while the other parameters were considered to be constant. The extraction recovery of more than 95% was obtained for 2-4-D in the presence of potentially interfering agent because of the high selectivity of synthesized MIP-NPs that allows its potential application as a sample preparation and clean up technique for analysis of 2,4-D in different matrices in the presence of interfering agents.

Comparison of MIP and NIP

In order to compare MIP and NIP, two extractions by both MIP and NIP in water sample were assessed under the optimal conditions. As it has shown (Table 3), because of the high capacity of MIP for extraction of 2,4-D in comparison with NIP, the extraction recovery of MIP is more than that of NIP. The obtained results can prove the successful engineering of cavity for 2,4-D in the structure of synthesized MIP-NPs. In order to evaluate the maximum adsorption capacity, the difference between concentration of the solution before extraction and the concentration of the solution after extraction was calculated. The sorption capacities of the MIP and NIP were calculated to be 89.2 mg g^{-1} and 12.1 mg g^{-1}, respectively.

The effect of interfering agent

The effect of interfering agents on the extraction recovery of 2,4-D were investigated in the presence of atrazine, 3,4-Dichlorophenol and 2,4,6-Trichlorophenol with tenfold concentration as interfering agents separately, while, the other parameters were considered to be constant. The extraction recovery of more than 95% was obtained for 2,4-D in the presence of potentially interfering agents because of the high selectivity of MIP that allows its potential application as a sample preparation tool for analysis of 2,4-D extracted from environmental and biological samples.

Statistical and calibration parameters

Under optimized conditions that have been described, the MIP-NPs-SPE showed a linear calibration curve within concentration ranging from 5 to 800 μg L^{-1}. The least

Table 4 Determination of 2,4-D in urine and different water samples

Sample	Analyte	C_{added}	$C_{founded}$	RSD % $_{Intra\text{-}day}$ (N = 3)	RSD % $_{Inter\text{-}day}$ (N = 3)	Relative recovery (%)
Distilled water	2,4-D	---	---	---	---	---
		50.0 μg L^{-1}	49.3 μg L^{-1}	3.1	3.6	98.6
Tap water	2,4-D	---	---	---	---	---
		50.0 μg L^{-1}	49.2 μg L^{-1}	3.4	3.7	98.4
Siahrood river water	2,4-D	---	---	---	---	---
		50.0 μg L^{-1}	49.4 μg L^{-1}	3.5	4.3	98.8
Derka river water	2,4-D	---	1.9 μg L^{-1}	---	---	---
		50.0 μg L^{-1}	51.4 μg L^{-1}	4.1	4.4	99.0
Sea water	2,4-D	---	---	---	---	---
		50.0 μg L^{-1}	49.1 μg L^{-1}	4.2	4.5	98.2
Urine	2,4-D	---	---	---	---	---
		50.0 μg L^{-1}	48.9 μg L^{-1}	4.1	4.6	97.8

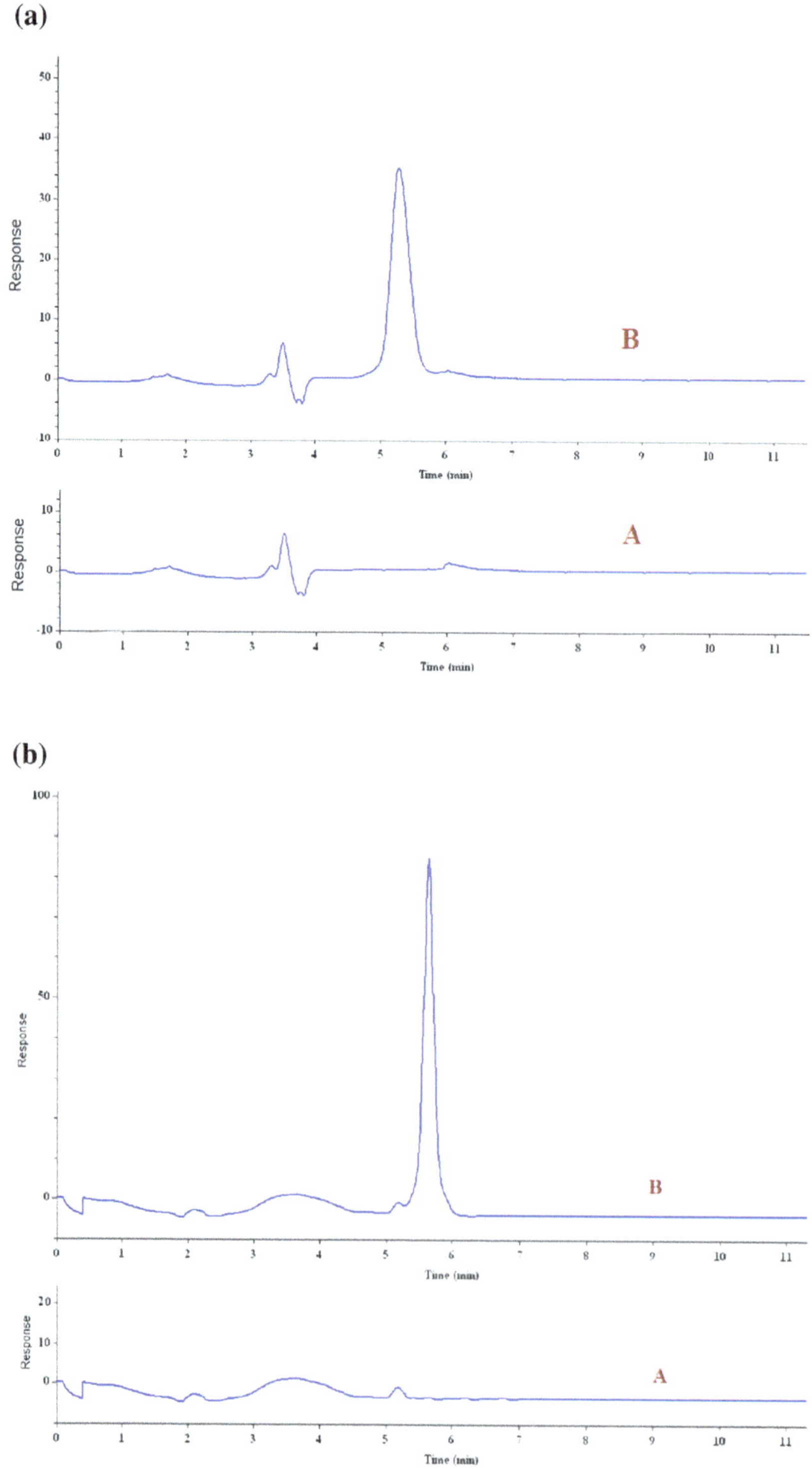

Figure 7 The chromatograms of the (A) non-spiked and (B) spiked (100 μgL^{-1}) sea water sample after extraction under optimum conditions (a) and the chromatograms of the (A) non-spiked and (B) spiked (100 μgL^{-1}) urine sample after extraction under optimum conditions (b).

square equations at above linear dynamic range for water and urine samples were as follows:

$$\text{Peak area} = 0.949\,C^{a}(\mu g\,L^{-1}) + 0.579,\quad (R^2 = 0.99)\ {}^{a}\text{Concentration of 2,4–D (For water)}$$

$$\text{Peak area} = 0.939\,C^{a}(\mu g\,L^{-1}) + 0.655,\quad (R^2 = 0.99)\ {}^{a}\text{Concentration of 2,4–D (For urine)}$$

The limits of detections, defined as $C_{LOD} = 3S_b/m$, where S_b is the standard deviation of seven replicate blank signals and m is the slope of the linear section of calibration curve after preconcentration, for a sample volume of 10 mL, were found to be 1.25 $\mu g\ L^{-1}$ and 1.80 $\mu g\ L^{-1}$ for 2,4-D in water and urine samples, respectively. Also, the relative standard deviations for eight separate batch experiments with 50 mg of sorbent for determination of 0.1 μg 2,4-D in 10 mL of water were calculated to be 4.2% and 4.7% in water and urine samples, respectively.

Determination of 2,4-D in different water and urine samples

In order to evaluate the analytical applicability of the proposed method, determination of 2,4-D in urine and different water samples such as distilled water, tap water (Tehran, Iran), river waters obtained from Siahrood river and Derka river (Ghaemshahr, Iran) and sea water (Caspian Sea, Sari, Iran) was carried out. Table 4 shows that the results of three replicate analyses of each real sample obtained by the method are in good agreement with the spiking amounts. The repeatability of the method was demonstrated by the mean relative standard deviation (R.S.D.). Also, the relative recovery is defined as following equation:

$$RR = (C_{found} - C_{real}/C_{added}) \times 100$$

Where C_{found}, C_{real}, and C_{added} are the concentrations of analyte after addition of known amount of standard in the real sample, the concentration of analyte in real sample and the concentration of known amount of standard which was spiked to the real sample, respectively. 2,4-D trace determination in water and urine samples, using MIP-NPs-SPE as a reliable sample treatment technique can be conducted. Figure 7 provides chromatograms for determination of 2,4-D in spiked urine and sea water samples.

Conclusion

The molecular imprinted polymer is a selective sample preparation technique for preconcentration of molecules such as 2,4-D from aqueous solutions. The MIP-NPs has been synthesized by precipitation polymerization technique. The analytical characteristics such as good precision and preconcentration factor, high quantities of recoveries, wide dynamic linear range, and low detection of limit were achieved due to the powerful efficiency of the MIP-NPs-SPE method. Other advantages of suggested method are: lack of matrix effect, low consumption of organic solvent, environmentally friendly, safe, simplicity and selectivity. The synthesized MIP-NPs can be used repeatedly (7 times) with no significant decrease in its binding affinities. Due to relatively high preconcentration factor, trace amount of 2,4-D at $\mu g\ L^{-1}$ levels can be determined and separated by MIP-NPs.

Competing interests

The authors declare that they have no competing interests.

Authors' contributions

The overall implementation of this study including design, experiments and data analysis, and manuscript preparation were the results of efforts by all of the authors. All authors have made extensive contribution into the review and finalization of this manuscript. All authors read and approved the final manuscript.

Acknowledgements

The authors would like to appreciate Tehran University of Medical Sciences for funding and supporting this project. The authors also thank Mr Mirghani Seyed-Someh and Mrs Safora Arefian for their kind technical assistance through this study. The authors declare that there is no conflict of interests.

Author details

[1]Department of Occupational Health Engineering, School of Public Health, Shahroud University of Medical Sciences, Shahroud, Iran. [2]Department of Chemistry, Shahid Beheshti University, Tehran, Iran. [3]Department of Occupational Health, School of Public Health, Tehran University of Medical Sciences, Tehran, Iran. [4]Department of Occupational Health Engineering, School of Public Health and Institute for Environmental Research, Tehran University of Medical Sciences, Tehran, Iran.

References

1. Garabrant DH, Philbert MA: **Review of 2, 4-dichlorophenoxyacetic acid (2, 4-D) epidemiology and toxicology.** *CRC Crit Rev Toxicol* 2002, **32**(4):233–257.
2. Chaudhary AJ, M-u H, Grimes SM: **Simultaneous recovery of metals and degradation of organic species: copper and 2, 4, 5-trichlorophenoxyacetic acid (2, 4, 5-T).** *J Hazard Mater* 2009, **165**(1):825–831.
3. de Lipthay JR, Sørensen SR, Aamand J: **Effect of herbicide concentration and organic and inorganic nutrient amendment on the mineralization of mecoprop, 2, 4-D and 2, 4, 5-T in soil and aquifer samples.** *Environ Pollut* 2007, **148**(1):83–93.
4. IARC: *IARC monographs on the evaluation of carcinogenic risksto humans: chlorophenoxy herbicides*. 1998, available on line http://www-cie.iarc.fr.
5. EPA (US Environmental Protection Agency): *Reregistration Eligibility Decision for 2,4-D. EPA 738-R-05-002*; 2005.
6. Kohli J, Khanna R, Gupta B, Dhar M, Tandon J, Sircar K: **Absorption and excretion of 2, 4-dichlorophenoxyacetic acid in man.** *Xenobiotica* 1974, **4**(2):97–100.
7. Sauerhoff M, Braun W, Blau G, Gehring P: **The fate of 2, 4-dichlorophenoxyacetic acid (2, 4-D) following oral administration to man.** *Toxicology* 1977, **8**(1):3–11.
8. Irons RD (Ed): *Toxicology of the Blood and Bone Marrow*. New York: Raven Press; 1985.
9. Harris S, Solomon K, Stephenson G: **Exposure of homeowners and bystanders to 2, 4-dichlorophenoxyacetic acid (2, 4-D).** *J Environ Sci Health B* 1992, **27**(1):23–38.
10. *National Primary Drinking Water Regulations, Office of Water, U.S. Environmental Protection Agency, Washington, DC.*; 2009.

11. Hamilton D, Ambrus A, Dieterle R, Felsot A, Harris C, Holland P, Katayama A, Kurihara N, Linders J, Unsworth J, Wong S: Regulatory limits for pesticide residues in water (IUPAC Technical Report). *Pure Appl Chem* 2003, **75**(8):1123–1155.
12. Rodríguez I, Rubí E, González R, Quintana JB, Cela R: On-fibre silylation following solid-phase microextraction for the determination of acidic herbicides in water samples by gas chromatography. *Anal Chim Acta* 2005, **537**(1–2):259–266.
13. Biesaga M, Jankowska A, Pyrzyńska K: Comparison of different sorbents for solid-phase extraction of phenoxyalkanoic acid herbicides. *Microchim Acta* 2005, **150**(3–4):317–322.
14. Catalina MI, Dallüge J, Vreuls RJ, Brinkman UAT: Determination of chlorophenoxy acid herbicides in water by in situ esterification followed by in-vial liquid–liquid extraction combined with large-volume on-column injection and gas chromatography–mass spectrometry. *J Chromatogr A* 2000, **877**(1):153–166.
15. Jing T, Wang Y, Dai Q, Xia H, Niu J, Hao Q, Mei S, Zhou Y: Preparation of mixed-templates molecularly imprinted polymers and investigation of the recognition ability for tetracycline antibiotics. *Biosens Bioelectron* 2010, **25**(10):2218–2224.
16. Behbahani M, Salarian M, Bagheri A, Tabani H, Omidi F, Fakhari A: Synthesis, characterization and analytical application of Zn (II)-imprinted polymer as an efficient solid-phase extraction technique for trace determination of zinc ions in food samples. *J Food Compos Anal* 2014, **34**:81–89.
17. Hoshina K, Horiyama S, Matsunaga H, Haginaka J: Molecularly imprinted polymers for simultaneous determination of antiepileptics in river water samples by liquid chromatography–tandem mass spectrometry. *J Chromatogr A* 2009, **1216**(25):4957–4962.
18. Behbahani M, Barati M, Bojdi MK, Pourali AR, Bagheri A, Tapeh NAG: A nanosized cadmium (II)-imprinted polymer for use in selective trace determination of cadmium in complex matrices. *Microchim Acta* 2013, **180**(11–12):1117–1125.
19. Prieto A, Schrader S, Bauer C, Möder M: Synthesis of a molecularly imprinted polymer and its application for microextraction by packed sorbent for the determination of fluoroquinolone related compounds in water. *Anal Chim Acta* 2011, **685**(2):146–152.
20. Lucci P, Núñez O, Galceran MT: Solid-phase extraction using molecularly imprinted polymer for selective extraction of natural and synthetic estrogens from aqueous samples. *J Chromatogr A* 2011, **1218**(30):4828–4833.
21. Behbahani M, Bagheri S, Amini MM, Sadeghi Abandansari H, Moazami HR, Bagheri A: Application of a magnetic molecularly imprinted polymer for the selective extraction and trace detection of lamotrigine in urine and plasma samples. *J Sep Sci* 2014, **37**:1610–1616.
22. Shahtaheri S, Katmeh M, Kwasowski P, Stevenson D: Development and optimisation of an immunoaffinity-based solid-phase extraction for chlortoluron. *J Chromatogr A* 1995, **697**(1):131–136.
23. Koohpaei A, Shahtaheri S, Ganjali M, Forushani AR, Golbabaei F: Application of multivariate analysis to the screening of molecularly imprinted polymers (MIPs) for ametryn. *Talanta* 2008, **75**(4):978–986.
24. Koohpaei A, Shahtaheri S, Ganjali M, Forushani AR, Golbabaei F: Optimization of solid-phase extraction using developed modern sorbent for trace determination of ametryn in environmental matrices. *J Hazard Mater* 2009, **170**(2):1247–1255.
25. Bulut VN, Gundogdu A, Duran C, Senturk HB, Soylak M, Elci L, Tufekci M: A multi-element solid-phase extraction method for trace metals determination in environmental samples on Amberlite XAD-2000. *J Hazard Mater* 2007, **146**(1–2):155–163.
26. Soylak M, Ercan O: Selective separation and preconcentration of copper (II) in environmental samples by the solid phase extraction on multi-walled carbon nanotubes. *J Hazard Mater* 2009, **168**(2–3):1527–1531.
27. Ebrahimzadeh H, Behbahani M: A novel lead imprinted polymer as the selective solid phase for extraction and trace detection of lead ions by flame atomic absorption spectrophotometry: synthesis, characterization and analytical application. *Arab J CHEM* 2013, doi:10.1016/j.arabjc.2013.09.017.
28. Omidi F, Behbahani M, Samadi S, Sedighi A, Shahtaheri SJ: Coupling of molecular imprinted polymer nanoparticles by high performance liquid chromatography as an efficient technique for sensitive and selective trace determination of 4-chloro-2-methylphenoxy acetic acid in complex matrices. *Iranian J Publ Health* 2014, **43**(5):645–657.
29. Wang T, Tong J, Sun M, Chen L: Fast and selective extraction of chloramphenicol from soil by matrix solid-phase dispersion using molecularly imprinted polymer as dispersant. *J Sep Sci* 2011, **34**(15):1886–1892.
30. Tamayo FG, Casillas JL, Martin-Esteban A: Highly selective fenuron-imprinted polymer with a homogeneous binding site distribution prepared by precipitation polymerisation and its application to the clean-up of fenuron in plant samples. *Anal Chim Acta* 2003, **482**(2):165–173.
31. Haginaka J, Sanbe H: Uniform-sized molecularly imprinted polymers for 2-arylpropionic acid derivatives selectively modified with hydrophilic external layer and their applications to direct serum injection analysis. *Anal Chem* 2000, **72**(21):5206–5210.
32. Turiel E, Martín-Esteban A, Tadeo JL: Molecular imprinting-based separation methods for selective analysis of fluoroquinolones in soils. *J Chromatogr A* 2007, **1172**(2):97–104.
33. He J, Lv R, Zhu J, Lu K: Selective solid-phase extraction of dibutyl phthalate from soybean milk using molecular imprinted polymers. *Anal Chim Acta* 2010, **661**(2):215–221.
34. Yan H, Qiao J, Pei Y, Long T, Ding W, Xie K: Molecularly imprinted solid-phase extraction coupled to liquid chromatography for determination of Sudan dyes in preserved beancurds. *Food Chem* 2012, **132**(1):649–654.
35. Djozan D, Ebrahimi B: Preparation of new solid phase micro extraction fiber on the basis of atrazine-molecular imprinted polymer: application for GC and GC/MS screening of triazine herbicides in water, rice and onion. *Anal Chim Acta* 2008, **616**(2):152–159.
36. Akiyama T, Hishiya T, Asanuma H, Komiyama M: Molecular imprinting of cyclodextrin on silica-gel support for the stationary phase of high-performance-liquid-chromatography. *J Inclusion Phenom Macrocyclic Chem* 2001, **41**(1–4):149–153.
37. Zhang H, Dramou P, He H, Tan S, Pham-Huy C, Pan H: Molecularly imprinted stationary phase prepared by reverse micro-emulsion polymerization for selective recognition of gatifloxacin in aqueous media. *J Chromatogr Sci* 2012, **50**(6):499–508.
38. Kan X, Zhao Y, Geng Z, Wang Z, Zhu J-J: Composites of multiwalled carbon nanotubes and molecularly imprinted polymers for dopamine recognition. *J Phys Chem C* 2008, **112**(13):4849–4854.
39. Ye L, Mosbach K, Spivak DA, Sibrian-Vazquez M: *Molecularly Imprinted Materials: Towards the Next Generation. Materials Research Society Symposium Proceedings*. Cambridge Univ Press; 2002.
40. Tokonami S, Shiigi H, Nagaoka T: Review: micro- and nanosized molecularly imprinted polymers for high-throughput analytical applications. *Anal Chim Acta* 2009, **641**(1–2):7–13.
41. Haginaka J: Monodispersed, molecularly imprinted polymers as affinity-based chromatography media. *J Chromatogr B* 2008, **866**(1–2):3–13.
42. Ye L, Cormack PA, Mosbach K: Molecularly imprinted monodisperse microspheres for competitive radioassay. *Anal Commun* 1999, **36**(2):35–38.

Biogas production experimental research using algae

Pranas Baltrėnas and Antonas Misevičius*

Abstract

The current study is on the the use of macro-algae as feedstock for biogas production. Three types of macro-algae, *Cladophora glomerata* (CG), *Chara fragilis* (CF), and *Spirogyra neglecta* (SN), were chosen for this research. The experimental studies on biogas production were carried out with these algae in a batch bioreactor. In the bioreactor was maintained 35 ± 1°C temperature. The results showed that the most appropriate macro-algae for biogas production are *Spirogyra neglecta* (SN) and *Cladophora glomerata* (CG). The average amount of biogas obtained from the processing of SN – 0.23 m^3/m^3d, CG – 0.20 m^3/m^3d, and CF – 0.12 m^3/m^3d. Considering the concentration of methane obtained during the processing of SN and CG, which after eight days and until the end of the experiment exceeded 60%, it can be claimed that biogas produced using these algae is valuable. When processing CF, the concentration of methane reached the level of 50% only by the final day of the experiment, which indicates that this alga is less suitable for biogas production.

Keywords: Biogas, Methane, Algae, Batch reactor, Anaerobic digestion

Introduction

Although algae are beneficial to the production of oxygen, but their rapid spread to minus. The spread of algae in water bodies is an important environmental problem, which results in disappearance of the water bodies. After the review of the Lithuanian and foreign scientific literature on the use of algae, it can be noted that algae are mainly used for the production of biofuels including biogas, in medicine and in food industries [1-3].

Algae can be unicellular, multicellular, and acellular. They can live alone or in colonies. Algae can be divided into micro-algae (microscopic cells 3-10μm in size) and macro-algae. Depending on the type of algae, usually a half of its nutritional value is protein, less than a third - carbohydrates, and the remaining compounds are fats, vitamins and trace elements. Factors influencing more like algal production are:

- High water temperature (depends on solar radiation, topography, currents, water sources);
- Nutrients (depend on the ecosystem, sediments, and the shoreline);
- Water pH;
- Low oxygen levels;
- Anthropogenic pollution;
- The physical parameters of the water body (the speed of current, the cross-section area, the discharge, the steepness of coasts);
- Soil for entrenchment;
- Other factors (including the mechanic effect of sediments, bottom shifts, species and the spread of plants, fauna).

The anaerobic processing of organic waste and its utilization for energy production is encouraged by stringent environmental regulations, growing waste disposal costs and rising prices of energy resources [4]. The use of algae as a feedstock could address two major environmental problems. First, to use algae as a feedstock for biogas production, it should be extracted from water, thus, the water body would be cleaned and, at the same time, protected from eutrophication. Second, the air pollution would be reduced and the climate change

* Correspondence: antonas.misevicius@gmail.com
Institute of Environmental Protection, Vilnius Gediminas Technical University, Vilnius, Lithuania

stabilized. The biological decomposition of organic waste produces gases that consist of methane, carbon dioxide, hydrogen, hydrogen sulphide. Methane is the gas that has the 21-times-stronger impact on the greenhouse effect than carbon dioxide [5-7]. Having these two issues solved could, at the same time, produce economic benefits. Biogas, obtained during the bioreactor treatment of accumulated algae, could be used as fuel for the production of electricity and/or thermal energy [8,9].

Razon and Tan [1] cultivated algae in the photo-bioreactors and used one part of the cultivated algae for biodiesel production and the other part for biogas production [1]. Harun et al. [10] analyzed the possibility of using micro-algae for biogas, biodiesel and bioethanol production. These researchers argue that it is most useful to process algae for biogas and biodiesel production, because most of the energy, i.e. 16.14 $MJkg^{-1}$, is produced when doing so [10]. Zhong et al. [11] studied the biogas productivity with five organic waste mixtures, i.e. blue algae and corn silage. The scientist argues that the best yield of biogas is when the C/N (carbon/nitrogen) ratio is 20/1; then the biogas production rate is 0.6 m^3/kg DW, and methane concentrations were about 55% [11]. Mussgnung et al. [12] conducted biogas production experimental studies with six species of micro-algae [12]. The results of the studies demonstrate that the biogas production rate is from 0.28 to 0.65 m^3/kg DW (DW – dry weight) and methane concentrations range from 54 to 67% [12]. Salermo et al. [13] have also conducted biogas production studies using algae, however, the scientists have been mixing algae in different proportions with soybean oil and glycerin [13]. The amount of biogas ranged from 0.3 to 0.5 ml/mld, and methane averaged in 68% [13]. Vergara-Fernandez et al. [14] used two types of algae for biogas production by dissolving the algae in the batch bioreactor. Their results indicate that biogas production reached 0.18 m^3/kg DW, and methane concentration was 65% [14]. The analysis of literature shows that various types of micro-algae are used for biogas production. However, there is no information on the use of freshwater macro-algae for biogas production. It is therefore relevant to examine the efficiency of macro-algae for energy production.

The aim of the current research is to analyze what amount of biogas and its main component -methane - is emitted during the anaerobic processing of three types of macro-algae at the mesophilic mode in the batch bioreactor. Also, the research aims at identifying which type of the three tested algae species is the most efficient raw material for biogas production.

Materials and methods

Waste characteristics

The amount of used algae for the analysis and algae moisture are presented in Table 1. The same amount of each type of algae, i.e. 2000 grams, was taken for the analysis. The dry material volume in the bioreactor was calculated measuring algae moisture according to the formula.

Experimental set-up

Figure 1 present the algae which were carried out experimental studies of biogas production. *Cladophora glomerata* [15], *Chara fragilis* [16] *Spirogyra neglecta* algae were selected according to their occurrence in water bodies. Distribution of algae in water bodies is one of the biggest.

The analyses were carried out in batch reactors (Figure 2) with a total volume of 5 L and a the working volume of 3 L (in the bioreactor substrate amounted to 3 L). The bioreactors, which worked at the mesophilic mode, were filled with three species of algae and were maintained at 35 ± 1°C. Mesophilic mode was chosen because it is the most optimal and most frequently not only in the laboratory but also in industrial bioreactors. At this temperature mode of substrates digestion is more stable and faster [17].

Reactor operation

The batch bioreactors were loaded with substrate through substrate intake; the substrate was removed through the same opening after the experiment (Figure 2).

In the bioreactor was maintained at 35 ± 1°C temperature. To know the current temperature in the container with water, the temperature gauge was built-in. If the temperature falls below the set temperature, the temperature sensor goes off and the electronic heating element automatically heats the water in the container and the substrate in the bioreactor to the required temperature. This type of bioreactor does not have any mixing equipment; also, because of the low volume mixing is not necessary. Bioreactor every day was mechanically shaken. The bioreactor is placed on the shaker

Table 1 Algae, quantity and moisture content

Algae	Moisture content, %	Dry matter, g/kg	Amount of algae in bioreactor, g DW
Cladophora glomerata	92.4	76	152
Chara fragilis	90.6	94	188
Spirogyra neglecta	90.1	99	198

DW – dry weight.

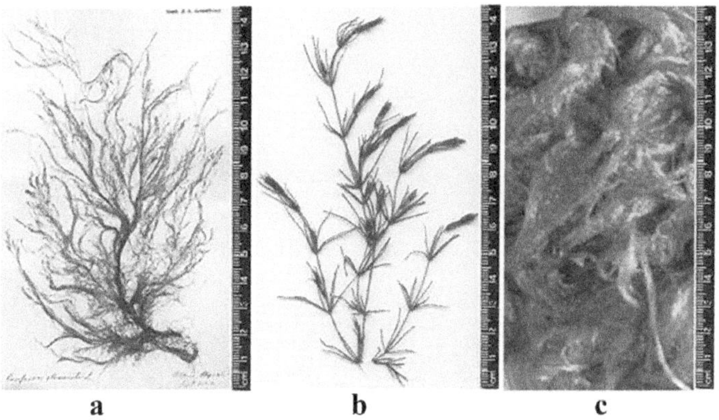

Figure 1 Macro algae (a– *Cladophora glomerata*, b – *Chara fragilis*, c – *Spirogyra neglecta*).

and shake for 10-15 minutes, the substrate is evenly mixed. To know the amount of gas, 4,5 liter biogas accumulation vessel, hoses and sleeves for fixing, and a ruler, was constructed. The biogas storage tank was connected to the biogas analyzer by means of the flexible hose. When the device is turned on, the biogas storage tank valve is opened simultaneously to allow biogas flow into the analyzer. The biogas composition measurement lasts nine minutes. At the end of measuring, the device presents the average biogas composition values.

Analytical methods

For the measurement of moisture, 10 grams of the test material was weighed. The material was placed in the thermostatic drying box and was dried at 105°C ± 2°C for three hours. After drying, the container with the test

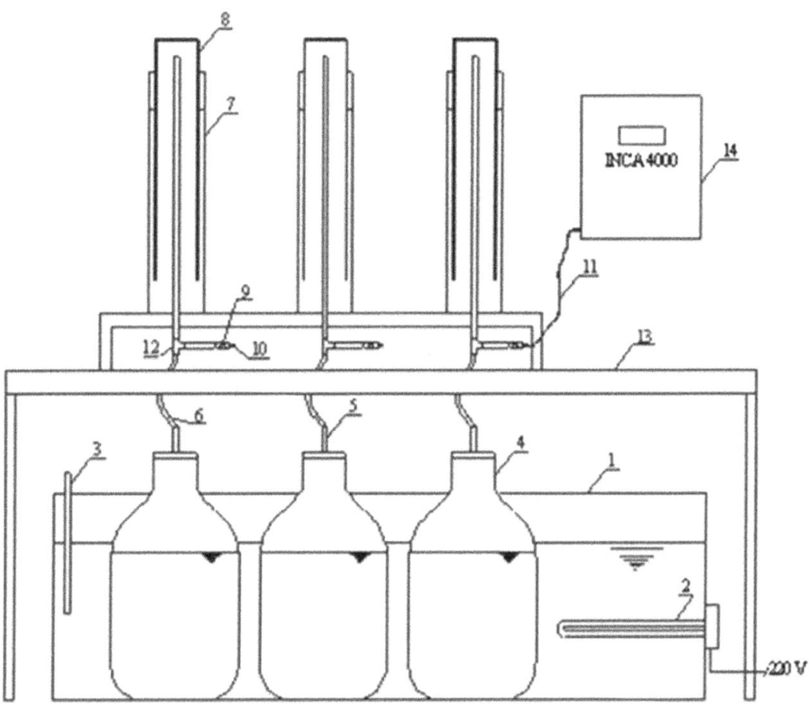

Figure 2 Scheme of the batch bio-reactor stand: 1 – vessel with water, 2 – substrate heating device, 3 – temperature sensor, 4 – bio-reactor, 5 – branch pipe for hose fixing, 6 – flexible hose, 7 – vessel with water, 8 – biogas accumulation vessel (PVC pipe), 9 – valve, 10 – branch pipe for gas discharge, 11 – elastic hose, 12 – T-socket, 13 – table, 14 – gas analyser.

material was placed in the dessicator for 45 minutes to cool down. After the test material cooled down, its moisture was calculated according to the formula:

$$Wa = ((Gw - Ga)/Ga)^{*}100, \% \qquad (1)$$

here:

Wa – material moisture content,%;
Gw – wet weight of the material, g;
Ga – absolute dry weight, g.

Measurements were carried out with the analyser INCA 4000 which measures methane (%), carbon dioxide (%) oxygen (%) concentration and the concentration of hydrogen sulphide in (ppm). The measurable ranges are: for oxygen – 0–25% (±1%); hydrogen sulphide – 0–100 ppm (±5%); methane – 0–100% (±1%); carbon dioxide – 0–100% (±1%). The analyser INCA 4000 works at an ambient air temperature range from -5°C to +40°C, and relative humidity from 0 to 95%. Substrate pH was determined at the beginning and end of the experiment using. pH meter measuring range from 0 to 14 (±0.1) units.

Results and discussion

Three experimental 15-days studies with macro-algae were conducted at 35 ± 1°C. The results of the studies are presented in Figures 3, 4, and 5. The amount of biogas and its main component – methane – are presented in the results. Although other components were measured, their graphic results are not presented, but are mentioned in the text. As shown in Figure 3, the biogas production had a tendency to rise up to day 8 of the experiment and reached 0.387 m^3/m^3d. Later, the amount of biogas decreased to 0.039 m^3/m^3d at the end of the experiment. The experimental studies was conducted using 152 g of dry weight of macro-algae - *Cladophora glomerata* - can produce 0.06 m3 of biogas during 15 days. Each plant or waste type has its own organic composition. In terms of the anaerobic processing, the biomass is evaluated with respect to the amount of fat, protein and carbohydrates in it. Given different quantities of these elements, a different amount of biogas and the concentration of methane is obtained. If there are more carbohydrates in the substrate, the biogas production process is faster, because of the faster decomposition of carbohydrates, and the concentration of methane can reach 50-60% [18]. However, if there is more fat or protein, the biogas production is slower, but the concentration of methane is higher. It can range from 75-90% [19]. Algae are the source of oils, carbohydrates and protein. Therefore, by knowing the chemical composition, the biogas and methane production capacity can be determined. In this case, with regard to the concentration of methane in biogas, it can be assumed that during the processing of *Cladophora glomerata*, the amount of protein was the biggest, because the concentration of methane was 70%. The decrease of biogas may occur due to several reasons. Without the supply of substrate in bioreactor, microorganisms do not get the nutrients, as a result, the biogas production is slowing down. Therefore, it can be concluded that on the 8-9 day of the experiment it is necessary to add some substrate. pH could also change, as at the beginning of the experiment the pH value was 6.8 ± 0.1, but at the end it decreased to 6.3 ± 0.1. When pH drops below 6.5, the biogas and methane production slows down [20-22]. In biogas the amount of oxygen ranged from 4.2% at the beginning of

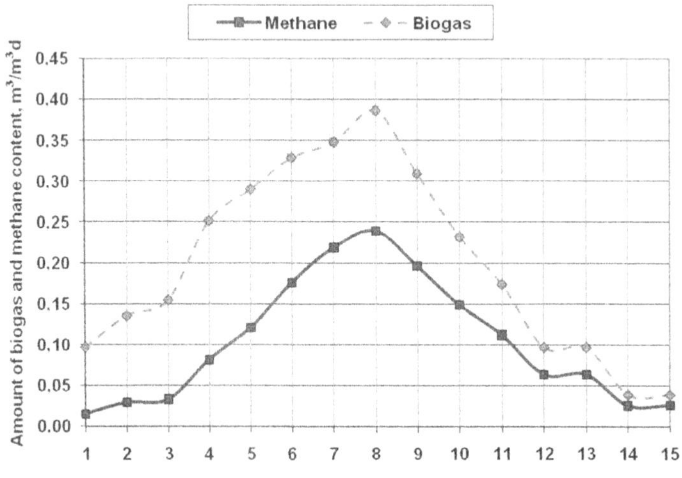

Figure 3 **The amount of biogas (m^3/m^3d), methane content (m^3/m^3d) in the anaerobic digestion of macro algae - *Cladophora glomerata* under batch reactor mesophilic conditions.**

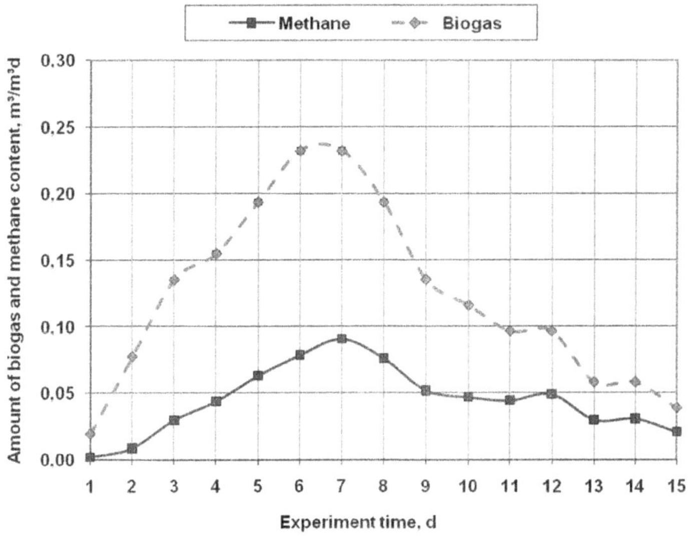

Figure 4 The amount of biogas (m^3/m^3d), methane content (m^3/m^3d) in the anaerobic digestion of macro algae - *Chara fragilis* under batch reactor mesophilic conditions.

the experiment, and then fell, reaching only 0.1%. The concentration of hydrogen sulfide in biogas varied in the range from 3 ppm to 35 ppm, therefore, the biogas purification of this pollutant is not necessary.

The anaerobic decomposition of *Chara fragilis* in the bioreactor, biogas and methane variation was similar to the previously mentioned case. The emission of biogas increased from 0.019 m^3/m^3d at the beginning of the experiment to 0.232 m^3/m^3d on day 6. Then, the amount of biogas was gradually decreasing until the final day of the experiment. Until day 7 of the experiment, the concentration of methane was increasing and reached 0.09 m^3/m^3d (i.e. 38.9% of the biogas volume), later, the concentration was stable for several days, and since day 10, was increasing again and reached 0.021 m^3/m^3d (53.1% of the biogas volume) on the final day of the experiment. Compared to other research results [1,2,10], the results of the current research suggest that during the processing of macro- and micro-algae, the concentration of methane in biogas in some cases is similar, and in some

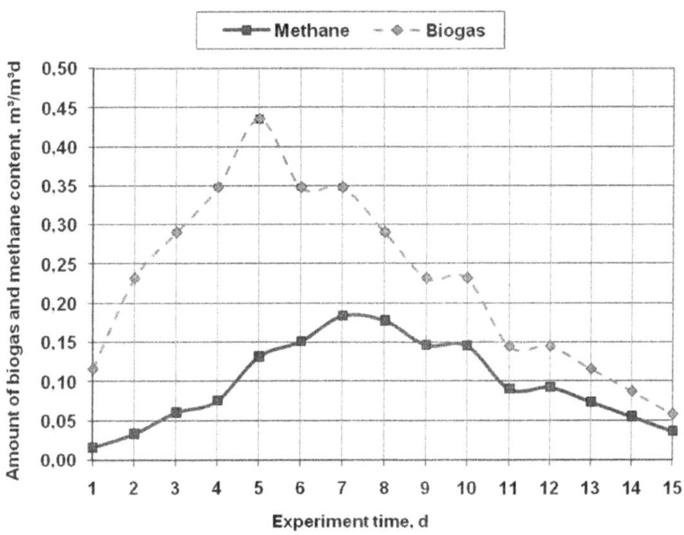

Figure 5 The amount of biogas (m^3/m^3d), methane content (m^3/m^3d) in the anaerobic digestion of macro algae - *Spirogyra neglecta* under batch reactor mesophilic conditions.

cases the obtained concentration is 10-15% higher. This fluctuation may occur due to the protein and carbohydrate amount in algae. Given the fact that the experiment lasted 15 days, it can be maintained that algae decomposed much faster during the anaerobic processing. The faster decomposition is conditioned by the fact that the walls of algae are easily destroyed, there is almost no lignin, thus algae is more technological in the production of biogas as compared with terrestrial plants [23]. The level of pH at the beginning of the experiment was 6.5 ± 0.1, while at the end it dropped to 6.2 ± 0.1. The anaerobic decomposition process was also influenced by pH. In biogas the amount of oxygen ranged from 2.8% at the beginning of the experiment, and later, at the end, it dropped to 0%. The concentration of hydrogen sulfide in biogas varied in the range from 24 ppm to 60 ppm, therefore, the biogas purification of this pollutant is not necessary.

During the processing of the macro-algae - *Spirogyra neglecta* - the upward trend in the emissions up to day 5 and then a downward trend until the end of the experiment could be observed. At the beginning of the experiment, the amount of biogas reached 0.12 m^3/m^3d, later, it increased to 0.44 m^3/m^3d and at the end of the experiment it dropped to 0.06 m^3/m^3d. In this case, the decrease in biogas amount can be observed after day 5 of the experiment, then, the decreased amount remains the same; later, it decreases again and the process repeats three times. This trend may occur due to the intensity change of the acetogenesis and methanogenesis processes [24]. The bacteria that produce methane during the process of methanogenesis cannot decompose acetates produced during the acetogenesis process. Therefore, when the amount of acetates increases, the substrate acidifies, and slows down the biogas production process. At the beginning of the experiment, the level of pH was 6.4 ± 0.1, while at the end it dropped to 6.2 ± 0.1.

The concentration of methane in biogas was increasing since day 4 at the rate of 10% up to day 8 of the experiment and that day it reached 0.178 m^3/m^3d (i.e. 61.3% of biogas volume). Since day 8, the concentration of methane stabilized and until the final day of the experiment only slight change in the concentration could be observed. The range is from 0.036 m^3/m^3d to 0.092 m^3/m^3d. Biogas, containing such levels of methane, is a valuable fuel and can be used for the production of energy or as a motor fuel, as the concentration of methane is 60% [25]. At the beginning of the experiment, the level of pH reached 6.4 ± 0.1, while at the end it dropped to 6.35 ± 0.1. During the experiment, the anaerobic conditions were secured, as the amount of oxygen ranged from 3.1% at the beginning of the experiment and later, at the end, it dropped to 0.1%. The concentration of hydrogen sulfide in biogas varied in the range from 15 ppm to 72 ppm, therefore, the biogas purification of this pollutant is not necessary.

Conclusions

1. The biggest average amount of biogas was measured during the processing of macro-algae *spirogyra neglecta* and reached 0,23 m^3/m^3d.
2. The highest average methane concentration in biogas was gauged during the decomposition of *cladophora glomerata* and reached 51,4%; during the processing of other algae (*spirogyra neglecta* and *chara fragilis*), the gauged concentration of methane was 46,5% and 36,9% respectively.
3. The assessment of both parameters, i.e. the amount of biogas and methane concentration, indicates that the most suitable algae for the production of energy are both *spirogyra neglecta* and *cladophora glomerata.*
4. During all the conducted experiments of processing all three kinds of algae, the anaerobic conditions were secured, and hydrogen sulfide concentrations were below 100 ppm. Therefore, biogas purification of this pollutant is not necessary.
5. The comparison of the emitted biogas and methane concentration during the processing of macro-algae with other biodegradable waste indicates that macro-algae is a suitable raw material for the production of biogas. During the processing of algae, the amount of biogas fluctuates between 0,64 and 1,32 m^3/m^3d, and the volume of methane ranges from 0,24 to 0,68 m^3/m^3d. During the decomposition of other biodegradable waste, the amount of biogas reaches from 0,9 to 1,67 m^3/m^3d. However, the concentration of methane is lower as compared with that obtained from macro-algae.

Competing interests

The authors declare that they have no competing interests.

Authors' contributions

PB participated in the conception of the study, interpretation of data and in the given final approval of the version to be published; AM responsible for experimental research, data analysis and Helped to draft the manuscript. Both authors read and approved the final manuscript.

Acknowledgments

Acknowledgement express Vilnius Gediminas Technical University Institute of Environmental Protection for the opportunity to use existing equipment and the possibility to carry out experimental studies.

References

1. Razon LF, Tan RR. Net energy analysis of the production of biodiesel and biogas from the microalgae. *Haematococcus pluvialis* and *Nannochloropsis*. Appl Energy. 2011;88:3507–14.
2. Vinogradova T, Danaher M, Baxter A, Moloney M, Victory D, Haughey SA. Rapid surface plasmon resonance immunobiosensor assay for microcystin toxins in blue-green algae food supplements. Talanta. 2011;84:638–43.

3. Sardi L, Martelli G, Lambertini L, Parisini P, Mordenti A. Effects of a dietary supplement of DHA-rich marine algae on Italian heavy pig production parameters. Livest Sci. 2006;103:95–103.
4. Navickas K, Župerka V, Venslauskas K. Gyvūninės kilmės šalutinių produktų anaerobinis perdirbimas į biodujas (Anaerobic treatment of animal by-products tobiogas). Res Pap IAg Eng LUA & LU Ag. 2007;39:60–8.
5. Baltrėnas P, Jankaitė A, Raistenskis E. Natūralių biodegradacijos procesų, vykstančių maisto atliekose eksperimentiniai tyrimai (Natural biodegradation processes occurring in food waste experimental research). J Environ Enginee Land Manag. 2005;13:167–76.
6. Zigmontienė A, Zuokaitė E. Investigation into emissions of gaseous pollutants during sewage sludge composting with wood waste. J Environ Enginee Land Manag. 2010;18:128–36.
7. Babaee A, Shayegan J, Roshani A. Anaerobic slurry co-digestion of poultry manure and straw: effect of organic loading and temperature. Iran J Environ Heal Scien Engineer. 2013;11: doi: 10.1186/2052-336X-11-15.
8. Kvasauskas M, Baltrėnas P. Research on anaerobically treated organic waste suitability for soil fertilization. J Environ Enginee Land Manag. 2009;17:205–11.
9. Ojolo SJ, Oke SA, Animasahun K, Adesuyi BK. Utilization of poultry, cow and kitchen wastes for biogas production: comparative analyses. Iran J Environ Heal Scien Engineer. 2007;4:223–8.
10. Harun R, Davidson M, Doyle M, Gopiraj R, Danquah M, Forde G. Technoeconomic analysis of an integrated microalgae photobioreactor, biodiesel and biogas production facility. Biom Bioener. 2011;35:741–7.
11. Zhong WZ, Zhang ZZ, Luo YJ, Qiao W, Xiao M, Zhang M. Biogas productivity by codigesting Taihu blue algae with corn straw as an external carbon source. Biores Technol. 2012;114:281–6.
12. Mussgnug JH, Klassen V, Schlüter A, Kruse O. Microalgae as substrates for fermentative biogas production in a combined biorefinery concept. J Biotechnol. 2010;150:51–6.
13. Salermo M, Nurdogan Y, Lundquist TJ. Biogas Production from Algae Biomass Harvested at Wastewater Treatment Ponds. In Proceedings of the 2009 Bioenergy Engineering Conference: 11-14 October 2009; Bellevue, Washington. ASABE Paper Number Bio098023.
14. Vergara-Fernández A, Vargas G, Alarcón N, Velasco A. Evaluation of marine algae as a source of biogas in a two-stage anaerobic reactor system. Biom Bioener. 2008;32:338–44.
15. Cladophora. [Available online at: http://en.wikipedia.org/wiki/Cladophora]. (accessed 10 March 2013).
16. Chara (alga). [Available online at: http://en.wikipedia.org/wiki/Chara_%28alga %29] (accessed 10 March 2013).
17. Golkowska K, Greger M. Anaerobic digestion of maize and cellulose under thermophilic and mesophilic conditions: a comparative study. Biom Bioener. 2013;56:545–54.
18. Misevičius A, Baltrėnas P. Experimental investigation of biogas production using biodegradable municipal waste. J Environ Enginee Land Manag. 2011;19:167–77.
19. Budrys R. Wastewater treatment sludge (WTS), and biodegradable waste (BW) processing. In 9th Conference of Young Scientists "Science-Lithuanian Future": 30 March 2006; Vilnius, Lithuania:30–9.
20. Schön M. Numerical modelling of anaerobic digestion processes in agricultural biogas plants. Innsbruck, Austria. 2010.
21. Weiland P. Biogas production: current state and perspectives. Appl Microb Biotechnol. 2009;85:849–60.
22. Al Seadi T, Rutz D, Prassl H, Köttner M, Finsterwalder T, Volk S, et al. Biogas handbook. Niels Bohrs Vej 9-10, DK-6700 Esbjerg, Denmark: University of Southern Denmark Esbjerg; 2008. ISBN: 978-87-992962-0-0.2008.
23. Algae. [Available online at: http://www.mokslasirtechnika.lt/mokslo-naujienos/zalioji-energija-is-mikrodumbli-daug-zadantis-alternatyvus-ateities-kuras.html]. (Accessed 13 March 2015).
24. Baltrėnas P, Kvasauskas M. Experimental invest tigation of biogas production using fatty waste. J Environ Enginee Land Manag. 2008;16:178–87.
25. Kalpokas V. Experimental investigation on biogas production using pig manure and slaughterhouse waste. In 8th International Conference "Environmental Engineering": 19-20 May 2011; Vilnius, Lithuania. Collection of articles: 150–4.

Spatial distribution of heavy metals in soil, water, and vegetables of farms in Sanandaj, Kurdistan, Iran

Afshin Maleki[1], Hassan Amini[2,3,1*], Shahrokh Nazmara[4], Shiva Zandi[1] and Amir Hossein Mahvi[4,5]

Abstract

Background: Heavy metals are ubiquitous elsewhere in nature and their measurement in environment is necessary to develop health management strategies. In this study, we aimed to find out concentrations and spatial patterns of heavy metals in main farms of Sanandaj in Kurdistan, Iran.

Methods: Over May to October 2012, six farms were selected to analyze concentrations and spatial patterns of several heavy metals, namely aluminum (Al), arsenic (As), cadmium (Cd), cobalt (Co), chromium (Cr), copper (Cu), nickel (Ni), lead (Pb), and zinc (Zn) in their soil, irrigation water, and edible vegetables. Overall, 36 samples of soil and water and 72 samples of vegetables including coriander (*Coriandrum sativum*), dill (*Anethum graveolens*), radish (*Raphanus sativus*) root and radish leaf were collected. The concentrations of metals were determined by inductively coupled plasma optical emission spectrometry. The spatial surfaces of heavy metals were created using geospatial information system.

Results: The order of metals in soil was Al > Zn > Ni > Cu > Cr > Pb > Co > As > Cd while in water it was Cr > Co > Zn > Pb > Cu > Ni > Al = As = Cd. The order of heavy metals in vegetables was Al > Zn > Cu > Cr > Ni > Pb > Co > As > Cd. Totally, the minimum concentrations of Al, Cu, Pb, and Zn were found in radish root while the maximum of Al, Co, Cr, and Ni were found in radish leaf. The minimum concentrations of Cd and Cr and maximum concentrations of Cu and Zn were also deciphered in dill. Noteworthy, coriander had the minimum concentrations of Co and Ni. The concentrations of Cr and Pb in vegetables were more than maximum allowable limits of the Food and Agriculture Organization (FAO) and the World Health Organization (WHO).

Conclusion: In summary, albeit the concentrations of heavy metals in soil and water samples were below FAO and the WHO standards, vegetables were contaminated by chromium and lead.

Keywords: Coriander, Dill, GIS, Heavy metals, Iran, Mapping, Radish, Soil, Vegetables, Water

Background

Heavy metals—those with specific density of about 4-5 g/cm^3 or higher—are actually ubiquitous elsewhere in nature. In fact, there are several sources of contamination, namely natural, agricultural, domestic, atmospheric, and other sources [1]. However, tremendous application and utilization of heavy metals in more recent years through industries caused steep emissions to our environment [2]. The main pathways of humans' exposure to these elements are through air, water, soil and hence agricultural crops [3].

The health effects of heavy metals have been known since ancient history [2]. In essence, toxicity and/or carcinogenicity of heavy metals, such as lead, arsenic, mercury, cadmium, and nickel have been reported in numerous studies [4-10], even in low dose exposures [11]. In brief, they may cause kidney, lung, nervous system, and skeletal damages, such as itai-itai disease [12-15]. Diminished intellectual capacity, gastrointestinal symptoms, coronary heart disease, variety of cancers, such as renal, skin, and bladder cancers, and even death have been

* Correspondence: Hassan.Amini@unibas.ch
[2]Department of Epidemiology and Public Health, Swiss Tropical and Public Health Institute (Swiss TPH), Socinstrasse 57, 4002 Basel, Switzerland
[3]University of Basel, Petersplatz 1, 4003 Basel, Switzerland
Full list of author information is available at the end of the article

also associated with chronic and/or acute exposures to heavy metals [3,16-18].

Some of heavy metals, such as iron, copper, and zinc are present in trace amounts (10 mg/kg, or mg/l) or ultra-trace amounts (1 μg/kg, or μg/l) in environmental matrices as they are essential for biochemical and/or physiological functions. However, quantities beyond the requirement of living organism may lead to its toxicity [1].

Overall, majority of heavy metals daily intake in humans is from diet, mainly through crop plants [8,19]. It is well recognized now that certain species of plants tend to bioaccumulate heavy metals [20-23]. For instance, Maleki and Alasvand Zarasvand [24] reported that lead, copper, chromium, and cadmium were present in edible vegetables, such as leek, sweet basil, parsley, garden cress, and tarragon in Sanandaj, Iran beyond the allowable national standards. In addition, Mohajer et al. [25] declared that most plants grown in Isfahan, Iran had heavy metals more than international standards in which 48 and 75 percent of vegetable samples had concentrations of cadmium and lead beyond the Food and Agriculture Organization (FAO) and the World Health Organization (WHO) guidelines. Eslami et al. [26] determined high levels of cadmium and lead in parsley, leek, radish leaves and roots, and sweet basil, which were well above the maximum threshold values recommended by FAO and the WHO. Pourang and Noori [27] also analyzed heavy metals in various plant species of an agricultural area near Tehran and reported that chromium, cadmium, and lead were substantially above national and international guidelines in most of vegetables, especially in onions. Cadmium and lead were again principal culprits in cucumbers and bell peppers grown in greenhouses of Qom, Iran [28]. Besides, there are many similar studies from China, Ghana, and other countries that measured heavy metals in agricultural soils, irrigation water and/or their crops [29-33].

The excess presence of heavy metals in edible vegetables that people consume, as reported by numerous researchers, may pose a health threat to general population. Therefore, it is essential to monitor their concentrations in vegetables. Moreover, measurement of heavy metals in irrigation water and also agricultural soil may help to better understand sources of contamination and consequently develop effective management strategies. The application of Geospatial Information System (GIS) technology also has been proposed by other researchers to identify spatial distribution of trace elements and sources of pollution [34,35]. Therefore, in this study, the authors aimed to decipher levels and spatial patterns of heavy metals in soil, irrigation water, and edible vegetables of farms in Sanandaj, Kurdistan, Iran.

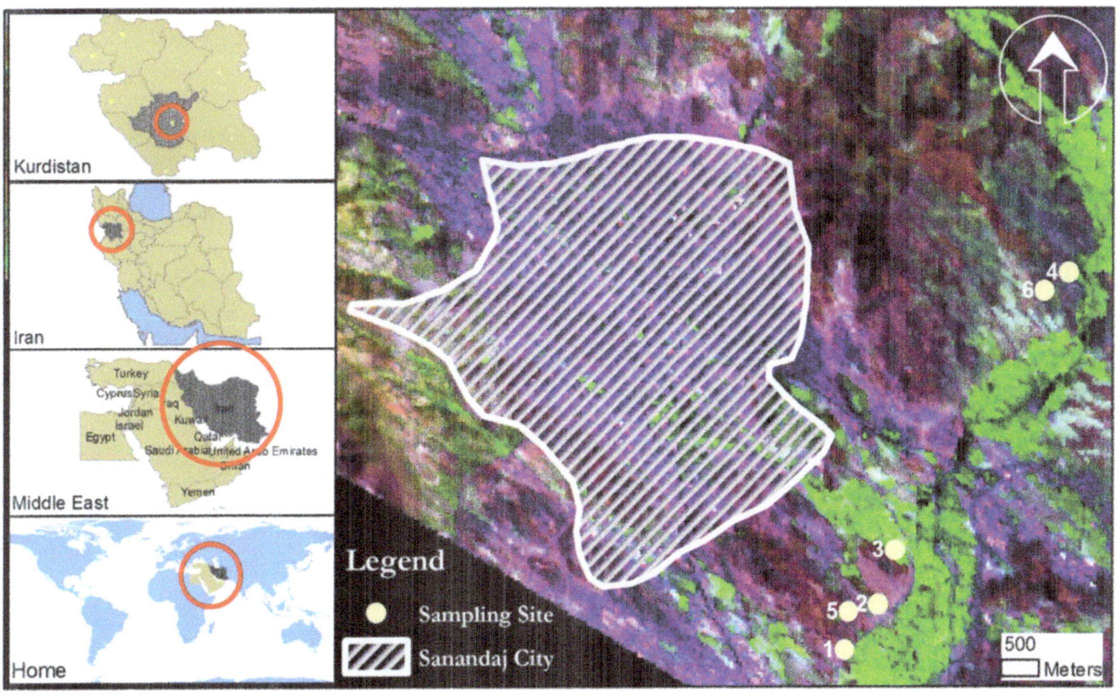

Figure 1 Study area and location of sampling sites in Sanandaj, Kurdistan, Iran.

Table 1 Descriptive statistics of heavy metals in Sanandaj's soil samples and the international maximum allowable standards

Heavy metal (mg/kg)	Al	As	Cd	Co	Cr	Cu	Ni	Pb	Zn
Mean	4139.5	3.8	0.10	14.8	28.7	42.6	47.9	25.4	77.2
Median	4126.5	3.8	0.10	14.3	29.1	38.7	48.1	26.6	77.8
Standard deviation	84.9	0.6	0.06	1.5	1.9	14.9	2.7	3.1	21.6
Min	4045.0	3.0	0.00	13.4	25.7	27.9	43.3	21.3	52.9
Max	4278.0	4.6	0.20	17.4	30.6	61.1	51.7	28.2	100.6
Austria standard [41]	-	50	5	50	100	100	100	100	300
The European Union standard [42]	-	-	3	-	150	140	75	300	300

Materials and methods

Study area and sampling sites

Sanandaj is capital of Kurdistan province in North West of Iran. The city is developing and non-industrialized [36]. However, there are various small industries and workshops, such as welding of metals and plating, small tanning industries, etc., which are mainly located in southeast region. There are several farmland areas in outskirts of the city near Sanandaj's small river, located also in southeast region (Figure 1). Nevertheless, there are six major farms for cultivating vegetables around the city and we included all of them in the study. Over May to October 2012, we selected these six farms to analyze levels and spatial distribution of several heavy metals, namely aluminum (Al), arsenic (As), cadmium (Cd), cobalt (Co), chromium (Cr), copper (Cu), nickel (Ni), lead (Pb), and zinc (Zn) in soil, irrigation water, and edible vegetables that they produce. The sampling was done over this period as it is suitable for planting and harvesting of vegetables in Sanandaj.

Soil sampling

Overall, 18 samples of soil were collected bimonthly during study period (6 farms × 3 times). For each sample at each farm, a mixture of sub-samples was collected to form a composite soil sample to be representative of the whole farm. In detail, a hole of 25 cm was dug using a clean stainless steel trowel and three to four slices of soil from top to bottom were sampled and preserved in a clean bag. The bag was labeled and transferred to the laboratory [37,38].

Irrigation water sampling

The farms were irrigated by groundwater. Overall, 18 samples of water were collected bimonthly during study period. In detail, sampling was done using a 500 ml washed polypropylene bottle. Noteworthy, 1 ml of nitric acid was added to the samples to avoid microbial activity [38,39].

Vegetable sampling

The four commonly produced vegetables of these farms were selected for sampling including coriander (*Coriandrum sativum*), dill (*Anethum graveolens*), radish (*Raphanus sativus*) root and radish leaf. Overall, 72 samples of vegetable were compiled bimonthly during study period (6 farms × 4 vegetables × 3 times). A mixture of six sub-samples at various distances (10 m, 30 m, 50 m, 70 m, 120 m and 140 m) was collected for each sample to form a composite sample of vegetables at each farm [40].

Analytical methods

The soil samples were oven dried at 80°C at laboratory until stable weights were obtained. Thereafter, they were crushed using a porcelain mortar with a pestle and mixed thoroughly until they could be sifted through a 10 mesh sieve. For heavy metal analyses, about 100 g of each soil sample was separated out, transferred to a beaker, and as stated in the SW-846, 3050 method of EPA, analytical degree of HNO_3 and H_2O_2 (30%) were applied for soil digestion.

Table 2 Physicochemical characteristics of soil samples in farms of Sanandaj, Kurdistan, Iran

Site	pH	EC (dS/m)	Total neutralizing value (%)	Organic carbon (%)	K (ppm)	P (ppm)	Soil texture	Bulk density (g/cm^3)	Soil particle percent (%)		
									Clay	Silt	Sand
1	8.1	0.622	9.75	1.54	261	11.7	Silty clay	-	47.5	50.7	1.8
2	7.9	0.954	13.5	1.9	323	29.2	Silty clay	1.25	42.5	43.2	14.3
3	7.9	0.726	12.25	0.2	527	25.2	Silty clay	1.21	50	41.6	8.4
4	7.9	0.711	11.5	1.3	512	22.7	Silty clay	1.21	49.2	43.7	7.1
5	7.8	0.610	24.25	1.47	302	10.14	Clay	1.26	47.5	23.2	29.3
6	7.8	0.625	25.45	1.2	337	12.2	Clay	1.25	48	24.5	27.5

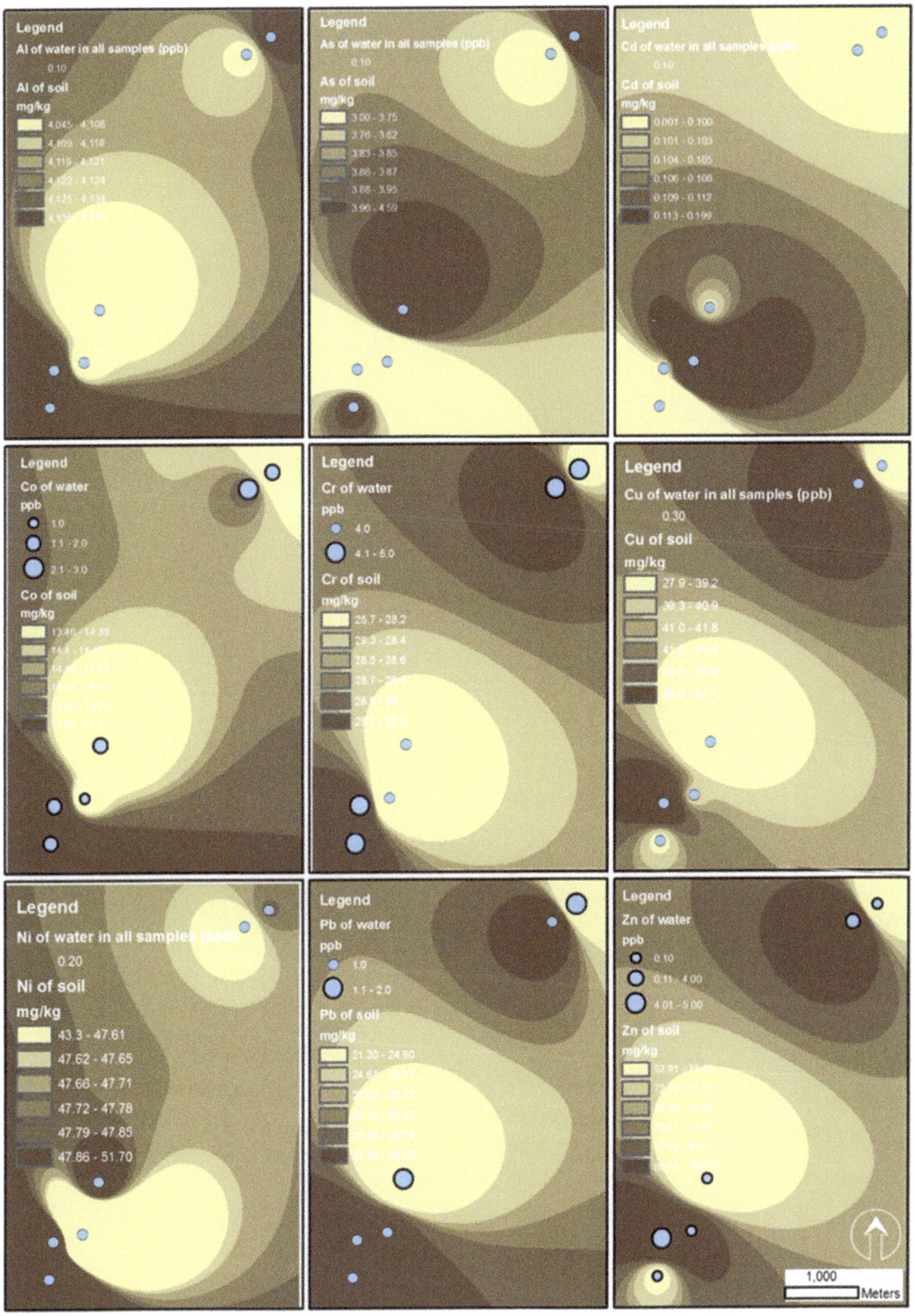

Figure 2 Spatial patterns of heavy metals in soil and irrigation water of farms in Sanandaj, Kurdistan, Iran.

The vegetable samples were transferred to laboratory and washed with distilled water to remove mulch or soil. In order to remove excess moisture, samples were air dried for approximately two weeks. Afterwards, using a porcelain mortar and a pestle, samples were grounded until they could be sifted through a 10 mesh sieve. For heavy metal analyses, about 1 g of each sample was separated out and transferred to a Pyrex beaker. Then, 10 ml of mixture of acids including HNO_3, $HClO_4$ and H_2SO_4 in ratio of 1:1:1 was added to the beaker and maintained at laboratory for 24 hours. After this lag, the beaker was heated at 95°C on hot plate until volume was reduced to 10 ml. Again, 10 ml of acid mixture was added and until reaching to 4 ml was heated. Afterwards, 50 ml of deionized water was added and the digest was filtered. Finally, 100 ml of solution was made by adding double deionized water [38,40].

The concentration of heavy metals in soil, irrigation water, and vegetables were determined by inductively coupled plasma optical emission spectrometry (ICP-OES) (Model SPECTRO ARCOS, SPECTRO Inc.; Germany). In detail, torch type of apparatus was flared end EOP Torch 2.5 mm; detector was CCD; nebulizer type was cross flow; nebulizer flow was 0.85 l/min; plasma power was 1400 W; coolant flow was 14.5 l/min; and pump rate was 30 RPM. Meanwhile, physicochemical characteristics of soil including pH, EC, total neutralizing value, organic carbon, K, P, soil texture, bulk density, and soil particle percent were analyzed according to the standard methods.

The GIS analysis

All geographic coordinates of sampling points were recorded using a Global Positioning System (GPS) device (Garmin, Garmin International Inc.; Kansas, USA). Next, a GIS was established and using Spatial Analyst extension to ESRI's ArcMap 9.3 GIS (ESRI, Redlands, CA, USA), spatial surfaces of heavy metals in soil and vegetables were created by interpolation method. The applied interpolation method was Inverse Distance Weighted (IDW).

Statistical analysis

Descriptive statistics, such as minimum, 25%ile, median, 75%ile, and maximum were presented by box plots. In addition, mean and standard deviation were calculated. We calculated all statistical analyses by STATA software (STATA Corp., TX, USA).

Results

Soil heavy metals

The concentrations of heavy metals in soil samples including Al, As, Cd, Co, Cr, Cu, Ni, Pb, and Zn are shown in Table 1.

The order of heavy metals presence in soil samples was as follow: Al > Zn > Ni > Cu > Cr > Pb > Co > As > Cd. Interestingly, heavy metals of soil in none of the cases exceeded international standard levels, such as Austria, and the European Union standards (Table 1). Results of physicochemical characteristics of soil samples are shown in Table 2. Importantly, pH of soil samples in all cases was circum-neutral to alkaline with the minimum of 7.8 and the maximum of 8.1 (Table 2). Figure 2, meanwhile, shows spatial pattern of measured heavy metals in soil samples of farms in Sanandaj, Kurdistan, Iran.

Irrigation water heavy metals

Table 3 shows the concentrations of heavy metals in water samples of farms in Sanandaj, Kurdistan, Iran. The order of heavy metals presence in water samples was as follow: Cr > Co > Zn > Pb > Cu > Ni > Al = As = Cd. The concentrations of Al, As, Cd, Cu, and Ni were similar for the six farms. As shown in Table 3, heavy metals of water samples in none of the cases exceeded international standard levels, such as Austria standard. Additionally, results of physicochemical characteristics are shown in Table 4. The pH of water samples in all cases was also circum-neutral to alkaline with the minimum of 7.6 and the maximum of 8.1 (Table 4). Meanwhile, spatial patterns of measured heavy metals in water samples of farms are shown in Figure 2 by graduate symbols.

Vegetables heavy metals

Table 5 tabulated the mean concentrations of heavy metals in vegetable samples of farms in Sanandaj, Kurdistan, Iran. Besides, descriptive statistics including the minimum, 25%ile, median, 75%ile, and maximum of heavy metals in vegetables are illustrated in Figure 3 as box plots. The order of heavy metals presence in coriander and dill samples were similar and as follow: Al > Zn > Cu > Cr > Ni > Pb > Co > As > Cd. The order in radish leaf was as Al > Zn > Cr > Cu > Ni > Pb > Co > As > Cd and in radish root samples was as Al > Zn > Cr > Cu > Ni > Co > Pb > As > Cd. Overall, the order of heavy metals for vegetables was as follow: Al > Zn > Cu > Cr > Ni > Pb > Co >

Table 3 Descriptive statistics of heavy metals in Sanandaj's irrigation water samples and the international maximum allowable standards

Heavy metal (ppb)	Al	As	Cd	Co	Cr	Cu	Ni	Pb	Zn
Mean	0.1	0.1	0.1	2.0	4.7	0.3	0.2	1.3	1.6
Median	0.1	0.1	0.1	2.0	5.0	0.3	0.2	1.0	0.1
Standard deviation	0.0	0.0	0.0	0.6	0.5	0.0	0.0	0.5	2.3
Min	0.1	0.1	0.1	1.0	4.0	0.3	0.2	1.0	0.1
Max	0.1	0.1	0.1	3.0	5.0	0.3	0.2	2.0	5.0
Austria standard [41]	5000	100	10	50	100	200	200	5000	2000

Table 4 Physicochemical characteristics of irrigation water samples in farms of Sanandaj, Kurdistan, Iran[a]

Site	pH	EC (μS/cm)	TDS (mg/l)	Total hardness (mg/l $CaCO_3$)	Turbidity (NTU)	Total alkalinity (mg/l $CaCO_3$)
1	8.1	585	379	280	5.0	126
2	7.9	479	312	208	3.1	130
3	7.6	610	396	312	2.5	140
4	7.6	600	388	300	2.4	137
5	7.6	732	477	440	1.2	166
6	7.7	715	465	432	1.0	170

[a]Reprint from Maleki et al. [43] with written permission. *Abbreviations: EC* Electrical Conductivity, *TDS* Total Dissolved Solids, *NTU* Nephelometric Turbidity Units.

As > Cd. In general, the minimum concentrations of Al, Cu, Pb, and Zn were found in radish root while the maximum of Al, Co, Cr, and Ni were found in radish leaf. The minimum concentrations of Cd and Cr and the maximum concentrations of Cu and Zn also were deciphered in dill. Noteworthy, coriander had the minimum concentrations of Co and Ni (Table 5). Figure 4 shows spatial distribution of measured heavy metals in vegetable samples of farms in Sanandaj, Kurdistan, Iran.

Discussion

In this research, we characterized the concentrations of several important heavy metals in agricultural soil, irrigation water, and vegetable crops of six farms in Sanandaj, Kurdistan, Iran. We further depicted spatial distribution of these heavy elements in the studied area.

In general, we know now from our wide literature that levels of each heavy metal in soil is controlled by several interactive complex factors, such as pH, organic matter, cation exchange capacity, clay constitute of soil, and concentrations of aluminum and iron content [45]. More importantly, these factors, especially pH, would affect bioaccessibility and bioaccumulation of these heavy elements in plants. While aluminum is one of the most abundant elements in soil, its availability for crops is dependent on pH [46,47]. It is believed that soluble aluminum, which is absorbable by plants, is present in soil pH below 5.0, where rarely this pH is suitable for agriculture [48]. Noteworthy, aluminum has been classified as a *contaminant of potential concern* only in soils with a pH of 5.5 or less [46]. This may be the reason why no standard have been set for aluminum in soil (Table 1). However, the unexpected result was that aluminum became the first rank in vegetables of Sanandaj (Table 5 and Figure 3) while pH of soil was circum-neutral to alkaline (Table 2), which means aluminum has been absorbable in soil pH above 5.5. Meanwhile, the minimum and the maximum concentrations of aluminum among the four tested vegetables, respectively, were found in radish root and radish leaf, which means radish leaf may contribute to the maximum intake of aluminum to Sanandaj's residents through consumption of tested vegetables. Interestingly, the concentration of aluminum in irrigation water samples, which was 0.1 ppm, is much lower than Austria's standard for irrigation water (5000 ppm).

The concentrations of all measured heavy metals in soil and irrigation water were below maximum allowable international standards, while in vegetables the concentrations of chromium (4.2 mg/kg) and lead (0.4 mg/kg) were more than the allowable limits, which are 2.3 and 0.3 mg/kg, respectively (Table 5). The presence of small industries/workshops in the proximity of the farms may be sources of these contaminations. However, this interpretation will be dubious as the concentrations of all heavy metals in soil and water were below the maximum allowable standards. Another reason for lead contamination of vegetables may be that these farms are located near major roads, which may cause air pollution and produce fine particles containing lead. However, it is more than 10 years that pb has been removed from

Table 5 Mean concentrations of heavy metals in Sanandaj's vegetable samples and maximum allowable standard[a]

Vegetable	Mean heavy metal (mg/kg)								
	Al	As	Cd	Co	Cr	Cu	Ni	Pb	Zn
Coriander	55.8	0.10	0.010	0.2	4.2	8.9	2.6	0.4	20.9
Dill	57.0	0.10	0.005	0.2	3.8	10.6	2.8	0.4	27.6
Radish leaf	73.3	0.10	0.010	0.5	4.7	4.2	3.0	0.4	20.7
Radish root	47.8	0.10	0.010	0.6	3.9	3.0	2.6	0.3	17.0
Total	58.5	0.10	0.010	0.4	4.2	6.7	2.8	0.4	21.5
FAO and the WHO standard [44]	-	0.43	0.200	50	2.3	73.5	67.9	0.3	99.4

[a]Partly reprint from Maleki et al. [43] with written permission.

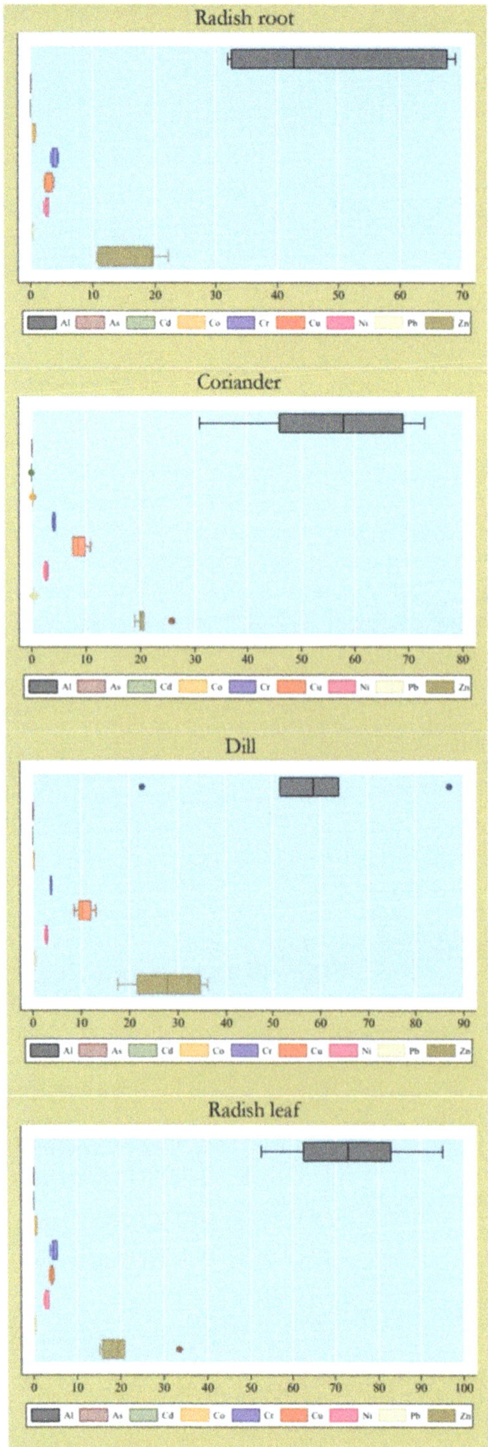

Figure 3 **Heavy metals of vegetables in farms of Sanandaj, Kurdistan, Iran.**

petrol of Iran because of health-related issues [49]. The other interpretation, which is more credible, is presence of Middle Eastern Dust (MED) events in this region [36,50]. In fact, during last decade the welkin of about 11 provinces of Western and South Western Iran have dramatically changed because of MEDs, which is believed originate from deserts of Iraq and Syria [50,51]. Although we could not find any study to date in Sanandaj that evaluate ionic composition of the MEDs, especially heavy metal composition, and as the samples of soil and water were not contaminated by heavy metals, the contamination of vegetables by chromium and lead may be due to the MEDs. In any case, chromium is toxic for most plants and affect seed germination [52,53]. Moreover, chromium compounds have been considered as carcinogen for humans [54]. Long-term exposure to lead, also, is associated with decreases of intelligence capacity in children [49]. Thus, it is essential to inform Sanandaj's population that chromium and lead contaminated vegetables of these farms. In detail, none of the sampled vegetables was safe to human consumption. However, the order of presence for chromium in vegetables was radish leaf > coriander > radish root > dill. For lead, the order was dill = coriander = radish leaf > radish root and radish root had a boundary standard lead content for consumption (Table 5). Overall, radish root and dill had lower concentrations of heavy metals than radish leaf and coriander in Sanandaj. On the other hand, Finster et al. [55] have found that lead tends to concentrate more in radish roots rather than shoots in Chicago, USA. However, the same was not found in Sanandaj [55]. As shown in Table 5, coriander and dill absorb copper at higher rates than chromium, while for radish root and radish leaf it was reverse. All of the vegetables, except radish root, absorb lead at higher rates rather than cobalt. Meanwhile, all of the vegetables were poor absorber of arsenic and cadmium. It is noteworthy that Sipter et al. [56] have found that sorrel, carrot, and onion absorb cadmium and zinc at higher rates than lead. Although zinc was the most absorbed heavy metal after aluminum in Sanandaj's sampled vegetables, lead and cobalt were absorbed at higher rates than cadmium. As illustrated in Figure 4, the vegetables of northeastern farms had more concentrations of aluminum, chromium, copper, and nickel while other measured heavy elements were lower in southwestern sites.

Conclusions

In conclusion, despite the concentrations of measured heavy metals in soil and irrigation water were below the international standards, the concentrations of chromium and lead in vegetables were higher than FAO and the WHO standards.

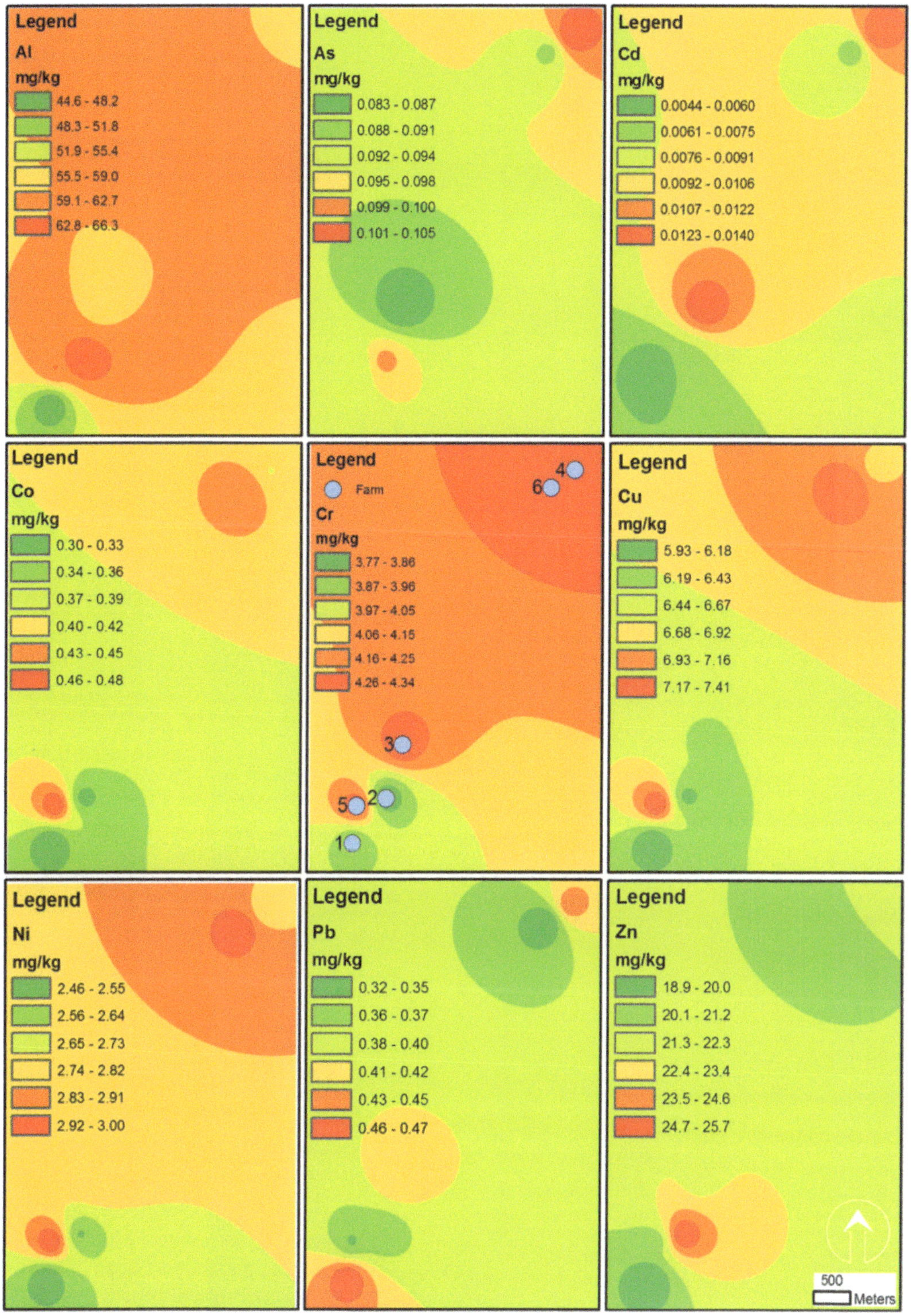

Figure 4 Spatial patterns of heavy metals in vegetables of farms in Sanandaj, Kurdistan, Iran.

Competing interest
The authors declare that they have no competing interest.

Authors' contributions
AM designed the study, supervised the sampling and analyses, and revised the manuscript. HA conducted statistical and GIS analyses, and drafted the manuscript. SN and SZ conducted experimental analyses in laboratory. AHM supervised the study. All authors read and approved the final manuscript.

Acknowledgements
The authors would like to thank staff of the laboratory at Faculty of Health, Kurdistan University of Medical Sciences, for their wholehearted cooperation. This research was financially supported by Kurdistan University of Medical Sciences; thereby we acknowledge.

Author details
[1]Kurdistan Environmental Health Research Center, Kurdistan University of Medical Sciences, Sanandaj, Iran. [2]Department of Epidemiology and Public Health, Swiss Tropical and Public Health Institute (Swiss TPH), Socinstrasse 57, 4002 Basel, Switzerland. [3]University of Basel, Petersplatz 1, 4003 Basel, Switzerland. [4]Department of Environmental Health Engineering, School of Public Health, Tehran University of Medical Sciences, Tehran, Iran. [5]Center for Solid Waste Research (CSWR), Institute for Environmental Research (IER), Tehran University of Medical Sciences, Tehran, Iran.

References
1. Nagajyoti P, Lee K, Sreekanth T: **Heavy metals, occurrence and toxicity for plants: a review.** *Environ Chem Lett* 2010, **8**:199–216.
2. Nriagu JO: **History of global metal pollution.** *Science* 1996, **272**:223–224.
3. Järup L: **Hazards of heavy metal contamination.** *Br Med Bull* 2003, **68**:167–182.
4. Tong S, von Schirnding YE, Prapamontol T: **Environmental lead exposure: a public health problem of global dimensions.** *Bull World Health Organ* 2000, **78**:1068–1077.
5. Neff JM: **Ecotoxicology of arsenic in the marine environment.** *Environ Toxicol Chem* 1997, **16**:917–927.
6. Duker AA, Carranza E, Hale M: **Arsenic geochemistry and health.** *Environ Int* 2005, **31**:631–641.
7. Thompson J, Bannigan J: **Cadmium: toxic effects on the reproductive system and the embryo.** *Reprod Toxicol* 2008, **25**:304–315.
8. Wagner GJ: **Accumulation of cadmium in crop plants and its consequences to human health.** *Adv Agron* 1993, **51**:173–212.
9. Waisberg M, Joseph P, Hale B, Beyersmann D: **Molecular and cellular mechanisms of cadmium carcinogenesis.** *Toxicology* 2003, **192**:95–117.
10. Denkhaus E, Salnikow K: **Nickel essentiality, toxicity, and carcinogenicity.** *Crit Rev Oncol Hematol* 2002, **42**:35–56.
11. Zahir F, Rizwi SJ, Haq SK, Khan RH: **Low dose mercury toxicity and human health.** *Environ Toxicol Pharmacol* 2005, **20**:351–360.
12. Nishijo M, Nakagawa H, Morikawa Y, Tabata M, Senma M, Miura K, Takahara H, Kawano S, Nishi M, Mizukoshi K: **Mortality of inhabitants in an area polluted by cadmium: 15 year follow up.** *Occup Environ Med* 1995, **52**:181–184.
13. Hayashi C, Koizumi N, Nishio H, Koizumi N, Ikeda M: **Cadmium and other metal levels in autopsy samples from a cadmium-polluted area and Non-polluted control areas in Japan.** *Biol Trace Elem Res* 2012, **145**:10–22.
14. Weiss B, Clarkson TW, Simon W: **Silent latency periods in methylmercury poisoning and in neurodegenerative disease.** *Environ Health Perspect* 2002, **110**:851.
15. Staessen JA, Roels HA, Emelianov D, Kuznetsova T, Thijs L, Vangronsveld J, Fagard R: **Environmental exposure to cadmium, forearm bone density, and risk of fractures: prospective population study. Public health and environmental exposure to cadmium (PheeCad) study group.** *Lancet* 1999, **353**:1140.
16. Kolonel LN: **Association of cadmium with renal cancer.** *Cancer* 1976, **37**:1782–1787.
17. Lanphear BP, Hornung R, Khoury J, Yolton K, Baghurst P, Bellinger DC, Canfield RL, Dietrich KN, Bornschein R, Greene T: **Low-level environmental lead exposure and children's intellectual function: an international pooled analysis.** *Environ Health Perspect* 2005, **113**:894.
18. Liu J-X, Zhou G-B, Chen S-J, Chen Z: **Arsenic compounds: revived ancient remedies in the fight against human malignancies.** *Curr Opin Chem Biol* 2012, **16**:92–98.
19. Clemens S: **Toxic metal accumulation, responses to exposure and mechanisms of tolerance in plants.** *Biochimie* 2006, **88**:1707–1719.
20. Volesky B, Holan Z: **Biosorption of heavy metals.** *Biotechnol Prog* 1995, **11**:235–250.
21. Veglio F, Beolchini F: **Removal of metals by biosorption: a review.** *Hydrometallurgy* 1997, **44**:301–316.
22. QuSheng L, ShaSha C, CeHui M, Bei C, LiHua P, FangBing Y: **Toxic effects of heavy metals and their accumulation in vegetables grown in a saline soil.** *Ecotoxicol Environ Saf* 2010, **73**:84–88.
23. Clemens S, Palmgren MG, Krämer U: **A long way ahead: understanding and engineering plant metal accumulation.** *Trends Plant Sci* 2002, **7**:309–315.
24. Maleki A, Zarasvand Alasvand M: **Heavy metals in selected edible vegetables and estimation of their daily intake in Sanandaj, Iran.** *Southeast Asian J Trop Med Public Health* 2008, **39**:335–340.
25. Mohajer R, Salehi M, Mohammadi J: **Accumulation of cadmium and lead in soils and vegetables of Lenjanat Region in Isfahan Province, Iran.** *Int J Agronomy Plant Product* 2012, **3**:576–578.
26. Eslami A, Khaniki GJ, Nurani M, Mehrasbi M, Peyda M, Azimi R: **Heavy metals in edible green vegetables grown along the sites of the Zanjanrood river in Zanjan, Iran.** *J Biol Sci* 2007, **7**:943–948.
27. Pourang N, Noori AS: **Assessment of metals in fourteen species of vegetables and crops cultivated in a suburban area using multivariate analyses.** *Toxicol Environ Chem* 2012, **94**:694–712.
28. Aghili F, Khoshgoftarmanesh A, Afyuni M, Schulin R: **Health risks of heavy metals through consumption of greenhouse vegetables grown in central Iran.** *Hum Ecol Risk Assess* 2009, **15**:999–1015.
29. Wang L, Guo Z, Xiao X, Chen T, Liao X, Song J, Wu B: **Heavy metal pollution of soils and vegetables in the midstream and downstream of the Xiangjiang River, Hunan Province.** *J Geogr Sci* 2008, **18**:353–362.
30. Wei B, Yang L: **A review of heavy metal contaminations in urban soils, urban road dusts and agricultural soils from China.** *Microchem J* 2010, **94**:99–107.
31. Akrong MO, Cobbina SJ, Ampofo JA: **Assessment of heavy metals in lettuce grown in soils irrigated with different water sources in the Accra metropolis.** *Res J Environ Earth Sci* 2012, **4**:576–582.
32. Wang XL, Sato T, Xing BS, Tao S: **Health risks of heavy metals to the general public in Tianjin, China via consumption of vegetables and fish.** *Sci Total Environ* 2005, **350**:28–37.
33. Bahemuka TE, Mubofu EB: **Heavy metals in edible green vegetables grown along the sites of the Sinza and Msimbazi rivers in Dar es Salaam, Tanzania.** *Food Chem* 1999, **66**:63–66.
34. Karyab H, Mahvi AH, Nazmara S, Bahojb A: **Determination of water sources contamination to diazinon and malathion and spatial pollution patterns in Qazvin, Iran.** *Bull Environ Contam Toxicol* 2013, **90**:126–131.
35. Amini H, Taghavi-Shahri SM, Henderson SB, Naddafi K, Nabizadeh R, Yunesian M: **Land use regression models to estimate the annual and seasonal spatial variability of sulfur dioxide and particulate matter in Tehran, Iran.** *Sci Total Environ* 2014, **488**:343–353.
36. Hosseini G, Maleki A, Amini H, Mohammadi S, Hassanvand MS, Giahi O, Gharibi F: **Health impact assessment of particulate matter in Sanandaj, Kurdistan, Iran.** *J Adv Environ Health Res* 2014, **2**:54–62.
37. Sridhara Chary N, Kamala C, Samuel Suman Raj D: **Assessing risk of heavy metals from consuming food grown on sewage irrigated soils and food chain transfer.** *Ecotoxicol Environ Saf* 2008, **69**:513–524.
38. Weldegebriel Y, Chandravanshi BS, Wondimu T: **Concentration levels of metals in vegetables grown in soils irrigated with river water in Addis Ababa, Ethiopia.** *Ecotoxicol Environ Saf* 2012, **77**:57–63.
39. Rice E, Baird R, Eaton A, Clesceri L: *Standard Methods for the Examination of Water and Waste Water.* 22nd edition. Baltimore: American Public Health Association, American Water Works Association, Water Environment Federation; 2012.
40. Tiwari K, Singh N, Patel M, Tiwari M, Rai U: **Metal contamination of soil and translocation in vegetables growing under industrial wastewater irrigated agricultural field of Vadodara, Gujarat, India.** *Ecotoxicol Environ Saf* 2011, **74**:1670–1677.
41. El Bassam N, Tietjen C: **Municipal sludge as organic fertilizer with special reference to the heavy metals constituents.** In *Soil Organic Matter Studies,* Volume 2. Vienna: IAEA; 1977.

42. McGrath S, Chang A, Page A, Witter E: **Land application of sewage sludge: scientific perspectives of heavy metal loading limits in Europe and the United States.** *Environ Rev* 1994, **2**:108–118.
43. Maleki A, Gharibi F, Alimohammadi M, Daraei H, Zandsalimi Y: **Concentration levels of heavy metals in irrigation water and vegetables grown in peri-urban areas of Sanandaj, Iran.** *J Adv Environ Health Res* 2014, **1**:81–88.
44. Codex Alimentarius Commission (FAO/WHO): *Food Additives and Contaminants*, ALINORM 01/12A. 2001:1–289.
45. Hernandez L, Probst A, Probst J, Ulrich E: **Heavy metal distribution in some French forest soils: evidence for atmospheric contamination.** *Sci Total Environ* 2003, **312**:195–219.
46. US Environmental Protection Agency: **Ecological soil screening level for aluminum. Interim final.** OSWER Directive 9285. Washington, DC: 2003:7–60.
47. Basta N, Ryan J, Chaney R: **Trace element chemistry in residual-treated soil.** *J Environ Qual* 2005, **34**:49–63.
48. Mulder J, Rasmussen L, Driscoll C: **Aluminum chemistry of acidic sandy soils with various inputs of acidic deposition in The Netherlands and in Denmark.** In *Environmental Chemistry and Toxicology of Aluminum.* Edited by Lewis T. CRC Press; 1989:171–194.
49. Finkelstein Y, Markowitz ME, Rosen JF: **Low-level lead-induced neurotoxicity in children: an update on central nervous system effects.** *Brain Res Rev* 1998, **27**:168–176.
50. Givehchi R, Arhami M, Tajrishy M: **Contribution of the Middle Eastern dust source areas to PM10 Levels in urban receptors: case study of Tehran, Iran.** *Atmos Environ* 2013, **75**:287–295.
51. Gharehchahi E, Mahvi AH, Amini H, Nabizadeh R, Akhlaghi AA, Shamsipour M, Yunesian M: **Health impact assessment of air pollution in Shiraz, Iran: a two-part study.** *J Environ Health Sci Eng* 2013, **11**:1–8.
52. Singh HP, Mahajan P, Kaur S, Batish DR, Kohli RK: **Chromium toxicity and tolerance in plants.** *Environ Chem Lett* 2013, 1–26.
53. Shanker AK, Cervantes C, Loza-Tavera H, Avudainayagam S: **Chromium toxicity in plants.** *Environ Int* 2005, **31**:739–753.
54. Costa M, Klein CB: **Toxicity and carcinogenicity of chromium compounds in humans.** *CRC Crit Rev Toxicol* 2006, **36**:155–163.
55. Finster ME, Gray KA, Binns HJ: **Lead levels of edibles grown in contaminated residential soils: a field survey.** *Sci Total Environ* 2004, **320**:245–257.
56. Sipter E, Rózsa E, Gruiz K, Tátrai E, Morvai V: **Site-specific risk assessment in contaminated vegetable gardens.** *Chemosphere* 2008, **71**:1301–1307.

5

Influence of dissolved organic matter in natural and simulated water on the photochemical decomposition of butylparaben

Marta Gmurek*, Magdalena Olak-Kucharczyk and Stanisław Ledakowicz

Abstract

Background: In the last few decades the quality of natural water has often deteriorated as a variety of novel pollutants have contaminated rivers and lakes. Trace amounts of some man-made chemicals can be hazardous to plants, animals as well as human health as carcinogens, mutagens or endocrine disruptors. Light radiation may help in its decomposition, aided by naturally occurring colored organic compounds (humic substances) in the water. The aim of these studies was to check the influence of presence of organic and inorganic matter on the removal of endocrine disrupting compound - butylparaben (BP) from water.

Methods: Photochemical decomposition of BP in aqueous solution using: photolysis by ultraviolet-C (UVC) and visible (VIS) irradiation, advanced oxidation in H_2O_2/UV system and photosensitized oxidation was examined. The degradation processes were carried out in different type of water matrix: natural water from Sulejow Reservoir, simulated natural water with humic acids and buffered solution.

Results: The presence of dissolved organic matter in water did not influence much on UVC photolysis and increases only about 8% of BP depletion rate in H_2O_2/UV system. While during visible light photolysis and photosensitized oxidation the addition of natural water matrix causes the acceleration of reaction rate by 16% and 36%, respectively. Moreover BP degradation proceeds via singlet oxygen generated from humic substances.

Conclusions: Butylparaben undergoes both direct and indirect photodegradation in aqueous solution under UVC and visible radiation. The efficiency of the H_2O_2/UV process, photolysis as well as photosensitized oxidation processes is strongly dependent on composition of the water.

Keywords: Photochemical degradation, Natural and synthetic water, Butylparaben, Humic acid, Hydroxyl radicals, Singlet oxygen

Background

In the last few decades the quality of natural water has often worsened owing to contamination with man-made trace organic chemicals. These are sometimes carcinogens, mutagens or endocrine disruptors. Such substances are often not removed in traditional wastewater treatment, are not easily biodegradable, and may accumulate in organisms [1-4]. Polluted water is a threat to human and environmental health. Contaminations have also influence on the condition and population sizes of animals and plants in natural waters. Therefore, the discovery of efficient degradation methods for these pollutants is of wide interest [5-8].

Photochemical degradation of these substances has been attempted and may be influenced by the array of dissolved organic matter (DOM), e.g., humic and fulvic acids, and by nitrate as well as other inorganic ions [9]. Hydrogen peroxide is also present in natural water, and generated mostly by solar radiation and microbial processes with concentrations in the range 10^{-6} - 10^{-5} M [10]. Reactive oxygen species (ROS) are also generated in the environment through photochemical processes and may be crucial to photochemical degradation. They include singlet oxygen ($^1O_2$), hydroxyl radical ($^{\bullet}OH$), superoxide

* Correspondence: marta.gmurek@p.lodz.pl
Faculty of Process and Environmental Engineering, Department of Bioprocess Engineering, Lodz University of Technology, Wolczanska 213, 90-924 Lodz, Poland

radicals ($HO_2^•/O_2^•$), and peroxyl radical (•OOR) as well as non-ROS transients, e.g., carbon radicals ($CH_3^•$) and triplet exited states of DOM ($^3DOM^*$) [11-15]. The production of these diverse array of reactive species is driven primarily by abiotic photochemical reactions involving naturally occurring organic and sometimes inorganic coloured substances (chromophores) [16].

The absorption of solar radiation between UVB and visible wavelengths by DOM in natural waters initiates a series of complex photochemical reactions that improve water -purification. The chromophores present within DOM become excited from their singlet ground state to their first excited singlet stated ($^1DOM^*$). Upon absorption of light, undergo intersystem crossing (ISC) to form their triplet excited state ($^3DOM^*$), and then interact with molecular oxygen to form either singlet oxygen ($^1O_2$) or superoxide ($O_2^{-•}$). Hydroxyl radicals (•OH), another common reactive oxygen species, can be formed from the interaction of water with $^3DOM^*$, the photolysis of hydrogen peroxide (H_2O_2), or the photolysis of nitrate (NO_3^-) [16].

As a result of the reactions described in Figure 1., concentrations of reactive oxygen species in natural waters have been detected in the range between 10^{-15} - 5×10^{-13} M, 10^{-15} - 10^{-12} M, 10^{-9} - 10^{-8} M, 10^{-18}- 2×10^{-16} M, for $^3DOM^*$, $^1O_2$, $O_2^{-•}$, and •OH, respectively [16]. The ROS can help to purify the aquatic environment of bioactive pollutants derived from human activities e.g. pharmaceuticals and personal care products, or, in some instances, convert them to less toxic substances. The reaction sequences followed by well-established concepts of direct and sensitized photooxidations, also potentially coupled to thermal autooxidation processes [16]. Although the role of reactive oxygen species in water purification is known, the mechanism of these processes is still not entirely clear. This work examined degradation of an endocrine disrupting compound (butylparaben (BP)) in aqueous solution using photolysis by Ultraviolet C and visible irradiation, advanced oxidation in a H_2O_2/UV system and photosensitized oxidation (POx). Degradation was carried out in different waters matrix: natural water from Sulejow Reservoir, simulated natural water with humic acids (HA), and buffered solution. The aim was to establish the influence of organic and inorganic matter on the removal of butylparaben from the water.

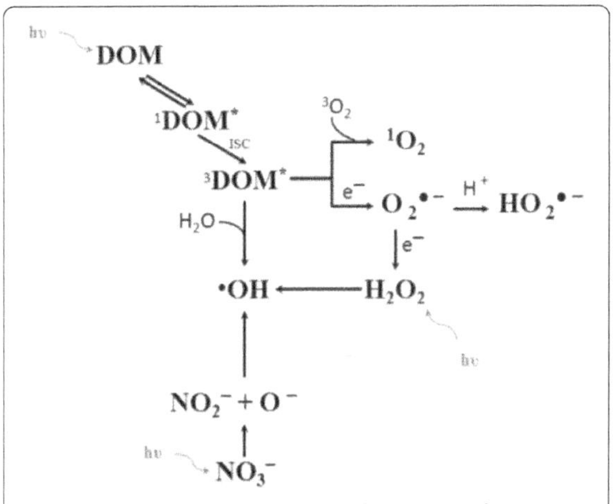

Figure 1 The pathways of photochemical generation of reactive oxygen species in natural water.

Materials and methods

Chemicals and reagents

Butylparaben (BP) (>99%, Table 1), synthetic humic acid (HA, technical), tert-butanol and sodium azide (99%) were purchased from Fluka. Hydrogen peroxide (30%), disodium phosphate (Na_2HPO_4), monopotassium phosphate (KH_2PO_4) and potassium nitrate (KNO_3) all p.a. were purchased from POCh, Poland. Meso-tetra (4-sulphonatophenyl)porphin ($TPPS_4$) was bought from Sigma-Aldrich. The element composition of Fluka humic acid (HA, cat. no. 53680) has been reported to contain 48.36% of C, 26.91% of O, 4.24% of H, 0.78%of N and 0.78% of S [17]. The atomic ratios described by Rodrigues et. al. [17], are 1.04 (H/C), 0.42 (O/C), and 0.012 (N/C) which are within the values reported in the literature for soil HA, with the exception of the N/C ratio. All chemicals were used as received.

Model solutions and natural water samples

Aqueous solutions of butylparaben were made by diluting it into: natural water from Sulejow Reservoir (RW), simulated natural water with humic acids ($SN1^{pH7}$ and $SN1^{pH9}$) or with nitrate ions (SN2) and buffered solution (BS). The concentration of butylparaben was 8×10^{-5} M. In experiments using the H_2O_2/UV system, an optimal concentration of hydrogen peroxide of 0.01 M was used. In buffer solution experiments with an xenon arc lamp (XBO), $TPPS_4$ was used as a photosensitizer at an optimal concentration of 2×10^{-5} M [18]. Buffer solutions were prepared from deionized water, purified using a Millipore Milli-Q Plus System (>18.2 MΩ). The pH of

Table 1 Physicochemical properties of butylparaben [19,20,23]

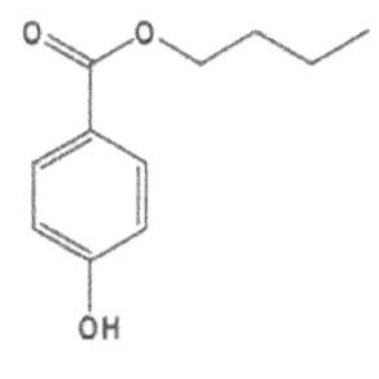	CAS No.	94-26-8
	molecular formula	$C_{11}H_{14}O_3$
	molar mass	194.23
	solubility in water	0.77 μM at 25°C; 7.5 μM at 80°C
	log K_{OW}	3.5
	pKa	8.24

the deionized solution was adjusted by adding phosphate buffer: Na_2HPO_4-KH_2PO_4. For more details, see [18,19]. Synthetic solutions with organic matter ($SN1^{pH7}$ and $SN1^{pH9}$) and nitrate (SN2) were made by diluting humic acids and potassium nitrate, respectively.

Natural water was collected in summer from the Sulejow Reservoir, situated in central Poland in the middle course of the Pilica River (latitude: 51°27.2′, longitude: 19°59.2′, area:27 km^2). Water for chemical analyses was filtered through Whatman GF/F (0.45 μm) filters and stored at 4°C before use. The pH of the reservoir water was 8.11, and its concentration of dissolved organic carbon (DOC) was 6.85 mg L^{-1}. The concentrations of major ions in the reservoir water were: Ca^{2+} (34.02 mg L^{-1}), K^+ (9.79 mg L^{-1}), Na^+ (6.51 mg L^{-1}), SO_4^{2-}(21.73 mg L^{-1}), Cl^- (12.34 mg L^{-1}), NO_3^- (0.46 mg L^{-1}). Mg^{2+}, NH_4^+, Li^+, F^-, NO_2^-, Br^-, PO_4^{3-} ions were detected at concentrations of: 0.969 mg L^{-1}, 0.044 mg L^{-1}, 0.003 mg L^{-1}, 0.112 mg L^{-1}, 0.025 mg L^{-1}, 0.007 mg L^{-1}, 0.003 mg L^{-1}, respectively.

The buffer solutions (BS) were prepared at three different pH values. BS1 had similar pH to the reservoir water (RW). BS2 was used at pH 7 to compare the influences of additives in the humic acid ($SN1^{pH7}$) and nitrate (SN2) treatments. Experiments with humic acids and visible-light irradiation were done at pH 9 (BS3 and $SN1^{pH9}$).

Photodegradation experiments

The photodegradation experiments were conducted using UVC and xenon arc lamps as sources of light. The UVC direct photolysis and degradation in a H_2O_2/UV system were carried out in a rotating device with quartz test tubes (10 mL), placed between two exposure panels, each of them consisting of three 7.2 W lamps. Low pressure lamps (LP, Luzchem) emitting mainly at a wavelength $\lambda = 254$ nm were used. For more details, see [19,20]. Photon flux rate entering the reaction space, calculated on the basis of actinometric experiments with uranyl oxalate [21] was equaled 1×10^{-5} einstein L^{-1} s^{-1}.

Photosensitizing oxidation experiments were carried out with an immersion xenon arc lamp located in a quartz well with cooling jacket. A 100 W xenon arc lamp (XBO, 100 W, Osram) served as the light source to simulate solar light irradiation. The lamp was surrounded by five plate reactors (volume 0.01 L), each placed 11 cm from the light source. Each reactor consisted of two glass plates (10 cm × 6 cm) bound with silicone seal such that the distance between the inner surfaces of the plates was 0.3 cm. The tested solutions were aerated and agitated by gas bubbling. The quantity of absorbed photons was calculated using Reinecke's actinometer for wavelengths ranging from 310 to 770 nm [22], and was 3.24×10^{-4} einstein L^{-1} s^{-1}. The 2×10^{-5} M solution of $TPPS_4$ absorbed 3.77×10^{-5} einstein L^{-1} s^{-1}.

Analysis

The butylparaben decay rate was monitored by high pressure liquid chromatography (HPLC) coupled with UV detection using a Waters apparatus. Analysis was performed with a Waters Nova-Pak C18 column (3.9 mm × 150 mm) using a mobile phase consisting of a degassed mixture (70/30, v/v %) of methanol and acidified water (0.01% orthophosphoric acid) at a constant flow of 1 mL min^{-1}. The detailed description of this analysis of BP is reported elsewhere [19,23]. The spectrophotometric analysis was performed on a Unicam UV 300 spectrophotometer. The dissolved organic carbon measurements were performed on a HACH IL 550TOC-TN apparatus. The ion concentrations were determined by an ion chromatograph (Dionex model ICS) on an IonPac CS18 (for cations) and an IonPac AS18 (for anions).

The performed experiments allowed us to estimate the extent of direct reaction of butylparaben with hydrogen peroxide in the absence of radiation, ("dark reaction").

Results indicated an insignificant role of the direct reaction of studied compounds with H_2O_2. The blank reaction was carried out to investigate the hydrolysis of BP. The experiments showed no decomposition of the investigated compound in the dark after 12 h, much longer time than used during the photodegradation.

Experiments were performed in duplicate to assure accurate data acquisition.

Results and discussion

For studies on photochemical degradation of butylparaben, the comparison of BP absorbance spectra in different reaction solutions with the emission spectra of the UVC and xenon arc (XBO) lamps were performed (Figure 2). Butylparaben in neutral solutions such as the humic acid and nitrate treatments, absorbs light mainly at low wavelengths up to 300 nm so its degradation by direct photolysis is expected to be higher using UVC systems. The degradation of butylparaben occurs by direct photolysis also in reservoir water (RW) and BS1, due to overlapping of the absorption spectrum of butylparaben with UVC and xenon arc lamps. In alkaline solution the direct photolysis of BP is likely as a results of occurring with xenon arc (XBO) irradiation.

The substances commonly found in natural waters, both organic and inorganic, may affect the photodegradation process of pollutants e.g. Cl^- ions accelerate the photodegradation of selected antibiotics under UV-Visible irradiation ($\lambda > 200$ nm), whereas simulated solar irradiation ($\lambda > 290$ nm) was incapable of antibiotics photodecomposition, irrespective of Cl^- [24].

Figure 3 shows the degradation of butyparaben in water collected from Sulejow Reservoir (RW). UVC photolysis of butylparaben proceeded slightly slower (about 6%) (Figure 3a) in natural water compared with photolysis in

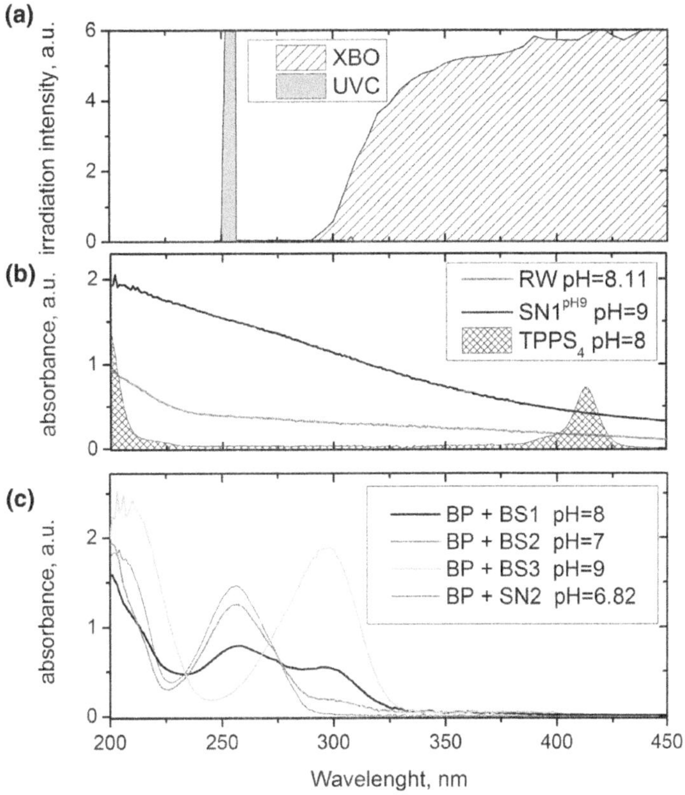

Figure 2 Emission spectra of lamps used in experiments **(a)**, absorption spectra of selected waters and $TPPS_4$ **(b)** ($C_{TPPS4} = 5 \times 10^{-6}$ M, $C_{HA} = 50$ mg L^{-1}) and BP solutions in different water matrix **(c)** ($C_{BP} = 8 \times 10^{-5}$ M).

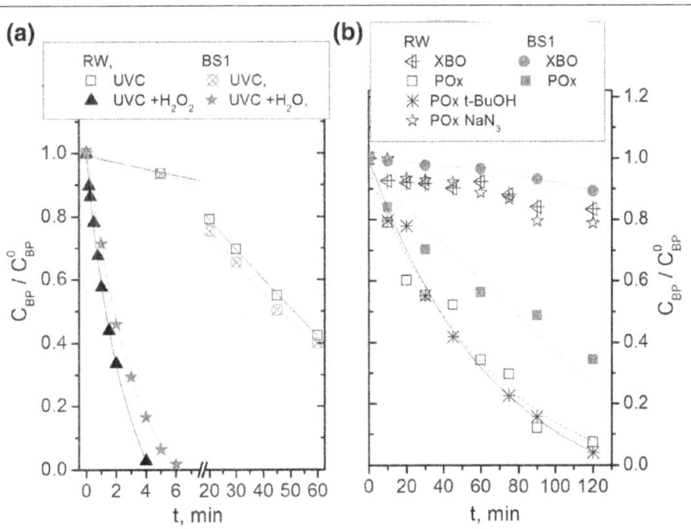

Figure 3 Changes of relative BP concentrations versus irradiation time during: UVC irradiation, and H_2O_2/UVC degradation **(a)**; VIS irradiation and photosensitized oxidation process (POx) **(b)** in natural water (pH = 8.11) and buffered solution (pH = 8.0) ($E_0^{UV} = 1 \times 10^{-5}$ einstein L^{-1} s^{-1}, $E_0^{VIS} = 3.24 \times 10^{-4}$ einstein L^{-1} s^{-1}, $C_{BP} = 8 \times 10^{-5}$ M, $C_{H2O2} = 0.02$ M, $C_{TPPS4} = 2 \times 10^{-5}$ M, $C_{t\text{-}BuOH} = 0.1$ M, $C_{NaN3} = 0.02$ M).

buffered solution (BS1), whereas, the advanced oxidation of butylparaben in a H_2O_2/UV system was about 18% (Figure 3a) faster in reservoir water than in BS1. Butylparaben degradation in a H_2O_2/UV system can take place through direct photolysis and reaction with hydroxyl radicals generated during hydrogen peroxide photodecomposition. Addition of H_2O_2 to the irradiated RW and BS1 shortened the BP degradation by about 40 and 30 times, respectively.

Preliminary examinations using a xenon arc lamp showed that during 2 h of irradiation of buffered solution without photosensitizer the same degree of butylparaben degradation was achieved as in an experiment without irradiation. This means that direct photolysis was not occurring, but decrease of butylparaben concentration during both experiments was a result of the adsorption of butylparaben on silicone tube in the reactor. After 2 h of irradiation of natural water without $TPPS_4$ the BP concentration decreased by 7% in comparison with experiments in buffered solutions (Figure 3b). Moreover in the dark, a decrease of butylparaben concentration was not observed if natural water was used. It is therefore possible that butylparaben decomposition occurs probably other than by adsorption. It is known that anions such as chloride, sulphate or carbonate have effects upon adsorption processes whilst phosphate and bicarbonate in the medium reduce the adsorption capacity [25,26].

Photolysis of organic compounds in water could be changed by the presence of naturally occurring organic and inorganic matter. Increasing the degree of butylparaben reduction by visible-light irradiation is presumably due to the natural dissolved constituents: humic acids, nitrate and chloride ions, where a strong influence on photolysis has been demonstrated [24,27]. Depending on quality and composition of water these elements can act as photosensitizers or conversely may exhibit quenching and scavenging effects [28,29].

Experiments using water from Sulejow reservoir showed that butylparaben concentration decreased by 93% after 2 h exposure in the reaction solution containing $TPPS_4$ to visible radiation.whilst in buffer solutions, butylparaben concentration fell by 66%. The large difference in the butylparaben decomposition in these experiments may be caused by reactions involving components of the Sulejow water, such as dissolved organic matter. Dissolved organic material, by absorbing light can generate reactive oxygen species [30,31], which increase the rate of butylparaben decay. The used of a free radical scavenger – *tert*-butanol (*t*-BuOH), reduced butylparaben decomposition by hydroxyl radicals (Figure 3b). Sodium azide, a quencher of singlet oxygen, confirmed the role of singlet oxygen in the reaction mechanism. It can therefore be assumed that the DOM found in natural water, which resulted in increased reaction rate, has the ability to generate singlet oxygen. Humic substances present in low concentrations, can lead to photosensitized oxidation in the aqueous environment [32,33]. The differences in the effects of direct photolysis were observed, probably also due to the compounds contained in the natural water. However, experiments carried out with sodium azide resulted in inhibition of degradation to the level of that of direct photolysis, and *t*-BuOH did not affect the reaction. But the acceleration of the

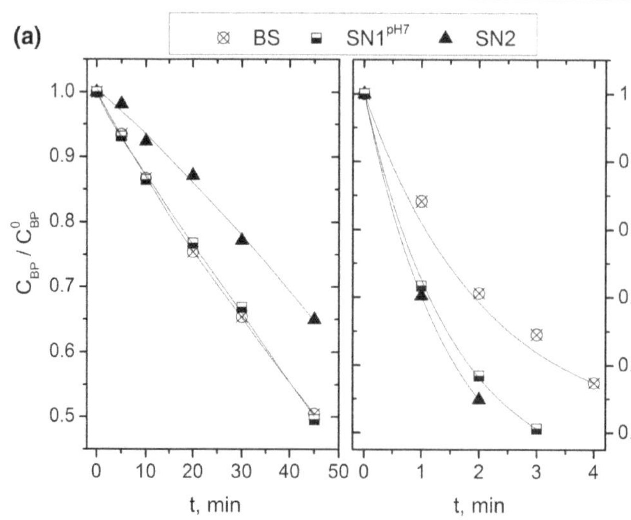

Figure 4 Changes of relative BP concentrations versus irradiation time upon degradation using UVC **(a)** and in H_2O_2/UVC system **(b)** in simulated natural water and buffered solution ($SN1^{pH7}$ pH = 6.47; SN2 pH = 6.82, BS2 pH = 7, $E_0^{UV} = 1 \times 10^{-5}$ einstein L^{-1} s^{-1}, $C_{BP} = 8 \times 10^{-5}$ M, $C_{H2O2} =$ 0.01 M, $C_{HA} = 4.4$ mg L^{-1}, $C_{NO3-} = 4.0$ mg L^{-1}).

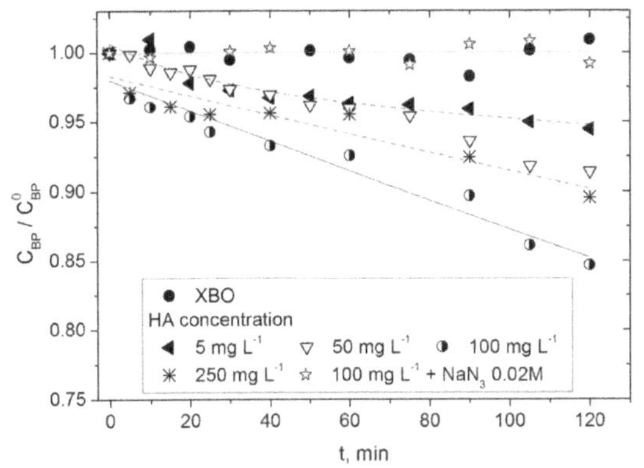

Figure 5 Changes of relative BP concentrations versus irradiation time upon degradation using visible light in simulated natural water (pH = 9, $E_0 = 3.24 \times 10^{-4}$ einstein L^{-1} s^{-1}, $C_{BP} = 8 \times 10^{-5}$ M, $C_{Na\ N3} = 0.02$ M).

direct photolysis compared with reactions in buffered solution was not related to hydroxyl radicals or singlet oxygen, but probably to the presence of organic radicals.

The influences of additives on UVC photolysis as well as H_2O_2/UV system were investigated. The presence of humic acid ($SN1^{pH7}$) in reaction solution upon UVC irradiation did not influence on butylparaben degradation, whilst the nitrate ions (SN2) inhibited BP decay (Figure 4a). Studies by Ge et al. [24], have shown that under UV-Visible irradiation ($\lambda > 200$ nm), NO_3^- ions are able to inhibit to some extent the photodegradation rates, mainly due to their photoshielding effects. Humic acids can behave in irradiated solution as sensitizers, light filters and quenchers of free radicals, and therefore their show distinct effects on photodegradation of pollutants under UV irradiation ($\lambda < 300$ nm) and simulated sunlight [27]. Humic acids absorb UVC radiation (Figure 2b), which should slow down the butylparaben degradation. However, studies have shown that these compounds did not undergo photolysis at a wavelength of 254 nm [34]. Photoexcitation of humic acids may lead to the generation of reactive oxygen species resulting in the intensification of the degradation process, but at the same time humic acids can quench reactive oxygen species, so their effect on butylparaben photolysis may be negligible.

In the case of the H_2O_2/UV system, the presence of humic acid ($SN1^{pH7}$) and nitrate ions (SN2) accelerated degradation of butylparaben by about 25% and 30%, respectively (Figure 4b). The increased decay rate of organic compounds in the presence of H_2O_2 and NO_3^- was also observed by Li et al. [35] during simulated sunlight irradiation.

The effects of humic acids in visible light on the degradation of butylparaben were examined (Figure 5) in a synthetic alkaline water (pH 9; BS3 and $SN1^{pH9}$). To avoid the adsorption of butylparaben, the silicone tubes from the reactor construction were removed. The

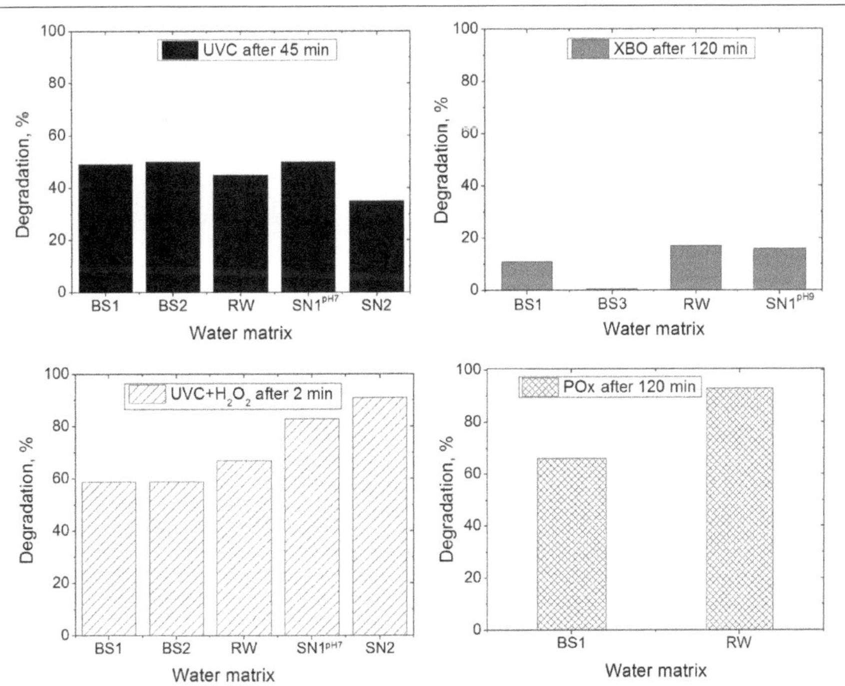

Figure 6 Influence of dissolved organic and inorganic matter in natural and simulated water on the BP photochemical degradation processes.

concentrations of humic acids (HA) were in the range: 5–250 mg L^{-1}. As can be seen in Figure 5, BP photolysis is depended on the humic acid concentration. At first, increasing humic acid concentrations resulted in acceleration of initial rate of butylparaben decay, with the highest rate at 100 mg L^{-1}. Further increase of humic acid concentrations reduced butylparaben decay primarily due to their light screening effect [36]. This process caused a decrease in efficiency of reactive oxygen species formation and butylparaben decomposition rate. It has been previously shown (Figure 1) that humic acids contain chromophores capable of sensitizing the generation of singlet oxygen. Therefore the excitation of humic acids leads to production of singlet oxygen. The experiments with azide anions, used as a singlet oxygen quencher, have indicated that singlet oxygen plays a dominant role in photodegradation of butylparaben, sensitized by humic substances. In summary, the photolysis rate of butylparaben can be enhanced by humic substances at low concentrations but could be inhibited at higher concentrations.

As can be seen from Figure 6, efficiency of the H_2O_2/UV, direct photolysis as well as photosensitized oxidation processes is strongly dependent on composition of the water.

It can be noticed that, the impact of dissolved organic and inorganic matter on the photochemical processes is related to light sources. Photolysis under xenon arc (XBO) radiation, and photosensitized oxidation in the presence of $TPPS_4$ was fastest in reservoir water.

Conclusions

Butylparaben undergoes both direct and indirect photodegradation in aqueous solution under UVC and visible radiation. The presence of dissolved organic matter in water did not influence on UVC photolysis and increases only about 8% of BP depletion rate in H_2O_2/UV system. While during visible light photolysis and photosensitized oxidation the addition of natural water matrix causes the acceleration of reaction rate by 16% and 36%, respectively.

The results indicate that butylparaben degradation proceeds via singlet oxygen, generated from humic substances. The presence of NO_3^- lead to the highest butylparaben degradation rate in the H_2O_2/UV system. In the case of UVC light, only slight influences of water composition were observed. It could be shown that the water matrix plays an important role on the efficiency of photodegradation processes. However, the obtained results enrich the existing knowledge of the photosensitized oxidation as well as advanced oxidation processes in natural waters.

Although, the H_2O_2/UV system gave the fastest degradation of butylparaben ,the possibility of using sunlight in the photosensitized oxidation makes this method more attractive from a practical and economical point of view in the treatment of drinking water.

Abbreviations

DOM: Dissolved organic substances; ROS: Reactive oxygen species; HA: Humic acids; O_2: Singlet oxygen; OH: Hydroxyl radical; POx: Photosensitized oxidation; BP: Butylparaben; $TPPS_4$: Meso-tetra (4-sulphonatophenyl)porphin; RW: Natural water from Sulejow Reservoir; $SN1^{pH7}$: Simulated natural water with humic acids at pH 7; $SN1^{pH9}$: Simulated natural water with humic acids at pH 9; SN2: Simulated natural water with nitrate ions; BS1: Buffered solution at pH 8; BS2: Buffered solution at pH 7; BS3: Buffered solution at pH 9; XBO: Xenon arc lamp.

Competing interests

The authors declare that they have no competing interests.

Authors' contributions

MG carried out the photosensitized oxidation, UV–vis photolysis as well as experiments with humic acid, participated in the analysis of the samples and drafted the manuscript. MOK carried out the H_2O_2/UV experiments and UV photolysis, participated in the analysis of the samples. SL conceived of the study, and participated in its design and coordination and helped to draft the manuscript. All authors read and approved the final manuscript.

Acknowledgements

Authors are thankful to the Regional European Center of Ecohydrology in Lodz (Poland) performing the analysis of ion analysis in natural water from Sulejow Reservoir. Marta Gmurek is grateful for a financial support from Foundation for Polish Science within the START scholarship.

References

1. Madsen T, Boyd BH, Nylén D, Pedersen R, Petersen GI, Simonsen F. Environmental and Health Assessment of Substances in Household Detergents and Cosmetic Detergent Products. CETOX, Danish Environmental Protection Agency, Environmental Project No. 615. 2001.
2. Vethaak AD, Rijs GBJ, Shrap SM, Ruiter H, Gerritsen A, Lahr J. Estrogens and xenoestrogens in the aquatic environment of the Netherlands. Occurrence, potency and biological effects. RIZA/RIKZ report no. 2002.001. 2002.
3. Campbell CG, Borglin SE, Green FB, Grayson A, Wozei E, Stringfellow WT. Biologically directed environmental monitoring, fate, and transport of estrogenic endocrine disrupting compounds in water: a review. Chemosphere. 2006;65:1265–80.
4. Caliman FA, Gavrilescu M. Pharmaceuticals, personal care products and endocrine disrupting agents in the environment–a review. Clean. 2009;37:277–303.
5. Legrini O, Oliveros E, Braun AM. Photochemical processes for water treatment. Chem Rev. 1993;93:671–98.
6. Gogate PR, Pandit AB. A review of imperative technologies for wastewater treatment I: oxidation technologies at ambient conditions. Adv Environ Res. 2004;8:501–51.
7. Pera–Titus M, Garcia-Molina V, Baños MA, Gimenez J, Esplugas S. Degradation of chlorophenols by means of advanced oxidation processes: a general review. App Catal B. 2004;47:219–56.
8. Ning B, Graham N, Zhang Y, Nakonechny M, El-Din MG. Degradation of endocrine disrupting chemicals by ozone/AOPs. Ozone Sci Eng. 2007;29:153–76.
9. Vaughan PP, Blough NV. Photochemical formation of hydroxyl radical by constituents of natural waters. Environ Sci Technol. 1998;32:2947–53.
10. Ostroumov SA. On Some issues of maintaining water quality and self-purification. Water Resour. 2005;32:305–13.
11. Canonica S, Freiburghaus M. Electron–rich phenols for probing the photochemical reactivity of freshwaters. Environ Sci Technol. 2001;35:690–5.
12. Davies–Colley RJ, Donnison AM, Speed DJ, Ross CM, Nagels JW. Inactivation of faecal indicator microorganisms in waste stabilisation ponds: interactions of environmental factors with sunlight. Wat Res. 1999;33:1220–30.
13. Kohn T, Nelson KL. Sunlight–mediated inactivation of MS2 coliphage via exogenous singlet oxygen produced by sensitizers in natural waters. Environ Sci Technol. 2007;41:192–7.
14. Boreen AL, Arnold WA, McNeill K. Photodegradation of pharmaceuticals in the aquatic environment: a review. Aq Sci. 2003;65:320–41.

15. Zafiriou OC, Joussot-Dubien J, Zepp RG, Zika RG. Photochemistry of natural waters. Environ Sci Technol. 1984;18:358–71.
16. Blough NV, Zepp RG. Reactive oxygen species in natural waters. In: Foote CS, editor. Active Oxygen in Chemistry. New York: Chapman and Hall; 1995. p. 280–333.
17. Rodrigues A, Brito A, Janknecht P, Proença MF, Nogueira R. Quantification of humic acids in surface water: effects of divalent cations, pH, and filtration. J Environ Monit. 2009;11:377–82.
18. Gmurek M, Miller JS. Photosensitised oxidation of a water pollutant using sulphonated porphyrin. Chem Pap. 2012;66:120–8.
19. Błędzka D, Gryglik D, Miller JS. Photodegradation of butylparaben in aqueous solutions. J Photochem Photobiol A Chem. 2009;203:131–6.
20. Błędzka D, Gryglik D, Olak M, Gębicki JL, Miller JS. Degradation of butylparaben and 4-tert-octylphenol in H2O2/UV system. Radiat Phys Chem. 2010;79:409–16.
21. Murov SL, Carmichael I, Hug GL. Handbook of photochemistry. 2nd ed. New York: Basel; 1993.
22. Wegner EE, Adamson AW. Photochemistry of complex ions. III. Absolute quantum yields for the photolysis of some aqueous chromium (III) complexes. Chemical actinometry in the long wavelength visible region. J Am Chem Soc. 1966;88:394–403.
23. Gryglik D, Lach M, Miller JS. The aqueous photosensitized degradation of butylparaben. Photochem Photobiol Sci. 2009;8:549–55.
24. Ge L, Chen J, Qiao X, Lin J, Cai X. Light-source-dependent effects of main water constituents on photodegradation of phenicol antibiotics: mechanism and kinetics. Environ Sci Technol. 2009;43:3101–7.
25. Liang H, Li X, Yang Y, Sze K. Effects of dissolved oxygen, pH, and anions on the 2,3-dichlorophenol degradation by photocatalytic reaction with anodic TiO2 nanotube films. Chemosphere. 2008;73:805–12.
26. Sujana MG, Soma G, Vasumathi N, Anand S. Studies on fluoride adsorption capacities of amorphous Fe/Al mixed hydroxides from aqueous solutions. J Fluorine Chem. 2009;130:749–54.
27. Chen Y, Zhang K, Zuo Y. Direct and indirect photodegradation of estriol in the presence of humic acid, nitrate and iron complexes in water solutions. Sci Total Environ. 2013;463–464:802–9.
28. Liu S, Li QX. Photolysis of spinosyns in seawater, stream water and various aqueous solutions. Chemosphere. 2004;56:1121–7.
29. Frimmel FH. Photochemical aspects related to humic substances. Environ Int. 1994;20:373–85.
30. Canonica S, Jans U, Stemmler K, Hoigne J. Transformation kinetics of phenols in water: photosensitization by dissolved natural organic material and aromatic ketones. Environ Sci Technol. 1995;29:1822–31.
31. Chin YP, Miller PI, Zeng L, Cawley K, Weavers LK. Photosensitized degradation of Bisphenol A by dissolved organic matter. Environ Sci Technol. 2004;38:5888–94.
32. Manjun Z, Xi Y, Hongshen Y, Lingren K. Effect of natural aquatic humic substances on the photodegradation of bisphenol A. Front Environ Sci Eng Chin. 2007;1:311–5.
33. Sakkas VA, Lambropoulou DA, Albanis TA. Study of chlorothalonil photodegradation in natural waters and in the presence of humic substances. Chemosphere. 2002;48:939–45.
34. Veselinović A, Bojić A, Purenović M, Bojić D, Andjelković T. Photodegradation of humic acids in the presence of hydrogen peroxide. Zbornik radova Tehnološkog fakulteta u Leskovcu. 2009;19:220–6.
35. Li Y, Duan X, Li X, Tang X. Mechanism study on photodegradation of nonylphenol in water by intermediate products analysis. Acta Chim Sin. 2012;70:1819–26.
36. Milne PJ, Zika RG. Luminescence quenching of dissolved organic matter in seawater. Mar Chem. 1989;27:147–64.

6

Biodegradation of naphthalene using Pseudomonas aeruginosa by up flow anoxic–aerobic continuous flow combined bioreactor

Behrooz Karimi[1,2*], Maryam Habibi[1*] and Mehry Esvand[1]

Abstract

Background: Naphthalene is a poly aromatic hydrocarbon (PAH) present in many sediment-water systems. The aim of this study was to evaluate the applicability of an anoxic/aerobic system for the biological treatment of water polluted by naphthalene by Pseudomonas aeruginosa PTCC 1707 to utilize naphthalene. The naphthalene elimination from wastewater was determined in anoxic–aerobic continuous flow combined bioreactor under continuously oxic and anoxic conditions. Experiments were conducted in continues mode, and naphthalene was administered in consecutive spike doses. Then Pseudomonas aeruginosa bacteria suspension with a specific turbidity (0.5-10 NTU) was prepared from growing bacteria on R_2A medium and injected to reactor.

Findings: At naphthalene concentration = 0.5-20 mg/L, 33–65.5% naphthalene removal efficiencies were observed. Mean COD removal efficiency in solid retention times of 2, 4, 6, and 8 days was 82.7, 92.45, 95.97 and 96.1%, respectively. Naphthalene removal efficiency by bacterium pseudomonas at pH 8 was 96% and at pH 4, 5.5, 7 and 9.5, 68, 80, 90 and 85%, respectively. As the initial concentration of naphthalene increased from 0.5 to 20 mg/L, the remaining concentration of naphthalene decreased from 33.4% to 65.5% after 3 days.

Conclusion: Based on experimental results, it was determined that this process can effectively reduce naphthalene under optimal conditions and this method can be used for the removal of similar compounds.

Keyword: Anoxic–aerobic continuous flow combined bioreactor, Biodegradation, Naphthalene, Pseudomonas aeruginosa

Introduction

Remediation of contaminated soil and groundwater is an important issue that is of concern among environmentalists and hydrogeologists [1]. Polycyclic aromatics hydrocarbons (PAHs, also known as polycyclic organic matter or POM) are chemical species with two to six fused benzene rings and are well known toxic hazardous pollutants and highly potent carcinogens that can cause tumors in some organisms [2]. PAHs originate from natural and anthropogenic sources. Anthropogenic sources include engine exhaust, industrial processes, crude oil, urban run-off, domestic heating systems, incinerators and smoke. Natural sources include terrestrial coal deposits, volcanic eruptions and forest fires. The main sources of PAHs in surface water are atmospheric deposition, run-off from contaminated soils and deposition from sewage discharges [3]. The main characterized of PAHs were high toxicity, concentrated substrate and salt (usually exceeding 3 wt.%), and poor decolorization and biodegradation.

Naphthalene is the simplest, most volatile and least toxic of the PAHs. In fact naphthalene has been used in several research laboratories as a model to develop catalysts and biological process with potential to effectively destroy PAHs [4]. Albeit naphthalene has a relative low solubility in water (32 mg/L) but it is highly hazardous. About 5% of all naphthalene disposed into the environment is released into water. Studies of naphthalene degradation may be significant because naphthalene is a common pollutant that serves as a chemical model for the degradation of PAHs [5]. The range of naphthalene concentration in wastewaters

* Correspondence: karimibehroz@yahoo.com; M.habibi1992@yahoo.com
[1]Department of Environmental Health Engineering, School of Health, Arak University of Medical Sciences, Arak, Iran
[2]Department of Environmental Health Engineering, School of Health, Tehran University of Medical Sciences, Tehran, Iran
Full list of author information is available at the end of the article

is from ng/L to mg/L. Concentrations such as 1.65 mg/L were reported on wastewater samples from the radioisotope manufacturing facilities, 6–220 ng/L, in municipal wastewater, 285 mg/L (as naphthalene sulfonic acid), in effluents from ion-exchange resin towers, and 0.1–2.1 mg/L in dyeing and textile wastewater [6].

Various physical, chemical, biological, and their combined technologies have been attempted to remediate organic-contaminated waters. The in situ microbial degradation of PAHs is limited by their low bioavailability and low water-solubility [7]. Among various attempts made to treat such wastewater, such as, evaporation, polymeric absorption, solvent extraction, and conventional biological treatment, are proved ineffective due to the quite stable structure of the naphthalene ring and the high concentrations of salt and acid in the streams from the dye manufacturing process [8]. The methods for treating PAHs mainly include biodegradation, scrubber absorption, high-energy electron beam irradiation, ozonation, catalytic combustion volatilization, photo-oxidation, chemical oxidation and adsorption [9]. Most of the PAHs such as naphthalene are not aerobically degraded in activated sludge system, as the benzene rings is susceptible to reduction under low redox potential. The oxic/anoxic (O/A) system is an alternative to the traditional activated sludge process for treating high naphthalene solution [10].

Recently, a number of oxic/anoxic bacteria have been used to biodegrade naphthalene with several pathways and metabolic diversities described [11]. Bacteria such as Pseudomonas putida, Rhodococcusopacus, Mycobacterium sp., Nocardia otitidiscaviarum, and Bacillus pumilus have been reported to biodegrade naphthalene. Pseudomonas aeruginosa is an environmental bacterium that can be isolated from many different habitats, including water, soil, and plants, but it is also an opportunistic human pathogen causing serious nosocomial infections [12]. Pseudomonads are the best-known bacteria capable of utilizing hydrocarbons as carbon and energy sources and producing bio surfactants which enhance the uptake of such immiscible hydrophobic compounds.

The aim of this study was to evaluate the applicability of an anoxic/aerobic system for the biological treatment of naphthalene by P. aeruginosa to utilize hydrocarbons ranging from naphthalene to polycyclic aromatic hydrocarbons as a carbon source. Furthermore, P. aeruginosa growth conditions in anoxic-aerobic reactor, that constitute the most important factor affecting biodegrading efficiency, kinetics, and the biodegradation mechanism of naphthalene, have been investigated.

Methods

Chemical

Naphthalene (99.9% purity), was supplied by MERCK. The physicochemical properties of naphthalene used in this study are listed in Table 1. R_2A agar, Murashige and Skoog Basal Salt Mixture (MS salts), Benzyl-adenine and Indole-3-acetic acid (IAA) were purchased from Sigma–Aldrich (USA).

A minimal medium (MM) was composed of (L): KH_2PO_4 1.0 g, NaCl 5 g (NH_4) $_2SO_4$ 0.3 g, $MgSO_4 \cdot 7H_2O$ 0.3 g, $CaCl_2$ 20 mg, Sugar (2.5 g/L). MM also contained trace elements as follows: (L): $ZnSO_4$ 5.0 g, $FeCl_3$ 2.3 g, $MnSO_4$ 5.0 g, and (NH_4) $6Mo_7O_{24}$ 1.0 g. Solid MM plate was composed of (L MM): 20 g agar. Solid LB plate was composed of (L): 5 g NaCl, 10 g peptone, 5 g yeast extract, 20 g agar. Flasks containing the medium were sterilized by autoclaving at 121°C for 20 min. The pH of the medium was between 6.8 and 7.2. All chemicals used were of analytical grade and all reagents were used as supplied.

Bacterial enumeration

Pseudomonas aeruginosa was counted on R_2A medium (Figure 1) and MSM containing 30 mg/L naphthalene, according to Standard Plate Count Method. Pseudomonas aeruginosa bacteria PTCC 1707 growing on the above medium (with naphthalene and Sugar as the only carbon source) were defined as naphthalene degrading bacteria. Then bacterial suspension with a specific turbidity (0.5-10 NTU) was prepared from growing bacteria.

Synthetic wastewater

Ammonium and nitrite were supplemented to mineral medium as required in the form of $(NH_4)_2SO_4$ and $NaNO_2$, respectively. The composition of the mineral medium was (g/L except for trace element solution): KH_2PO_4 0.01, $CaC_{12}.2H_2O$ 0.00565, $MgSO_4.7H_2O$ 0.3, $KHCO_3$1.25, $FeSO_4$ 0.00625, EDTA 0.00625 and 1.25 mL/L of trace elements solution. The trace element solution contained (g/L): EDTA 15, H_3BO_4 0.014, $MnCl_2.4H_2O$ 0.99, $CuSO_4.5H_2O$0.25, ZnSO4.7H_2O 0.43, $NiCl_2.6H_2O$ 0.19, $NaSeO_4.10H_2O$ 0.21, $NaMoO_4.2H_2O$ 0.22 and $NaWO_4.2H_2O$ 0.050. Synthetic wastewater containing naphthalene was gradually entered into the reactor. Naphthalene was added to deionized water and stirred for 12–14 h to prepare a saturated solution. The naphthalene with

Table 1 Physico-chemical properties of naphthalene

Molecular weight	128.19
Formula	$C_{10}H_8$
Boiling point	218C
Melting point	80.5C
Solubility (at 20°C)	32 mg/l
Specific gravity	1.145
Henry's law constant	20 atmm^3 water/m^3 air
K_{ow}	2800

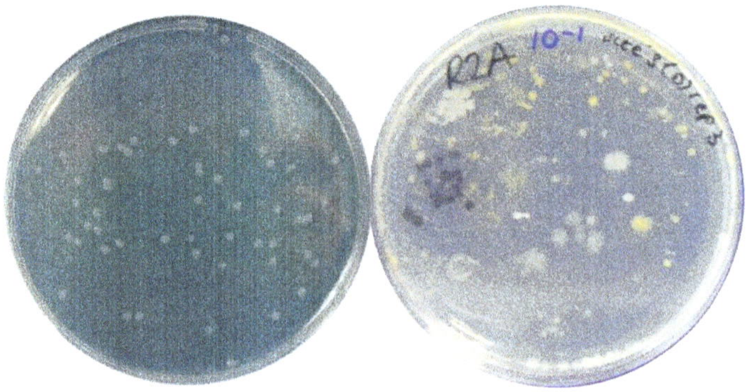

Figure 1 R_2A **medium was developed to growing the Pseudomonas aeruginosa.**

concentrations 0.5-20 mg/L was prepared and introduced in reactor. The pH was adjusted using either concentrated sulfuric acid or 0.25 N NaOH.

Biodegradation experiments

Various factors were examined for their influence on growth of selected strain and on the biodegradation of naphthalene. These included temperature, pH, nitrogen concentration, salinity, inoculum concentration, different naphthalene concentration and SCOD. Various conditions are briefly described: incubation temperatures of 20, 25, 30, 35 and 40°C; autoclaved medium pH of 5.5, 6.0, 6.5, 7.0, 7.5, 8.0 and 9.0 using 1 M HCl or 1 M NaOH; the C/N ratio of 0.7, 1.0, 1.3, 2.0, 4.0 and 20.0 using naphthalene and $(NH_4)_2SO_4$; the salinity of 0, 1, 5, 8, 10, 15 g/L with NaCl [11] and naphthalene at concentrations of 0.5, 1, 5, 10 and 20 mg/L were used for this experiment. The cultures were incubated in a shaking incubator at 150 rpm, 30°C. The naphthalene concentration after degraded in various samples was determined using gas chromatography. All experiments were carried out in triplicate. The degree of naphthalene degradation was calculated as:

$$\text{Degradation efficiency } (\%) = \frac{C_0 - C_t}{C_0} \times 100$$

Where C_0 and C_t stand for the naphthalene concentrations before and after degradation, respectively.

Reactor systems and experimental conditions

The experimental system employed in this study consisted of one reactor with two stages (anoxic and oxic) with a working volume of five liters in continues conditions with stirring (350 rpm), have a diameter and height of 10 and 80 cm, respectively. A schematic of the laboratory reactor system is provided in Figure 2.

After 4–6 h of incubation, turbidity 0.5(1.5×10^6 bacteria per ml), 1, 2, 5 and 10 NTU of the bacterial suspension (Pseudomonas aeruginosa) was obtained. The 20 mL of bacterial suspension was added per 1 L of synthetic wastewater. Reactors were filled with synthetic wastewater and bacterial suspension as biomass, with a useful volume of 5 L (Table 2). One dual-channel peristaltic pump was used to initially feed the reactors with a constant flow (0.28 L d^{-1}). The influent originated from container, was stored at 4°C during the entire process. The reactor's recycle flows were made by a peristaltic pump at a maximum flow rate of 0.55 L d^{-1}. The temperature was set at 35°C and the influent pH was controlled in the range of 6.8-7.0.

The anoxic condition was obtained when oxygen concentration reached 0mgL^{-1}. Aeration in the reactor was provided by filtered air using bubble diffusers. Oxygen concentrations were checked using oxygen probes maintained in the slurry throughout the experiment in all reactors. The temperature range during incubation was 20–27°C, pH was 6.4–7.7, and oxygen concentrations were over 2 mg L^{-1} in oxic section and 0 mg L^{-1} in the anoxic section. Samples were taken in triplicate for chemical analyses at 0, 2, 4, 6, 8, 12, 15, 20 and 23 days of incubation. Samples for GC analysis were withdrawn at the end of each experiment.

GC method for analysis

The sample was added into a 40 mL glass amber vial containing 9 mL nanopure water and 10 mL acetate buffer (0.1 M at pH 5.0). 50 L sodium tetra ethyl borate ($NaBEt_4$, 5%) and 20 L tetra butyltin (TeBT at 1 mg L^{-1}, as an internal standard) were then added. The vial was immediately placed on a magnetic stirrer to maintain a constant agitation. A SPME fiber coated with 30 m thickness poly dimethyl siloxane (PDMS) purchased from Supelco (Bellefonte, PA, USA) was exposed to the headspace over the vigorously stirred sample for 20 min at room temperature. The fiber was then placed in the GC injector, desorbed at 250°C for 3 min.

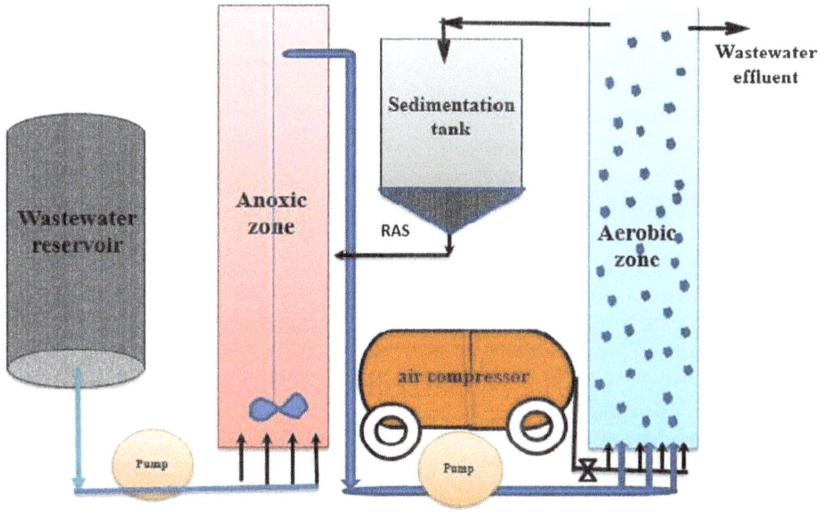

Figure 2 Schematic of the laboratory reactor system.

Themeasurements ofnaphthalenewere detailed inourpreviousstudy. Naphthalene was quantified using a Varian Model 3380 gas chromatograph equipped with a flame ionization detector, Chrompack capillary column (Select 624 CB D_f 1.8 μm, FS 30 × 0.32 mm ID), and an auto-sampler with a 100 μm PDMS coated SPME fiber assembly (Supelco, Bellefonte, PA).

The sample adsorption time with the SPME fiber was 10 min in agitate mode and desorption time was 2 min followed by a 1 min waiting period. The analysis was performed in split less mode with an injection temperature of 250°C, isothermal oven temperature of 180°C, and detector temperature of 275°C.

The data presented are the mean values ofthree measurements with the relative standard deviations of 6.7–10.2%. The pH was measured using an Ag/AgCl combination pH electrode attached to a pH meter (Ion Analyzer 220, Corning, Inc., Corning, NY).

Chemical oxygen demand (COD)

COD was measured in the supernatant fraction (soluble COD, CODs) according to the standard methods. By difference between COD and CODs, the particulated COD (CODp) was calculated. The COD solubilization (SCOD) represents the transfer of COD from the particulated fraction of the sludge to the soluble fraction. SCOD was calculated by using the difference between CODs after ultrasonic treatment and the initial CODs ($CODs_0$) in relation to the initial particulated COD (CODp):

$$\text{SCOD}\ (\%) = \frac{(COD_s - COD_{S0})}{(COD_p)} \times 100$$

The aimed total COD in the influents of reactor was 300 mg COD/L.

Table 2 Operation conditions of the anoxic and oxic reactors

	Anoxic zone	Aerobic zone	total
Volume reactor	2.5 L	2.5 L	5 L
Upflow velocity (mh^{-1})	1.00	1.00	1.00
Flow rate (Ld^{-1})	0.28	0.28	0.28
Total COD (mgL^{-1})	300	300	300
HRT (h)	24	24	24
$pH_{influent}$	4-8	4-8	4-8

Statistical analyses

Mean and standard deviation of the triplicates in each treatment are calculated. The differences among three nutrient groups were evaluated firstly by a parametric one-way analysis of variance (ANOVA). If significant difference was found at $p \leq 0.05$, multiple comparison test of Tukey–Kramer was employed. All statistical analyses were performed using SPSS ver 16.

Results and discussion

Initially, it was worked on the compatibility between bacterium pseudomonas aeruginosa and naphthalene for 3 months. For this purpose, glucose with 100 mg/L COD was used as the carbon source. In the next step, concentration of the input glucose to the system was gradually reduced, while increasing naphthalene dose. This course continued to the point where the bacterium became perfectly compatible with naphthalene, and in presence of naphthalene, COD concentration was brought within range of 30–40 mg/L.

Growth P. aeruginosa on anoxic–aerobic reactor

To examine the growth of P. aeruginosa (OD and CFU/mL) in vertical anoxic–aerobic continuous flow combined bioreactor and tolerance of naphthalene by P. aeruginosa, the cells were cultivated in nutrient broth with concentration of naphthalene. It appears that the cells were able to survive naphthalene concentration as high as 20 mg/L naphthalene. Figure 3 shows the growth curves of P. aeruginosaAT18 in the presence of naphthalene, this can be attributed to growth of biomass on naphthalene intermediates. Goel et al. [13] reported a similar observation of growth of naphthalene degrading culture on their catabolic intermediates.

Effect of retention times on naphthalene degradation during anoxic–aerobic process

Research results indicated a decline in the reactor efficiency, with increase of organic input load. Mean COD removal efficiency in solid retention times of 2, 4, 6, and 8 days was 82.7, 92.45, 95.97 and 96.1%, respectively. As can be seen in Figure 4, with increase of hydraulic retention time from 0 to 80 minutes, naphthalene removal efficiency increases so as with increase of naphthalene concentration, removal efficiency decreases. In Figure 5 is illustrated the naphthalene removal from water by bacterium pseudomonas aeruginosa. Naphthalene concentration from 20 mg/L came to 5.4 mg/L after lapse of 80 minutes. To verify the amount of naphthalene auto-decomposition, control reactor was used. At length, it was observed that anoxic/aerobic process was about 60% more effective than control reactor in naphthalene removal. Naphthalene removal in retention times of 20, 40, 60 and 80 min was 29%, 50%, 72% and 94%, respectively. In the control reactor, for the same retention times, removal efficiency was 60% lower, which can be attributed to auto-evaporation processes. The system bacterial counting in the beginning and end of this experiment was 6.5×10^3 bacteria per ml and 3.5×10^5 bacteria per ml, respectively. Results of this study indicated that during the anoxic/aerobic process bacterium pseudomonas aeruginosa was able to bring average naphthalene concentration from 20 mg/L to 5–7 mg/L, implying 55–64.3% removal efficiency.

Effect of solution flow rate on naphthalene degradation during anoxic–aerobic process

The biological degradation of naphthalene (10 mg/L) was conducted at the flow rate of 2.5, 3.5, 5.5, 7.7, 12, and 26 ml/min. The results are shown in Figure 6. As observed, the efficiency of naphthalene degradation was 88%, 82%, 80%, 66%, 52% and 31% at pH 8, respectively. The naphthalene concentration of each output was kept constant. It takes at least 12 h to completely degrade naphthalene. The residence time of the naphthalene solution was estimated by dividing the volume of the bioreactor (5 L) by the flow rate. The removal of naphthalene and COD decreases with increasing the flow rate, in other words, decreasing the residence time, as reported [14]. The effect is due to the decreasing residence time for microorganisms to contact with naphthalene and COD. Figure 6 also shows that the remained COD concentration becomes higher than naphthalene concentration with decreasing the flow rate of naphthalene solution. The degradation of COD requires a longer time than the degradation of naphthalene. On the other hand, naphthalene evaporation was increase with increasing the flow rate, as can be seen in control reactor (Figure 5). Accordance with this report, previous studies results have indicated that the COD still remained after naphthalene completely degradation [15].

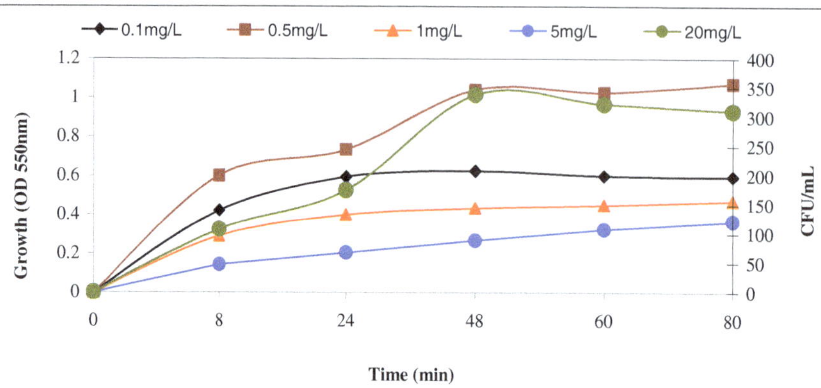

Figure 3 Growth of P. aeruginosa (OD and CFU/mL) in vertical anoxic–aerobic continuous flow combined bioreactor with 0.1, 0.5, 1, 5, 10 and 20 mg/L for naphthalene.

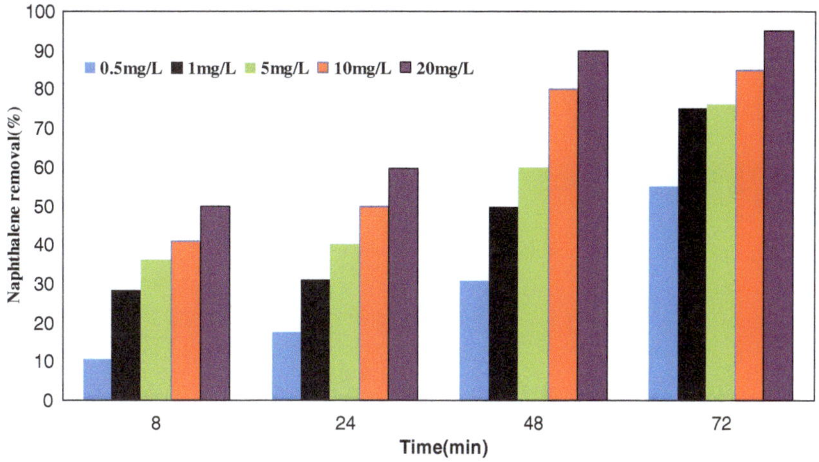

Figure 4 Effect of bacterial concentration on naphthalene degradation in hydraulic retention time of 20–80 minutes and in cellular retention time of 2–8 days.

Effect of solution pH on naphthalene degradation during anoxic–aerobic process

Among other effective parameters on naphthalene removal, pH level is important. In this study, effect of pH 4, 5.5, 7, 8 and 9.5 on naphthalene removal process was tested. Naphthalene removal efficiency by bacterium pseudomonas at pH 8 was 96% and at pH 4, 5.5, 7 and 9.5, 68, 80, 90 and 85%, respectively. COD removal efficiency at these pHs varied between 68-96%, and with pH increase, the system removal efficiency improved. Other results of the experiment are presented in Figure 7.

Effect of naphthalene concentration

The artificial wastewater containing the naphthalene, glucose and mineral medium was prepared with the naphthalene concentration of 0.5-20 mg/L and the initial COD 100 ± 18 mg/L. In Table 3, effect of the vertical anoxic–aerobic continuous flow combined bioreactor and control reactor on naphthalene and COD concentration and their removal efficiency is presented.

Effect of the turbidity formed by bacterial action on naphthalene removal efficiency

In this section, to investigate the effect of bacterium pseudomonas aeruginosa on naphthalene concentration, different turbidity levels produced by the bacterium was examined. Hence, after culture of the respective bacterium in R_2A environment, a bacterial suspension with 0.5-10 NTU was formed. Next, concentrations of 0.5-20 mg/L in each turbidity level were examined. The results are presented in Figure 8. At 0.5 mg/L concentration naphthalene, a removal efficiency of naphthalene 18-85% was obtained, so as at higher turbidity levels, higher removal efficiency was realized.

Pseudomonas is a gram-negative rod-shaped bacterium with high ability in decomposition of organic and

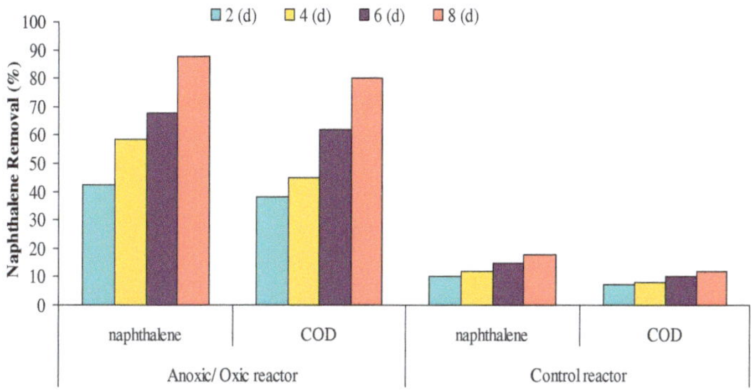

Figure 5 Naphthalene and COD removal from water by bacterium pseudomonas aeruginosa in vertical anoxic–aerobic continuous flow combined bioreactor and control reactor at cellular retention time 2-8d and 28°C.

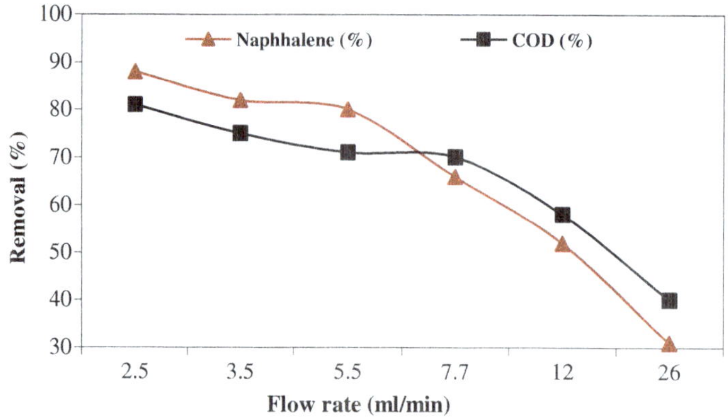

Figure 6 The biological degradation of naphthalene at the flow rate of 2.5, 3.5, 5.5, 7.7, 12, and 26 $mlmin^{-1}$ at pH 8.

oil pollutants, including naphthalene. Its ability depends on production of catalytic enzymes and formation of metabolic paths [16]. Due to presence of various degrading enzymes in bacteria, they have stronger effect on naphthalene degradation process relative to other microorganisms. In this study, following culture of bacterium pseudomonas aeruginosa and formation of the microbial suspension from it and having accomplished the compatibility process between this microorganism and naphthalene (which is the indicator of aromatic hydrocarbons), they were blended in a combined anoxic/aerobic reactor. As the solid retention time increased from 2 days to 8 days, COD and naphthalene removal efficiency gradually increased. On day 8, removal efficiency of naphthalene and COD reached 94 and 96.1%, respectively. Beklemishev et al. [17] using the extracted bacteria from soil reported a maximum degradation efficiency of 58-73% for 3 and 4-membered ring aromatic compounds after 7 days. Seoud et al. [18] by inseminating bacterium pseudomonas into a biological reactor within 5–7 days managed to achieve a naphthalene removal efficiency of about 60%. Kozlova et al. [19] using pseudomonas putida G7 investigated naphthalene degradation in the soil sample. They succeeded within 7 days to achieve removal efficiency of 95%. On day 4, naphthalene degradation in the soil sample was 85% and after 6 days 90% naphthalene was removed [19]. Feijoo–Siota et al. [20] using pseudomonas stutzeri reported a naphthalene biologic degradation of 93% within 6 days. A naphthalene degradation speed of 0.2 ml/L per hour was obtained by Pathak by injection of flavor bacterium strain in to a biological reactor. In addition, the produced enzymes in this process were identified by him [16].

The obtained results in laboratorial condition indicate feasibility of naphthalene degradation by injection of bacterium pseudomonas into a biological anoxic/aerobic reactor. Although auto-decomposition of such volatile hydrocarbon as naphthalene can also occur at environment temperature, this decomposition in vicinity of

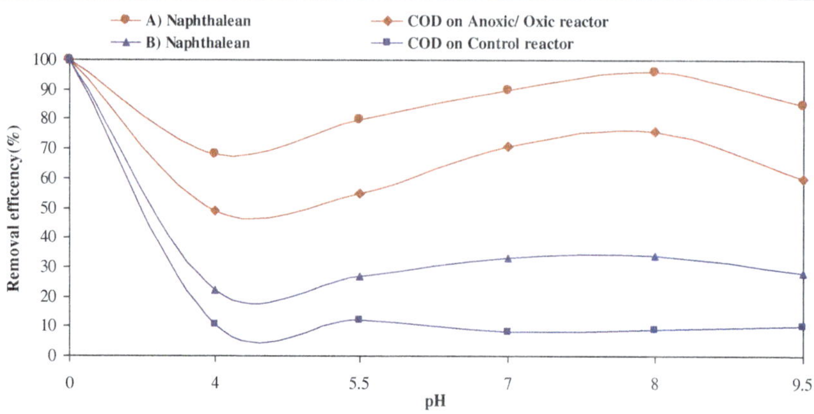

Figure 7 Naphthalene and COD removal efficiency in vertical anoxic–aerobic continuous flow combined bioreactor and control reactor at different pH levels, for cellular retention time of 8 days at 28°C and flow rate 2.5 $mlmin^{-1}$.

Table 3 effect of vertical anoxic–aerobic continuous flow combined bioreactor and control reactor on naphthalene and COD concentration and their removal efficiency

Naphthalene concentration		Naphthalene removal efficiency		COD
		Anoxic/Oxic reactor	Control reactor	
0.5 mg/l	(%)	66	27	78
	mg/l	0.17 ± 0.6	0.365 ± 0.01	0.11 ± 4.2
1 mg/l	(%)	58.4	21.5	94
	mg/l	0.416 ± 0.02	0.785 ± 0.05	0.06 ± 0.03
5 mg/l	(%)	51	26.5	90
	mg/l	2.45 ± 1.5	3.675 ± 0.21	0.5 ± 0.6
10 mg/l	(%)	44.5	19.5	92
	mg/l	5.55 ± 0.5	8.05 ± 2.15	0.8 ± 0.05
20 mg/l	(%)	32.5	17	89
	mg/l	13.5 ± 4.50	16.6 ± 5.48	2.2 ± 1.35

pseudomonas in a biological anoxic/aerobic reactor can be enhanced up to several times (in this study up to 60% [21]. During anoxic degradation process, biological metabolites such as diphenylmethane, cyclohexane, hydroxytoluene, and alpha-Cadinol are produced from degrading bacteria, which facilitate degradation process. These compounds, in naphthalene degradation, act like surfactants and effect on solution pH [22].

In addition, bacteria are able to change and adapt themselves to changes in environmental condition such as a change from anoxic to aerobic condition. In either anoxic or aerobic condition, bacterium pseudomonas heterotrophy is able to use naphthalene as the aromatic compounds indicator and as a source of carbon [23]. Change of bacterium metabolism from anoxic to aerobic helps it produce the required enzymes in shorter time. Among anoxic/aerobic advantages, it can be referred to lower utilization cost, less biomass production during anoxic process, and finally less slime decomposition. Lower cost of this method in aromatic hydrocarbons removal such as naphthalene is very beneficial. In nature, aromatic compounds decomposition is influenced by environmental parameters such as pH, temperature degree, and amount of injected bacterium [24].

From ANOVA analysis, effect of the five parameters on naphthalene degradation was examined. The results indicated the statistical significant of the five parameters ($p = 0.0023$, 0.0078, 0.0064, 0.0011 and < 0.0001), and for COD degradation (p-values are smaller than 0.05). The obtained R^2 is 0.92 which indicate that 92% of the information results are correct and 6% of these experiments have error (Table 4).

From this study and based on numerous studies, it was found that pH control within range of 7–8 could increase the process efficiency [25]. Base pH boundary 7.8-8.5 had the strongest effect on naphthalene degradation. pH can affect microbial activityand therefore investigations into the effect of enzyme activity, transport processes and the nutrient solubility were made. As shown in Figure 7, the highest removal efficacy and lowest remaining concentration of naphthalene was found at pH 8.0. More than 96% of naphthalene and 76 of COD was degraded when the pH of the bioreactor ranged from 7 to 8. Degradation efficiency however significantly declined when the pH was <6.0 or >8.5. These results are consistent with most studies, where microorganisms favoured growth at pH levelsranging from 6.0 to 8.0 [25,26]. It is likely that such acidic or alkalinecon-ditions affect bacterial activity, and hence naphthalene degradation [27].

In addition, the greatest naphthalene degradation was obtained at 25-37°C at constant bacterium injection doses. The amount of bacterium injection into the system was statistically significant ($p < 0.0001$) and relative

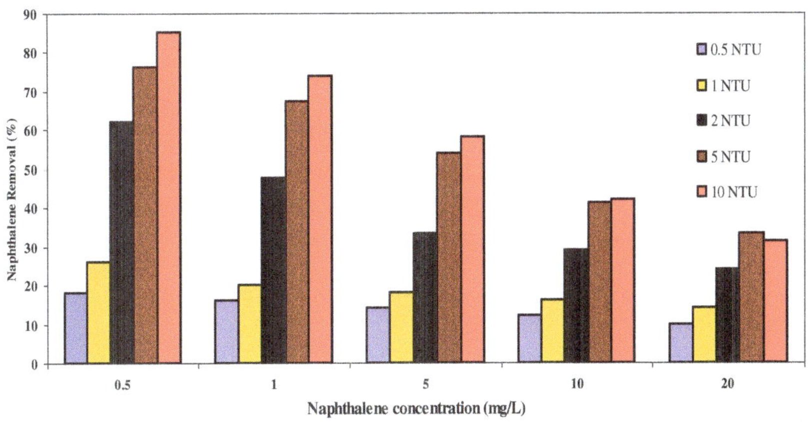

Figure 8 Naphthalene removal efficiency with produced turbidity by bacterium (in NTU), (cellular retention time of 8 days at 28°C; solution pH: 7 and flow rate 2.5 mlmin^{-1}).

Table 4 One-way ANOVA for naphthalene degradation at different pH, SRT, Flow rate and naphthalene concentration

Parameter	No. of groups	F	P-value	F crit
pH	5	13.05	0.0023	2.47
Time	4	16.4	0.0078	6.57
Flow rate	6	11.25	0.0064	4.65
Naphthalene concentration	5	11.5	0.0011	3.55
Bacterium injection	5	15.5	0.0001	4.88

$R^2 = 0.92$.

to other parameters its effect was found stronger. Increase in dose of bacterium injection into the system is goes along with increase of naphthalene degradation. At pH 8 and 10 NTU which is the greatest amount of bacterium injected to the system, the highest naphthalene removal efficiency was obtained. At lower pH, retention time and injection quantities, a minimum of 63% removal efficiency was obtained, where as at higher pH and retention time (80 min), removal efficiency could be brought to around 100%. The same result obtained from other studies [28].

As the initial concentration of naphthalene increased from 0.5 to 20 mg/L, the remaining concentration of naphthalene decreased from 33.4% to 65.5% after 3 days. The removed amount of naphthalene using strain P. aeruginosa however decreased as the initial concentration of naphthalene increase, which is due to the initial concentration that provides an important driving force to overcome all mass transfer resistances of the naphthalene between the aqueous and solid phases [29]. Consequently a lower initial concentration of naphthalene may enhance the process. This suggests that strain P. aeruginosa could survive and rapidly degrade a high concentration of naphthalene at 20 mg/L. Despite the substrate concentrations being high enough to support growth, this may cause toxic effects, and toxic metabolites may accumulate in the growth medium. However, the tolerated high concentration of naphthalene in the vertical anoxic–aerobic continuous flow combined bioreactor means that strain P. aeruginosa is a potential alternative strategy in naphthalene degradation [29].

Conclusions

This work highlights the link between the Pseudomonas aeruginosa and the degradation of naphthalene as PAH in a wastewater subjected to anoxic/oxic condition on vertical anoxic–aerobic continuous flow combined bioreactor. A novel Pseudomonas aeruginosa counted and injected on vertical anoxic–aerobic continuous flow combined bioreactor can be used to effectively biodegrade naphthalene. It emerged that the degradation of naphthalene rise to 94% within 8 days under optimum conditions (temperature 27°C, pH 8.0, and naphthalene concentration of 20 mg/L). Naphthalene concentration, retention times, flow rate, pH and turbidity formed by bacterial in the bioreactor have been shown to be of particular importance in the removal of naphthalene. Naphthalene degradation increased with the increasing naphthalene concentration to 20 mg/L. Alkaline pH [7,8] was favorable for Pseudomonas aeruginosa for naphthalene degradation. More than 96% of naphthalene and 76% of COD was degraded when the pH of the bioreactor ranged from 7 to 8. Increase in dose of bacterium injection into the system is goes along with increase of naphthalene degradation. At pH 8 and 10 NTU which is the greatest amount of bacterium injected to the system, the highest naphthalene removal efficiency was obtained. As the initial concentration of naphthalene increased from 0.5 to 20 mg/L, the remaining concentration of naphthalene decreased from 65.5% to 33.4% after 3 days. Based on experimental results, it was determined that this process can effectively reduce naphthalene under optimal conditions and this method can be used for the removal of similar compounds.

Abbreviations

(PAH): Poly aromatic hydrocarbon; (COD): Chemical oxygen demand; (POM): Polycyclic organic matter.

Competing interests

The authors declare that they have no competing interests.

Authors' contributions

BK administered data collection. All authors read and approved the final manuscript.

Acknowledgements

This article is approved by Arak university of Medical Sciences coded 573. I appreciate the research Deputy of university, and management of research projects for project funding and all those who without their cooperation, this study was not possible.

Author details

[1]Department of Environmental Health Engineering, School of Health, Arak University of Medical Sciences, Arak, Iran. [2]Department of Environmental Health Engineering, School of Health, Tehran University of Medical Sciences, Tehran, Iran.

References

1. Darvishi Cheshmeh Soltani R, Rezaee A, Safari M, Khataee AR, Karimi B. Photocatalytic degradation of formaldehyde in aqueous solution using ZnO nanoparticles immobilized on glass plates. Desalin Water Treat. 2013;53:1613–20.
2. Anbia M, Moradi SE. Removal of naphthalene from petrochemical wastewater streams using carbon nanoporous adsorbent. Appl Surf Sci. 2009;255:5041–7.
3. Karimi B, Ehrampoush MH, Ebrahimi A, Mokhtari M, Amin MM. Catalytic oxidation of hydrogen peroxide and the adsorption combinatory process in leachate waste pretreatment from composting factory. Int J Environ Health Eng. 2012;1:15.
4. Aranda A, López JM, Murillo R, Mastral AM, Dejoz A, Vázquez I. Total oxidation of naphthalene with high selectivity using a ceria catalyst

prepared by a combustion method employing ethylene glycol. J Hazard Mater. 2009;171:393–9.
5. Di Gennaro P, Moreno B, Annoni E, García-Rodríguez S, Bestetti G, Benitez E. Dynamic changes in bacterial community structure and in naphthalene dioxygenase expression in vermicompost-amended PAH-contaminated soils. J Hazard Mater. 2009;172:1464–9.
6. Nesterenko-Malkovskaya A, Kirzhner F, Zimmels Y, Armon R. Eichhornia crassipescapability to remove naphthalene from wastewater in the absence of bacteria. Chemosphere. 2012;125:124–8.
7. Badr T, Hanna K, De Brauer C. Enhanced solubilization and removal of naphthalene and phenanthrene by cyclodextrins from two contaminated soils. J Hazard Mater. 2004;112:215–23.
8. Gu L, Nie JY, Zhu N, Wang L, Yuan HP, Shou Z. Enhanced Fenton's degradation of real naphthalene dye intermediate wastewater containing 6-nitro-1-diazo-2-naphthol-4-sulfonic acid: A pilot scale study. Chem Eng J. 2012;45:22–8.
9. Chang CF, Chang CY, Chen KH, Tsai WT, Shie JL, Chen YH. Adsorption of naphthalene on zeolite from aqueous solution. J Colloid Interface Sci. 2004;277:29–34.
10. Karimi B, Rajaei M-S, Ganadzadeh MJ, Mashayekhi M, Jahanbakhsh M. Evaluation of nitrate removal from water by Fe/H2O2 and adsorption on activated carbon. Arak Med Univ J. 2013;15:67–76.
11. Akhtar S, Husain Q. Potential applications of immobilized bitter gourd (Momordica charantia) peroxidase in the removal of phenols from polluted water. Chemosphere. 2006;65:1228–35.
12. Soberon-Chavez G, Lepine F, Deziel E. Production of rhamnolipids by Pseudomonas aeruginosa. Appl Microbiol Biotechnol. 2005;68:718–25.
13. Goel RK, Flora JR, Ferry J. Mechanisms for naphthalene removal during electrolytic aeration. Water Res. 2003;37:891–901.
14. Karimi B, Ehrampoush MH, Ebrahimi A, Mokhtari M. The study of leachate treatment by using three advanced oxidation process based wet air oxidation. Iran J Environ health Sci Eng. 2013;10:1–7.
15. Maillacheruvu K, Safaai S. Naphthalene removal from aqueous systems by Sagittarius sp. J Environ Sci Health, Part A. 2002;37:845–61.
16. Pathak H, Kantharia D, Malpani A, Madamwar D. Naphthalene degradation by < i > Pseudomonas sp. HOB1: In vitro studies and assessment of naphthalene degradation efficiency in simulated microcosms. J Hazard Mater. 2009;166:1466–73.
17. Beklemishev M, Kozliak E. Bioremediation of concrete contaminated with n-hexadecane and naphthalene. Acta biotechnologica. 2003;23:197–210.
18. Seoud MA, Maachi R. Biodegradation of naphthalene by free and alginate entrapped Pseudomonas sp. Zeitschrift Fur Naturforsch C. 2003;58:726–31.
19. Kozlova E, Puntus I, Slepenkin A, Boronin A. Naphthalene degradation by Pseudomonas putida strains in soil model systems with arsenite. Process Biochem. 2004;39:1305–8.
20. Feijoo-Siota L, Rosa-Dos-Santos F, de Miguel T, Villa T. Biodegradation of Naphthalene by Pseudomonas stutzeri in Marine Environments: Testing Cells Entrapment in Calcium Alginate for Use in Water Detoxification. Bioremediation J. 2008;12:185–92.
21. Quantin C, Joner E, Portal J, Berthelin J. PAH dissipation in a contaminated river sediment under oxic and anoxic conditions. Environ Pollut. 2005;134:315–22.
22. Roslev P, King GM. Survival and recovery of methanotrophic bacteria starved under oxic and anoxic conditions. Appl Environ Microbiol. 1994;60:2602–8.
23. W-t Z, Huang X, Lee D-J. Enhanced treatment of coke plant wastewater using an anaerobic–anoxic–oxic membrane bioreactor system. Sep Purif Technol. 2009;66:279–86.
24. Karimi B, Ehrampoush MH, Jabary H. Indicator pathogens, organic matter and LAS detergent removal from wastewater by constructed subsurface wetlands. J Environ Health Sci Eng. 2014;12:52–9.
25. Tuomi PM, Salminen JM, Jørgensen KS. The abundance of nahAc genes correlates with the 14C-naphthalene mineralization potential in petroleum hydrocarbon-contaminated oxic soil layers. FEMS Microbiol Ecol. 2004;51:99–107.
26. Chang BV, Chang I, Yuan SY. Biodegradation of phenanthrene and pyrene from mangrove sediment in subtropical Taiwan. J Environ Sci Health Part A. 2008;43:233–8.
27. Blum P, Hunkeler D, Weede M, Beyer C, Grathwohl P, Morasch B. Quantification of biodegradation for xylene and naphthalene using first order decay models, Michaelis–Menten kinetics and stable carbon isotopes. J Contam Hydrol. 2009;105:118–30.
28. Wen Y, Ren Y, Wei C-H, Li K-Y, Lin F-M, Chen X-Y. A study on nitrogen removal efficiency of Pseudomonas stutzeri strains isolated from an anaerobic/anoxic/oxic wastewater treatment process. Afr J Biotechnol. 2010;9:869–73.
29. Sun HM, Tian WJ, Wang YM. Occurrence and Fate of Polycyclic Aromatic Hydrocarbons in the Anaerobic-Anoxic-Oxic Wastewater Treatment Process. Adv Mate Res. 2013;610:1722–5.

The estimation of per capita loadings of domestic wastewater in Tehran

Alireza Mesdaghinia[1], Simin Nasseri[1], Amir Hossein Mahvi[2,3], Hamid Reza Tashauoei[4] and Mahdi Hadi[1*]

Abstract

The amount of wastewater characteristics loading is one of the main parameters in the design of wastewater collection and treatment systems. The generation per capita per day (GPCD) of wastewater characteristics was estimated by analyzing the monthly data of nine wastewater treatment plants in Tehran, capital city of Iran. GPCD values were calculated from measured collected wastewater flow, the population and concentration data. The results indicated the values of 32.96 ± 1.91, 49.25 ± 2.49, 37.31 ± 2.44, 6.77 ± 0.53, 1.96 ± 0.11, 92.23 ± 5.68, 2.07 ± 0.39 and 128.96 ± 6.69 g/d.cap of GPCD for BOD_5, COD, TSS, TKN, P, TDS, ON and TS, respectively, for Tehran's wastewater. The per capita estimated for the wastewater production and treatment were determined to be 186.06 ± 7.85 and 136.72 ± 5.43 L/d.cap, respectively. It is estimated that about 504 m^3/d and 346 m^3/d of sludge, will be produced and waste as excrement raw sludge, respectively, in Tehran. Simple regression models were presented the relationships such as the change of collected and treated wastewater with population and changes of GPCD parameters with each other. It was revealed that the Tehran's wastewater may be classified as highly degradable, but during recent decades its Biodegradability Index (BI) has been reduced up to 15%. The new suggested revised per capita parameters can be used for design purposes in Tehran, and possibly, in areas with similar characteristics, substituting the classical values obtained from foreign textbooks. These values could help in designing more accurate treatment systems and may lower the required capacity for the treatment of wastewater up to 40% in Tehran.

Keywords: Domestic wastewater, Per capita loading, Wastewater treatment plant

Introduction

The amount of wastewater characteristics loading is one of the main parameters in the design of wastewater collection and treatment systems. The per capita loading of wastewater characteristics such as chemical oxygen demand (COD), Biological oxygen demand (BOD_5), nitrogen, phosphorus and solids have been considered as useful main functions in the design of wastewater collection systems and in the control of water resources pollution [1].

The pollutants per capita values can be used to estimate the present and the future pollution loading of wastewater produced from a population. These also are useful to estimate the equivalent population of an urban or industrial wastewater flow [2]. By expressing the wastewater pollution in terms of per capita values, the concept of pollution would be more understandable for the citizens and policy makers. However, the changes in mode and living standards [3] and the development of wastewater collection and treatment technologies, would suggest that a review and a re-examination of the pollution per capita loadings be made [1]. On the other hand, the discharge of these pollutants can cause considerable problems in environment [4]. Increased pollution of water-receiving bodies, and the imposition of restrictive limits by local administrations, led a need for new treatment technologies [5-9]. Thus it is very important that the properties of the discharged wastewater be assessed in order to be able to improve current technologies and provide adequate wastewater treatment [10].

Tehran, the capital city of Iran, has a population of over 7.5 million. There are nine public and 18 private wastewater treatment plant (WWTP) in Tehran those can treat more than 100 MCM of wastewater per year [11]. By construction of a new treatment plant system in the south of Tehran which can treat about 750 million cubic meters per year after project completion, the other

* Correspondence: hadi_rfm@yahoo.com
[1]Center for Water Quality Research (CWQR), Institute for Environmental Research (IER), Tehran University of Medical Sciences, Tehran, Iran
Full list of author information is available at the end of the article

treatment systems will be switched off gradually. Based on the current existing information of in-use domestic wastewater treatment plants in Tehran it may be possible to make an estimate of wastewater per capita parameters that can be used for design purposes and development programs of wastewater treatment systems in Tehran.

One of aims of the study reported in this paper is to re-establish the main wastewater pollution measures (including BOD_5, COD, TSS, TKN, P, TDS, ON(Organic Nitrogen) and TS) generation per capita per day (GPCD) according to the recorded data of nine public wastewater treatment systems in Tehran. The per capita loading of wastewater is an important parameter in the design process of a treatment plant's units. Iran's water and sewage utility (ABFA company) states that per capita water consumption in Tehran is currently about 378 liters per day [11]. Our study also sought to determine the amount of wastewater produced per capita per day or the conversion factor of water to wastewater. Pollutant discharge per capita (PDC; g/d.cap) with the wastewater treatment system in Tehran is another parameter that is important in the case of wastewater discharge in to receiving bodies. This parameter and the per capita of the producing sludge for domestic wastewater in Tehran would also be estimated in this study from wastewater treatment plants data. The later parameter may be useful in sludge treatment and management programs. The findings of this study can be used as basic data for the design of wastewater treatment systems in Tehran and possibly in areas with similar characteristics.

Materials and methods

The data were used in this study obtained from monthly reports (from 2007 to 2013) of nine wastewater treatment plants in Tehran including Sahebgharaniyeh, Mahallti, Zargandeh, Qeitariyeh, Qods, Shush, Ekbatan, Dowlatabadi and Jonoob. The data includes the quantitative information of wastewater production and characteristics data over 80 months from April 2007 to November 2013 for all domestic WWTPs in Tehran. The analysis of wastewater samples were done by the laboratory stuffs of WWTPs according to Standard Methods for the Examination of Water and Wastewater [12]. The parameters monitored were temperature, pH, Biological Oxygen Demand (BOD_5), Total Dissolved Solid (TDS), Total Solids (TS), Total Suspended Solid (TSS), Chemical Oxygen Demand (COD), Organic Nitrogen (ON), Total Phosphorous (TP) and Total Kjeldahl Nitrogen (TKN). Data analysis involved the data pre-processing and conducting some descriptive and analytical studies using Microsoft Excel 2007 and R software packages.

The study included data pre-processing and preparing them to make the estimates of desired parameters. Initial data processing, although is a time consuming step, but is very important part in the success of statistical analysis [13]. At this step, the raw data of nine in-use WWTPs collected during the recent years was assessed. The raw data was included 720 instances, although there were some outlier values. The data that appear to be very distant from the normal data distribution may be classified as being outliers. In certain instances however, this outlying value may be correct and is a natural product of the variables distribution [14]. All examples with missing values were represented with NA (not available). In this study, we took a normal distribution with a cutoff of three times of standard deviations around the mean to detect the outliers. Thus, the data that was more than $\mu \pm 3SD$ was considered as outliers.

The descriptive statistics of raw (720 instances) and pre-processed (499 instances) data are summarized in Tables 1 and 2, respectively.

The estimation of pollutant generation per capita per day (GCPD) values was conducted according to the following equations:

$$
\begin{aligned}
GCPD_{BOD5} &= ((Collect/30) \times BODin)/CurentPop \\
GCPD_{COD} &= ((Collect/30) \times CODin)/CurentPop \\
GCPD_{TSS} &= ((Collect/30) \times TSSin)/CurentPop \\
GCPD_{TKN} &= ((Collect/30) \times TKNin)/CurentPop \\
GCPD_{P} &= ((Collect/30) \times Pin)/CurentPop \\
GCPD_{TDS} &= ((Collect/30) \times TDSin)/CurentPop \\
GCPD_{OrgN} &= ((Collect/30) \times OrNin)/CurentPop \\
GCPD_{TS} &= ((Collect/30) \times TSin)/CurentPop \\
GCPD_{Slu_P} &= ((ProSlu/30)\ /CurentPop) \times 1000 \\
GCPD_{Slu_E} &= ((ExcSlu/30)\ /CurentPop) \times 1000 \\
Coll_{PerP} &= ((Collect/CurentPop)/30) \times 1000 \\
Tret_{PerP} &= ((Treat/CurentPop)/30) \times 1000
\end{aligned}
$$

The pollutant discharge per capita (PDC; g/d.cap) with the wastewater treatment system was defined and determined in terms of pollutant generation per capita (GCPD; g/d.cap) and pollutant removal efficiency (PRE; %) of the wastewater treatment systems as follow [15]:

$$PDC = GCPD \times [(100-PRE)/100]$$

Results and discussion

The total yearly averaged population covered by Tehran's nine municipal wastewater treatment plants from 2007 to 2013 was determined to be 4,502,065 persons per year. In average, out of 22,778,632 m^3/year estimated collected wastewater from 2007 to 2013, only 19,749,770 m^3/year of it were treated. In other words, about three MCM per year (13% of estimated collected wastewater from 2007 to 2013) were discharged into the environment without adequate treatment. The mathematical relationships between

Table 1 The statistics of raw data of wastewater characteristic for Tehran WWTPs

Parameter	Mean	SD	SE	Max.	Min.	UB	LB
Nomin	300670	281473	24756	900000	10500	325427	275914
Collect	458191	807439	85130	7445021	39000	543321	373060
Treat	397265	796648	83993	7445021	11395	481258	313272
ProSlu	88.16	77.63	6.83	225.00	1.00	94.99	81.34
ExcSlu	64.15	57.37	5.05	188.00	1.00	69.20	59.11
CurentPop	90558	172233	18159	1459808	7000	108717	72399
Tin	21.83	3.81	0.42	29.50	12.90	22.24	21.41
pHin	7.96	0.34	0.04	9.00	6.91	7.99	7.92
BODin	171.85	54.42	5.93	352.00	15.00	177.78	165.92
CODin	259.60	79.69	8.74	507.00	28.80	268.34	250.87
TSin	697.97	171.35	19.03	1280.00	246.00	716.99	678.94
TSSin	198.65	69.09	7.61	400.00	30.00	206.26	191.04
TDSin	494.88	145.66	17.72	985.00	185.00	512.60	477.16
Pin	11.24	4.68	0.53	29.70	3.92	11.77	10.72
OrNin	11.30	6.05	1.99	28.80	0.97	13.29	9.31
TKNin	35.16	12.33	1.55	79.38	12.00	36.71	33.61
Tout	20.94	4.13	0.45	28.20	10.00	21.39	20.49
pHout	7.39	0.35	0.04	9.00	6.50	7.43	7.35
BODout	11.90	8.96	0.98	72.28	2.40	12.88	10.93
CODout	23.95	12.83	1.41	98.50	6.40	25.36	22.54
TSout	482.38	135.12	15.03	934.50	3.00	497.41	467.35
TSSout	14.25	14.04	1.55	114.00	1.00	15.80	12.70
TDSout	465.12	128.18	15.59	902.00	214.00	480.71	449.52
Pout	4.24	1.60	0.18	12.97	0.05	4.42	4.06
OrNout	0.93	0.75	0.09	5.00	0.00	1.02	0.83
TKNout	4.28	4.33	0.57	23.85	0.04	4.85	3.71

SD, Standard deviation; SE, 1.96 × Standard error; Max., Maximum of observation; Min., Minimum of observation; UB, Upper bound of 95% confidence interval; LB, Lower bound of 95% confidence interval.

wastewater flows and population in Tehran were shown in Figure 1.

According to the latest report of the basic operational items of Tehran's wastewater company [16], a capacity of 675,000 m^3/d had been allocated for the treatment of wastewater produced by 3,150,000 persons up to June 2014. This means that the per capita loading of wastewater considered by designers for the design of a wastewater treatment plant in Tehran, is about 215 L/d. By a roughly estimation according to Figure 1(b), it is expected that for a population of 3,150,000 persons, the capacity of 455,822 m^3/d is a sufficient capacity that needs to be allocated. This capacity is about 40% lower than current allocated value. Therefore, the overestimated per capita loading value of 215 L/d in Tehran, leads the system to be designed for a capacity more than that is required.

The pattern changes of Tehran wastewater quality contents from 1984 to 2013 is another issue were assessed in Table 3. The most of the wastewater quality parameters have not shown considerable changes during this period. However, averaged value of TSS parameter in the influent wastewater of Tehran's WWTPs was considerably decreased from 353.33 in 1984 to 198.65 mg/L in 2013. It is clear that TSS content of Tehran domestic wastewater has been decreased by 56% of its value in 1984. This result indicates that the per capita generation of TSS parameter could also be reduced similarly.

The estimated per capita loadings for domestic wastewater of Tehran, as summarized from the results of this investigation, are presented in Table 4. The GPCD values of 32.96 ± 1.91, 49.25 ± 2.49, 37.31 ± 2.44, 6.77 ± 0.53, 1.96 ± 0.11, 92.23 ± 5.68, 2.07 ± 0.39 and 128.96 ± 6.69 g/d.cap were estimated for BOD_5, COD, TSS, TKN, P, TDS, ON and TS, respectively. In a study conducted by Azimi and Ameri [20] on the estimation of per capita loadings for domestic wastewater of Saheb-Gharanieh treatment plant in Tehran (based on the data collected

Table 2 The statistics of pre-processed data of wastewater characteristic for Tehran WWTPs

	Mean	SD	SE	Max.	Min.	UB	LB
Nomin	300670	281473	24757	900000	10500	325427	275914
Collect	458190	807439	85130	7445021	39000	543321	373060
Treat	397265	796648	83993	7445021	11395	481258	313273
ProSlu	88.16	77.63	6.83	225.00	1.00	94.99	81.34
ExcSlu	64.15	57.37	5.05	188.00	1.00	69.20	59.11
CurentPop	90558	172233	18159	1459808	7000	108717	72399
Tin	21.83	3.81	0.42	29.50	12.90	22.24	21.41
pHin	7.96	0.34	0.04	9.00	6.91	7.99	7.92
BODin	171.85	54.42	5.93	352.00	15.00	177.78	165.92
CODin	259.60	79.69	8.74	507.00	28.80	268.34	250.87
TSin	697.97	171.35	19.03	1280.00	246.00	716.99	678.94
TSSin	198.65	69.09	7.61	400.00	30.00	206.26	191.04
TDSin	494.88	145.66	17.72	985.00	185.00	512.60	477.16
Pin	11.24	4.68	0.53	29.70	3.92	11.77	10.72
OrNin	11.30	6.05	1.99	28.80	0.97	13.29	9.31
TKNin	35.16	12.33	1.55	79.38	12.00	36.71	33.61
Tout	20.94	4.13	0.45	28.20	10.00	21.39	20.49
pHout	7.39	0.35	0.04	9.00	6.50	7.43	7.35
BODout	11.90	8.96	0.98	72.28	2.40	12.88	10.93
CODout	23.95	12.83	1.41	98.50	6.40	25.36	22.54
TSout	482.38	135.12	15.03	934.50	3.00	497.41	467.35
TSSout	14.25	14.04	1.55	114.00	1.00	15.80	12.70
TDSout	465.12	128.18	15.59	902.00	214.00	480.71	449.52
Pout	4.24	1.60	0.18	12.97	0.05	4.42	4.06
OrNout	0.93	0.75	0.09	5.00	0.00	1.02	0.83
TKNout	4.28	4.33	0.57	23.85	0.04	4.85	3.71

SD, Standard deviation; SE, 1.96 × Standard Error; Max., Maximum of observation; Min., Minimum of observation; UB, Upper bound of 95% confidence interval; LB, Lower bound of 95% confidence interval.

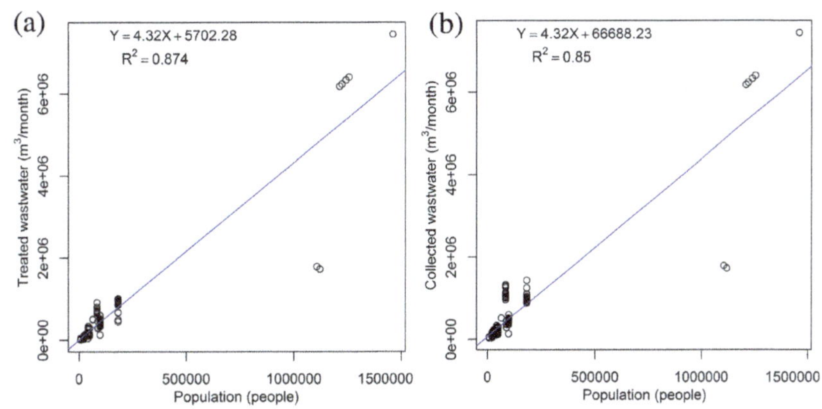

Figure 1 The flow of treated (a) and collected (b) wastewater versus population.

Table 3 Changes of Tehran wastewater quality contents from 1984 to 2013

Year	Parameters							Ref.
	pH	BOD_5	COD	TSS	TDS	P	TKN	
1984	n.a.	288.33	n.a.	353.33	495	25	n.a.	[17]
1993	7.43	184.47	261.87	256.03	n.a.	n.a.	45.56	[18]
1995	7.39	170	237.8	226.3	n.a.	9.9	39.37	[19]
1997	7.8	129.8	225	189.7	n.a.	2.7	38.3	[20]
2013	7.96	171.85	259.6	198.65	494.88	11.24	35.16	This study

n.a: not available.

in 1997), they were found GPCD values of 36, 62, 52, 10.5 and 0.74 g/d.cap for BOD_5, COD, TSS, TKN and P, respectively. Although their estimated values are not representative of all treatment plants, comparison of them with the GPCD estimated in our study show that the GPCD of BOD_5, TKN, and P were not considerably changed, but it was decreased by 71% and 79% of estimated values (in 1997) for TSS and COD parameters, respectively. This result is consistent with the pattern of TSS changes in Table 3.

Table 4 The estimated values of per capita parameters

Parameter	Mean	SD	SE	Max.	Min.	UB	LB
$GCPD_{Slu\_E}$	0.11	0.14	0.02	0.89	0.00	0.12	0.09
$GCPD_{Slu\_P}$	0.16	0.23	0.02	1.07	0.00	0.19	0.14
$GCPD_{TS}$	128.96	56.39	6.69	395.04	40.07	135.65	122.27
$GCPD_{OrgN}$	2.07	1.18	0.39	5.76	0.17	2.45	1.68
$GCPD_{TDS}$	92.23	43.03	5.68	303.75	27.98	97.90	86.55
$GCPD_P$	1.96	0.91	0.11	5.60	0.53	2.07	1.85
$GCPD_{TKN}$	6.77	3.88	0.53	31.14	2.19	7.30	6.24
$GCPD_{TSS}$	37.31	20.76	2.44	160.44	3.20	39.76	34.87
$GCPD_{COD}$	49.25	21.25	2.49	140.06	5.76	51.73	46.76
$GCPD_{BOD5}$	32.96	16.41	1.91	104.07	2.82	34.86	31.05
$(BOD_5/COD)_{out}$	0.41	1.06	0.12	7.25	0.95	2.51	2.27
$(BOD_5/COD)_{in}$	0.61	1.20	0.13	21.87	0.23	1.75	1.49
$Tret_{PerP}$	136.72	51.53	5.43	360.75	33.61	142.15	131.28
$Coll_{PerP}$	186.06	74.42	7.85	522.71	44.83	193.91	178.22
PDC_{TS}	89.49	38.92	4.63	283.05	0.39	94.12	84.86
PDC_{OrgN}	1.82	0.92	0.32	4.03	0.17	2.14	1.49
PDC_{TDS}	87.32	36.07	4.77	279.52	29.75	92.09	82.55
PDC_P	0.76	0.29	0.04	1.60	0.25	0.80	0.73
PDC_{TKN}	0.73	0.84	0.12	4.88	0.01	0.85	0.61
PDC_{TSS}	2.47	2.33	0.28	21.54	0.26	2.75	2.20
PDC_{COD}	4.46	2.93	0.34	25.51	0.84	4.81	4.12
PDC_{BOD}	2.15	1.60	0.19	15.31	0.36	2.34	1.96

SD, Standard deviation; SE, 1.96 × Standard Error; Max., Maximum of observation; Min., Minimum of observation; UB, Upper bound of 95% confidence interval; LB, Lower bound of 95% confidence interval.

For evaluating the biodegradability of Tehran's domestic wastewater the BOD_5/COD ratio, is called Biodegradability Index (BI), was determined. The BI Index varies from 0.4 to 0.8 for domestic wastewaters. If BOD_5/COD is > 0.6 then the waste is fairly biodegradable and can be effectively treated biologically. If BOD_5/COD ratio is between 0.3 and 0.6, then seeding is required to treat it biologically. If BOD_5/COD is < 0.3 then it cannot be treated biologically [21,22]. From data in the literature (Table 3) and the results of this study, the BI index was obtained to be 0.70, 0.71, 0.57 and 0.61 for the years of 1993, 1995, 1997 and 2013, respectively. Although these values reveal that the wastewater may be classified as highly biodegradable, BI values for later two years are almost 15% lower than those for previous years. This may be resulted from this fact that over the past 15-20 years a wide range of diverse industrial synthetic detergents which are mostly made from petroleum products and alcohols, has been produced and extensively used for cleaning and disinfection purposes and then discharged into sewage systems [23]. Many detergent compounds was found to be resistant to biodegradation by bacteria [24]. This may be the main reason of deceasing in the biodegradation potential of Tehran's wastewater according to the BI index.

Table 5 summarizes the mathematical simple relationships among the estimated GCPD parameters. The strongest relationship was found between $GCPD_{COD}$ and $GCPD_{BOD}$ ($R^2 = 0.74$). The next relationship with high correlation ($R^2 = 0.66$) was found between $GCPD_{BOD}$ and $GCPD_{TSS}$. These relationships may be useful for designers to help them to estimate the GPCD values from each other.

The per capita collected wastewater ($Coll_{PerP}$) was determined to be 186.06 ± 7.85 while the $Coll_{PerP}$ of 199.67 L/d.cap was estimated from the study's results of Sharifi Sistani [25]. This finding shows that this

Table 5 The main relationships between Tehran wastewater quality parameters

X	Y	Equation	R^2
$GCPD_{COD}$	$GCPD_{BOD}$	$Y = 0.66X + 0.16$	0.74
$GCPD_{BOD}$	$GCPD_{TSS}$	$Y = 1.03X + 3.61$	0.66
$GCPD_{COD}$	$GCPD_{TSS}$	$Y = 0.76X-0.15$	0.60
$GCPD_{BOD}$	$GCPD_{TDS}$	$Y = 2.03X + 25.88$	0.58
$GCPD_{COD}$	$GCPD_{TDS}$	$Y = 1.55X + 16.55$	0.56
$GCPD_{BOD}$	$GCPD_{TKN}$	$Y = 0.17X + 1.17$	0.52
$GCPD_{COD}$	$GCPD_{TKN}$	$Y = 0.12X + 0.62$	0.45
$GCPD_{TSS}$	$GCPD_{TKN}$	$Y = 0.12X + 2.31$	0.42
$GCPD_{COD}$	$GCPD_P$	$Y = 0.03X + 0.72$	0.35
$GCPD_{BOD}$	$GCPD_P$	$Y = 0.03X + 0.92$	0.33
$GCPD_{TSS}$	$GCPD_P$	$Y = 0.02X + 1.16$	0.30

parameter has been decreased in 2013 by 93% of its value in 2000. This seven percent decrease during recent thirteen years may be results from some reasons such as increasing the level of public awareness on water saving tips, using of treated water for construction purposes and cars or yards washing and probably increased use of fast foods instead of cooking meals at home.

Table 6 compares the per capita values of wastewater quality parameters estimated for Iran's domestic wastewater treatment plants in 2001. These values are drawn from a report of Department of Energy [26]. As shown in this table, different cities in Iran have different values for per capita loadings.

As shown in Table 6 the GCPD values of BOD_5, TSS, TKN and TP in 2001, according only to one wastewater treatment plant data (Zargandeh), were more than those for 2013 obtained to be 28.9, 32.3, 6.1 and 1.6 g/d.cap, respectively. The result indicates and confirms that the GCPD of TSS considerably reduced during the recent decade.

According to the technical criteria standard N. 3-129 [27], a new sewage treatment plant in Iran should be designed at least based on a per capita average of 40 to 50 g/d.cap BOD_5 and 50 to 60 g/d.cap of total suspended solids (TSS). These values have been universally used in the design of wastewater treatment systems and unchallenged since the publication of this standard in Iran. The recommended values of 40-50 g/d.cap for BOD_5 and 50-60 g/d.cap for TSS are more than the values of 31.05-34.86 and 34.87-39.76 g/d.cap estimated in this study, respectively. In another word, the estimated values of GCPD for BOD_5 and TSS for Tehran's wastewater are 27% and 32% lower than the mean of recommended values by Department of Energy, respectively. Using the guideline values recommended by Department of Energy for the design of wastewater treatment plant for the city of Tehran, with different living habits in different parts of the city, may results in considerable overestimations in the design process of new treatment plants. Thus, it is recommended that our estimated GPCDs be used in the design of new wastewater treatment plants in Tehran instead of recommended values by Department of Energy.

In Table 7, the GCPD values for main wastewater parameters in different countries were compared with the estimated GCPD values for Tehran's wastewater. The estimated values for Tehran are close to the per capita values obtained for countries such as Turkey, India, and Egypt. In these countries, the GCPD values are lower than that for European countries and United States. Low consumption of toilet papers in this countries and especially in Tehran may be one of the reasons for the low values of GCPD for BOD_5 and TSS [20].

It is estimated that over 90% of the treated wastewater effluent from treatment plants across Iran country is reused in some way; however, much of it is mixed with freshwater before further use, particularly in the suburban areas [29]. The direct use of untreated wastewater from sewage outlet, directly used for crop production is not a common scene in Iran. However, treated or partially treated wastewater used directly for irrigation without being mixed or diluted is more common. This is practiced in many treatment plants and there is no exact estimate about the amount used by this method to irrigate fodders, cereals, fruit trees, and vegetables eaten cooked or uncooked [29]. Thus the pollutants discharge per capita (PDC; g/d.cap) with the wastewater treatment systems is important parameter should be considered to be estimated.

The PDC with the wastewater treatment systems in Tehran was defined and determined in terms of GCPD and pollutant removal efficiency (PRE; %). The pollutants removal efficiency of wastewater treatment systems in Tehran ranged 92.11–93.41% for BOD_5, 89.65–90.97% for COD, 91.48–93.18% for TSS, 28.65-31.72% for TS, 1.73-2.76% for organic nitrogen (ON), 58.52-61.24% for P and 84.62-88.26% for TKN.

The ranges of estimated PDC summarized in Table 4, were compared with conventional domestic wastewater treatment systems in the United States [30] (Table 8). The generation per capita of BOD_5, COD, ON and TP of the United States wastewater treatment systems were almost thrice, four times, nine times and twice as those in Tehran, respectively. Conventional and nutrient removal activated sludge treatment systems are regarded as representative wastewater treatment processes in urban area of developed

Table 6 Basic characteristics of raw sewage intended for the design of wastewater treatment plants in Iran [26]

Paramater	Per capita parameters as g/d.cap for different plant or cities					
	Toiserkan	Zargandeh (Tehran)	Parkandabad (Mashhad)	Hovaizeh	Arak	Zabol
BOD_5	40	40	50	54	57	57
TSS	50	83	46	50	60	50
N(TKN)	-	14	-	-	5	-
TP	-	1	-	-	0.45	

Table 7 Comparison of per capita loadings (g/d.cap) of wastewater parameters in different countries with estimated values in Tehran

Parameter	BOD5	TSS	TKN	TP
Turkey[a]	27-50	41-68	8-14	0.4-2
India[a]	27-41	n.a.	n.a.	n.a.
Japan[a]	40-45	n.a.	1-3	0.2-0.4
Egypt[a]	27-41	41-68	8-14	0.4-0.6
Uganda[a]	55-68	41-55	8-14	0.4-0.6
Italy[a]	49-60	55-82	8-14	0.6-1
Germany[a]	55-68	82-96	11-16	1.2-1.6
Denmark[a]	55-68	82-96	14-19	1.5-2
Sweden[a]	68-82	82-96	11-16	0.8-1.2
Brazil[a]	55-68	55-68	8-14	0.6-1
United States[a]	50-120	60-150	9-22	2.7-4.5
Tehran (This study)	31-34	35-40	6.2-7.3	1.8-2

a: Adapted from *Wastewater engineering: treatment, disposal, and reuse* [28].

countries such as USA. PDCs with these treatment systems were estimated as 16.1 g-BOD_5/d.cap, 31.6 g-COD/d.cap, 4.9 g-ON/d.cap, and 3.2 g-TP/d.cap [30] while PDCs with Tehran's wastewater treatment systems were estimated as 2.15 ± 0.19 g-BOD_5/d.cap, 4.46 ± 0.34 g-COD/d.cap, 1.82 ± 0.32 g-ON/d.cap, and 0.76 ± 0.04 g-TP/d.cap. Deployment of larger removal efficiency treatment systems will decrease PDC with increase of PRE. When judging only from pollutant discharge reduction function of treatment systems, countries or cities with smaller GCPD and larger PDC-BOD_5 should be prioritized for investments on wastewater treatment measurements including assistances in order to improve ambient water quality [31].

The estimated PDC of some regions studied by Tsuzuki [15] were compared with that of Tehran and summarized in Table 9. When the criteria are applied, the group of countries in the Region of South China Sea and Tehran were found to be with higher and lower priority of BOD_5 discharge reduction from domestic wastewater, respectively (Table 9). The PDC of ROP-ME[a] sea area region, Red sea region and Gulf of Aden region is 2.5 g/d.cap and comparable with that obtained for Tehran (2.15 g/d.cap).

The comparatively low BOD_5-PDC in sewage treatment plants of Tehran may results from the fact that the per capita loading of BOD_5 in Tehran is lower than that for other countries and on the other hand the removal efficiency of BOD_5 in most of treatment plants are more than 90%.

Tajrishi [29] estimated that less than 40% of the total domestic sludge in Iran's wastewater treatment plants is being treated completely. In other words; of more than 200,000 cubic meters of daily produced sludge (2000 tons/d dry solids) of total fecal, septic and waste excrements sludge, only about 80,000 cubic meters (800 tons) is being digested and/or stabilized daily by different treatment methods. According to the finding of our study, the per capita values of 0.16 ± 0.02 and 0.11 ± 0.02 L sludge/d were determined for the produced and waste excrements sludge in Tehran's WWTPs, respectively. According to these values and the population covered by Tehran's WWTPs (3,150,000 persons/d), it is estimated that 504 m^3/d and 346 m^3/d of sludge will be produced and waste as excrement raw sludge, respectively, in Tehran. This high volume of sludge needs to be managed and discarded properly. The most common method of treatment for these sludge is digestion (aerobically and an aerobically). The lagooning, composting, and landfilling are the next methods of treatment. Mechanical dewatering may also be implemented as final treatment to reduce the volume of the stabilized sludge.

Conclusions

In this study, the basic characteristic data regarding to the nine main domestic wastewater treatment plants in Tehran was assessed and analyzed. The BOD_5 and TSS parameters of 32.96 ± 1.91, 37.31 ± 2.44 g/d.cap obtained in this study are considerably lower than the values of 40 to 50 and 50 to 60 g/d.cap, respectively, recommended by Department of Energy of Iran for the design of new treatment plants. The per capita loading of wastewater were used by designers for the design of a wastewater treatment plant in Tehran, was estimated to be 215 L/d.cap while the actual per capita collected wastewater according to the real data of treatment plants was determined to be 186.06 ± 7.85 L/d.cap. This disparity has interesting implication when these

Table 8 Comparison of GDPCs and PDCs of conventional activated sludge wastewater treatment systems in the USA [30] with those in Tehran

Country	Parameters	BOD5	COD	ON	TP
United States (Qasim, 1998)	GDPC (g/d.cap)	95	180	18	4
	Removal efficiency (%)	80-85	80-85	60-85	10-25
	PDC (g/d.cap)	16.1	30.6	4.9	3.2
Tehran (This study)	GDPC (g/d.cap)	31.0-34.8	46.7-51.7	1.6-2.4	1.8-2.0
	Removal efficiency (%)	92.1-93.4	89.6-90.9	1.7-2.7	58.5-61.2
	PDC ((g/d.cap)	1.96-2.3	4.1-4.8	1.4-2.1	0.7-0.8

Table 9 Comparison of PDC of other regions from 1998 to 2002 [15] with that of Tehran

Region/country	PDC (g/d.cap)	
	BOD	TP
South China Sea Region	43	n.a
Caspian Sea Region	24	n.a
Eastern African Region	11	n.a
Pacific Island Region	8.5	0.51
West and Central African (WACAF) Region	4.6	1.8
ROPME[a] sea area and Red sea and gulf of Aden region	2.50	1.10
Tehran (this study)	2.15	0.76

a: Regional Organization for the Protection of the Marine Environment.

estimated values are applied to the design of new wastewater treatment plant and calculation of an equivalent population for an industrial waste. The design of new treatment plant in Tehran with a per capita of 186.06 ± 7.85 L/d.cap may lower the required capacity for the treatment of wastewater up to 40%. The results of this study reveal that the Tehran's wastewater may be classified as highly degradable, but during recent decades the Biodegradability Index has been reduced up to 15%. This may be resulted from this fact that over the past 15-20 years, a wide range of diverse industrial synthetic detergents have been produced and extensively used for cleaning and disinfection purposes and then discharged into sewage systems. According to the PDC of BOD_5, Tehran was found to be with lower priority of BOD_5 discharge reduction from domestic wastewater. It is estimated that 504 m^3/d and 346 m^3/d of sludge will be produced and waste as excrement raw sludge, respectively, in Tehran.

In conclusion, the use of new revised per capita parameters obtained in this study could help in designing more efficient treatment systems and generating more reliable data for operational control of wastewater treatment process in Tehran. However, further research on wastewater quality and quantity assessment and adequate monitoring measures are required for existing and future treatment facilities in Tehran to ensure that they comply with safe operational and environmental standards.

Endnote

[a]Regional Organization for the Protection of the Marine Environment.

Nomenclature

Nomin; the nominal capacity of WWTP (m^3/month)
Collect; the collected volume of wastewater (m^3/month)
Treat; the treated volume of wastewater (m^3/month)
ProSlu; the produced sludge (m^3/month)
ExcSlu; the excess sludge (m^3/month)
CurentPop; the current covered population
Tin; the Influent temperature (C°)
pHin; the Influent pH
BODin; the Influent BOD_5 (mg/L)
CODin; the influent COD (mg/L)
TSin; the influent total solids (mg/L)
TSSin; the influent suspended solids (mg/L)
TDSin; the influent dissolved solids (mg/L)
Pin; the influent phosphorous (mg/L)
OrNin; the influent organic nitrogen (mg/L)
TKNin; the influent total Kjeldahl nitrogen (mg/L)
Tout; the effluent temperature (C°)
pHout; the effluent pH
BODout; the effluent BOD_5 (mg/L)
CODout; the effluent COD (mg/L)
TSout; the effluent total solids (mg/L)
TSSout; the effluent suspended solids (mg/L)
TDSout; the effluent dissolved solids (mg/L)
Pout; the effluent phosphorous (mg/L)
OrNout; the effluent organic nitrogen (mg/L)
TKNout; the effluent total Kjeldahl nitrogen (mg/L)
$GCPD_{Slu\_E}$; the generation per capita per day of excess sludge (L sudge/d.cap)
$GCPD_{Slu\_P}$; the generation per capita per day of produced sludge (L sludge /d.cap)
$GCPD_{TS}$; the generation per capita per day of total solids (g /d.cap)
$GCPD_{OrgN}$; the generation per capita per day of organic nitrigen (g /d.cap)
$GCPD_{TDS}$; the generation per capita per day of total dissolved solids (g /d.cap)
$GCPD_{P}$; the generation per capita per day of total phosphorous (g /d.cap)
$GCPD_{TKN}$; the generation per capita per day of total kjeldahl nitrogen (g /d.cap)
$GCPD_{TSS}$; the generation per capita per day of total suspended solids (g /d.cap)
$GCPD_{COD}$; the generation per capita per day of chemical oxygen demand (g /d.cap)
$GCPD_{BOD5}$; the generation per capita per day of biological oxygen demand (g /d.cap)
$(BOD_5/COD)_{out}$; the biodegradability index of effluent wastewater
$(BOD_5/COD)_{in}$; the biodegradability index of influent wastewater
$Tret_{PerP}$; the per capita per day of treated wastewater (L/d.cap)
$Coll_{PerP}$; the per capita per day of collected wastewater (L/d.cap)

Competing interests

The authors declare that they have no competing interests.

Authors' contributions

AM, SN and AHM contributed to drafting and editing the manuscript. HRT participated in raw data provision. MH contributed in the design of study, data analysis and drafting the manuscript. All authors read and approved the final manuscript.

Acknowledgements

The authors are grateful to the Center for Water Quality Research (CWQR) at the Institute for Environmental Research (IER) of Tehran University of Medical Sciences for providing facilities and supports for this research.

Author details

[1]Center for Water Quality Research (CWQR), Institute for Environmental Research (IER), Tehran University of Medical Sciences, Tehran, Iran. [2]Department of Environmental Health Engineering, Faculty of Health, Tehran University of Medical Sciences, Tehran, Iran. [3]Center for Solid Waste Research (CSWR), Institute for Environmental Research (IER), Tehran University of Medical Sciences, Tehran, Iran. [4]Department of Environmental Health Engineering, School of Public Health, Islamic Azad University-Tehran Medical Branch, Tehran, Iran.

References

1. Zanoni A, Rutkowski R. Per capita loadings of domestic wastewater. J Water Pollut Control Fed. 1972;44:1756–62.
2. Calvert C, Parks EH. The population equivalent of certain industrial wastes. Sewage Work J. 1934;6:1159–64.
3. Goldstein SN, Moberg WJ. Wastewater treatment systems for rural communities. DC: Washington; 1973.
4. Hadi M, Shokoohi R, Ebrahimzadeh Namvar A, Karimi M, Solaimany Aminabad M. Antibiotic resistance of isolated bacteria from urban and hospital wastewaters in Hamadan City. Iran J Health and Environ. 2011;4:105–14.
5. Hadi M, Samarghandi MR, McKay G. Simplified fixed bed design models for the adsorption of acid dyes on novel pine cone derived activated carbon. Water Air Soil Pollut. 2011;218:197–212.
6. Mahvi A. Sequencing batch reactor: a promising technology in wastewater treatment. Iran J Environ Health Sci Eng. 2008;5:79–90.
7. Mahvi A, Nabizadeh R, Pishrafti M. Evaluation of single stage USBF in removal of nitrogen and phosphorus from wastewater. Eur J Sci Res. 2008;23:204-211
8. Naghizadeh A, Mahvi A, Mesdaghinia A, Alimohammadi M. Application of MBR Technology in Municipal Wastewater Treatment. Arab J Sci Eng. 2011;36:3–10.
9. Naghizadeh A, Mahvi A, Vaezi F, Naddafi K. Evaluation of hollow fiber membrane bioreactor efficiency for municipal wastewater treatment. Iran J Environ Health Sci Eng. 2008;5:257–68.
10. Karagozoglu B, Altin A. Flow-rate and pollution characteristics of domestic wastewater. Int J Environ Pollut. 2003;19:259–70.
11. Tajrishy M, Cities S, Abdolghafoorian A, Abrishamchi A. Water reuse and wastewater recycling: Solutions to Tehran's growing water crisis. In: Quentin Grafton R, Wyrwoll P, White C, Allendes D, editors. Global Water: Issues and Insights. Australia: ANU Press; 2014. p. 223.
12. APHA, AWWA, WEF: *Standard methods for the examination of water and wastewater*. 22 edn: American Public Health Association (APHA), American Water Works Association (AWWA) & Water Environment Federation (WEF); 2012.
13. Teng CM. Correcting Noisy Data. In: Proceedings of 16th International Conference on Machine Learning; San Francisco. 1999. p. 239–48.
14. Masters T. Practical Neural Network Recipes in C++. San Diego: Academic Press; 1993.
15. Tsuzuki Y. Comparison of pollutant discharge per capita (PDC) and its relationships with economic development: An indicator for ambient water quality improvement as well as the Millennium Development Goals (MDGs) sanitation indicator. Ecol Indic. 2009;9:971–81.
16. Statistics and basic operational items of Tehran's wastewater company [http://ts.tpww.ir/abfa_content/media/image/2015/03/33358_orig.pdf]
17. Seyed Morteza H. Wastewater Quality and Quantity. Hoseinian: Tehran; 1974.
18. Sazeh Consultants Engineering & Construction Co.: Assessment the results of wastewater quality analyses of Tehran's Jonoob wastewater treatment plant. Sazeh Consultants Engineering & Construction Co. Tehran; 1993
19. Afshar J. Assessment of the quality and quantity of Tehran's wastewater. Master of Sciences Thesis: Tehran University of Medical Sciences, Department of Environmental Health Engineering; 1995.
20. Azimi AA, Ameri M. Determination of per capita flow rate and wastewater pollutants of saheb-gharanieh treatment plant in Tehran. J Environ Stud. 2002;28:93–100.
21. Rim-Rukeh A, Agbozu L. Impact of partially treated sewage effluent on the water quality of recipient Epie Creek Niger Delta, Nigeria using Malaysian Water Quality Index (WQI). J Appl Sci Environ Manag. 2013;17:5–12.
22. Srinivas T. Environmental biotechnology. New Delhi: New Age International Publishers; 2008
23. Matthijs E, Debaere G, Itrich N, Masscheleyn P, Rottiers A, Stalmans M, et al. The fate of detergent surfactants in sewer systems. Water Sci Technol. 1995;31:321–8.
24. Scott MJ, Jones MN. The biodegradation of surfactants in the environment. Biochim Biophys Acta Biomembr. 2000;1508:235–51.
25. Sharifi Sistani M. Wastewater treatment in Iran, past, present and future. Water Environ J. 2000;38:25–32.
26. Department of Energy: In Specialized workshop proceedings on assessment of wastewater treatment plants challenges; Shiraz. Water and Wastewater Company; 2001
27. Department of Energy. Technical criteria for reviewing and approval of urban sewage treatment projects, Standards No. 3-129. Tehran: Plan and Budget Organization, Office of Research and Technical Criteria; 1993.
28. Metcalf L, Eddy H, Tchobanoglous G: Wastewater engineering: treatment, disposal, and reuse. New York: McGraw-Hill; 2003
29. Tajrishy M. Wastewater Treatment and Reuse in Iran: Situation Analysis. Tehran: Departement of Civil Engineering, Sharif University of Technology, Environment and Water Research Center (EWRC); 2010.
30. Qasim SR: Wastewater treatment plants: planning, design, and operation. New York: CRC Press; 1998.
31. Tsuzuki Y. Relationships between pollutant discharges per capita (PDC) of domestic wastewater and the economic development indicators. J Environ Syst Eng. 2007;63:224–32.

Onion membrane: an efficient adsorbent for decoloring of wastewater

Samaneh Saber-Samandari* and Jalil Heydaripour

Abstract

Background: Recently, researchers have tried to design synthetic materials by replicating natural materials as an adsorbent for removing various types of environmental pollutants, which have reached to the risky levels in nature for many countries in the world. In this research, the potential of onion membrane obtained from intermediate of onion shells for adsorption of methylene blue (MB) as a model cationic dye was exhibited.

Methods: Before and after adsorption, the membrane was characterized by Fourier transform infrared spectroscopy (FTIR) and optical and scanning electron microscopy in order to prove its dye adsorption capability. The various experimental conditions affecting dye adsorption were explored to achieve maximum adsorption capacity.

Results: The dye adsorption capacity of the membrane was found to be 1.055 $g.g^{-1}$ with 84.45% efficiency after one hour and 1.202 $g.g^{-1}$ with 96.20% efficiency after eight hours in contact with the dye solution (0.3 $g.L^{-1}$). Moreover, the kinetic, thermodynamic and adsorption isotherm models were employed to described the MB adsorption processes. The results show that the data for adsorption of MB onto the membrane fitted well with the Freundlich isotherm and pseudo-second-order kinetic models. In addition, the MB adsorption from room temperature to ~50°C is spontaneous and thermodynamically favorable.

Conclusions: Evidently, the high efficiency and fast removal of methylene blue using onion membrane suggest the synthesis of polymer-based membranes with similar physical and chemical properties of onion membrane as a valuable and promising wastewater decoloring agents in water treatment.

Keywords: Adsorption, Cationic dye, Methylene blue, Onion membrane, Water treatment

Background

Many industrial production activities (e.g. dye, cosmetic, plastics, food, textile, planting, and mining) result in water pollution since they produce pollutants such as water-coloring agents and toxic heavy metals that are extremely harmful to people and the environment even at low concentrations. The removal of these compounds from wastewaters before discharging them into the environment is of great importance, since many dyes and their degradation products are toxic and carcinogenic, posing a serious hazard to the environment. The conventional methods used to treat colored effluents include photocatalytic degradation, microbiological decomposition, electrochemical oxidation, membrane filtration, and adsorption techniques [1]. Among these, adsorption is the most widely used method because of its efficiency, low cost, easy operation, simple design, less energy intensiveness, and non-toxicity. Recently, numerous approaches to develop adsorbents that are more effective have been studied [2]. Among these, adsorbents containing natural and synthetic polymeric materials, industrial by-products, agricultural wastes and biomass were applied for removal of dyes from aqueous solution [3-6].

Dyes can be classified into cationic, anionic and nonionic dyes. Cationic dyes are basic dyes while the anionic dyes include direct, acid, and reactive dyes [7]. However, cationic dyes are widely used in acrylic, wool, nylon, and silk dyeing, they considered as toxic colorants and can cause harmful effects such as allergic dermatitis, skin irritation, mutations and cancer [8]. Cationic dyes carry a positive charge in their molecule, furthermore they are water soluble and yield

* Correspondence: samaneh.saber@gmail.com
Department of Chemistry, Eastern Mediterranean University, TRNC via Mersin 10, Gazimagusa, Turkey

colored cations in solution [9]. Methylene blue, rhodamine B, and brilliant green are representative examples of cationic dyes [10]. Methylene blue (MB) is an important basic dye and widely used in the textile industry. Acute exposure to MB may cause increased heart rate, shock, vomiting, cyanosis, jaundice, quadriplegia, heinz body formation, and tissue necrosis in humans [11].

The main aim of this study is to exhibit the ability of dried onion membrane for removal of MB from aqueous solution. However, many researchers have studied the dye and metal adsorption capacity of several biomasses such as rice, corn and coconut husks [12-14], papaya seeds [15], watermelon [3] and onion skin [4], but to the best of our knowledge, there is no study relating the adsorption properties of onion membrane obtained from intermediate of onion shells. In this study, the adsorption of MB was confirmed using FTIR and optical and electron microscopy. In addition, the effect of various factors such as contact time, initial dye concentration, pH, temperature and adsorbent dose on the adsorption rate was examined. Finally, the adsorption of MB was analyzed by employing the adsorption kinetic, isotherm models, and thermodynamics.

Experimental procedures

Material

The onions were purchased from local markets in Famagusta (North Cyprus). Hydrochloric acid 37% (Merck), sodium hydroxide (Mediko Kimya), potassium chloride (Mediko Kimya), potassium hydrogen phthalate (Merck), sodium hydrogen carbonate (Aldrich), and potassium hydrogen phosphate (Merck) were used to prepare the buffer solutions with different pH values. Finally, MB (Aldrich) with a molecular formula of $C_{16}H_{18}ClN_3S$ was used without further purification.

Adsorbent preparation

The onions were peeled, chopped and then the membranes were removed from the leaves. 1 gram of onion membrane was obtained from approximately 250 g onion. The membranes (~4 g/kg of onion) were rinsed and washed with distilled water to remove impurities. Then, it was dried at 60°C in an oven for one day. After that, the dried adsorbent was kept in the desiccator to avoid moisture adsorption.

Swelling measurements

The swelling property of the membranes were investigated by immersing 0.06 g of membrane (15 × 15 mm^2) in 250 mL of distilled water at room temperature (±20°C) in atmospheric conditions until swelling equilibrium was reached. Following the removal from the water, they were blotted with filter paper and weighed. Then, the swelling capacity was calculated using the following equation [16,17]:

$$\text{Swelling } (\%) = \frac{W_2 - W_1}{W_1} \times 100 \quad (1)$$

where W_1 (g) and W_2 (g) are the weights of the dried and swollen membranes, respectively.

Dye adsorption

The initial aqueous MB solutions were prepared by dissolving 0.075 g of MB in 250 mL of deionized water (0.3 g.L^{-1}). Then, the 0.06 g of dried onion membranes (15 × 15 mm^2) were immersed in a prepared MB solution and shaken at 300 rpm for 10 hours at room temperature. During this period, 2 mL of solution was taken for further analysis frequently. Finally, the collected solutions were filtered and the amount of non-adsorbed dye ions in the solutions was determined spectrophotometrically using a UV-visible spectrophotometer at a wavelength of 668 nm [6]. The MB adsorption amount, capacity, and efficiency were calculated by the following equations:

$$\text{adsorption amount } \left(g.L^{-1}\right) = C_i - C_e \quad (2)$$

$$\text{adsorption capacity } \left(g.g^{-1}\right) = q_t = \frac{C_i - C_e}{W} \times V \quad (3)$$

$$\text{adsorption efficency } (\%) = \frac{C_i - C_e}{C_i} \times 100 \quad (4)$$

where W is the mass of adsorbent in g, V is the volume of MB solution in L, and C_i and C_e are the initial and equilibrium concentrations in g.L^{-1}, respectively.

In addition, the effect of variable conditions such as time, pH, adsorbent amount, and initial adsorbate concentration on the MB adsorption behavior of onion membranes was examined. For each case, one parameter was changed and analyzed and the other factors were kept constant. For instance, the influence of pH on adsorption was calculated by immersing 0.06 g of onion membrane in 250 mL of MB buffer solutions (0.3 g.L^{-1} concentration) with different pH values (3–11) and then shaken at room temperature (20°C) for eight hours (480 min).

Furthermore, the pH at point of zero charge (pHzpc), which shows the point that the acidic or basic functional groups do no contribute to the pH of the solution, was determined using the standard technique [18]. For this purpose, 50 mL of 0.01 mol.L^{-1} NaCl solution was placed in a 250 ml flask. The pH of the solutions in each flask was adjusted from 3–11 by adding either sodium hydroxide or hydrochloric acid solutions (0.1 mol.L^{-1}). Then, 0.06 g of onion membrane (15 × 15 mm^2) was immersed in each solution at 20°C and was allowed to equilibrate in an isothermal shaker. After a contact time of 24 hours, the suspensions were filtered through filter paper and the final pH values of supernatant were measured again using a pH meter. Lastly, the final pH values were plotted against the initial pH values. The pH at which the curve crosses the line final pH = initial pH was taken as the pHzpc of the onion membrane [19].

Methods of characterization

A UV/VIS spectrophotometer (Lambda 25 UV/VIS, Perkin-Elmer, Llantrisant, UK) was used to determine the MB adsorption amounts by the onion membranes. The pH values of the solutions, which were used to investigate the effect of pH on adsorption, were checked by a pH meter (WTW InoLab, accuracy ± 0.1). To prove the adsorption of MB by the onion membranes, the FTIR (Perkin-Elmer, Llantrisant, UK) spectra of membranes before and after adsorption were observed in the range of 500–4000 cm^{-1}. Images of the membranes were also taken with an optical microscope (MT9000 Polarizing Microscope, Meiji Techno Co. Ltd., Japan with Invenio 3S, Delta Pix Camera) and a scanning electron microscope (AIS2100, Seron Technology, Korea) operated at an acceleration voltage of 15 kV to study the change in surface morphology of the membrane after dye adsorption.

Results and discussion

Swelling properties of onion membrane

The dynamic swelling behavior of the onion membranes over 10 hours (600 min) of immersion in water is shown in Figure 1. The swelling percentage increased up to 1,106% and then plateaued, with no big differences in water uptake with further increases in time. Initially, the water molecules were in contact with the membrane, then, they attacked and penetrated into the onion membrane cells. Obviously, this swelling system cannot continue forever, and by the increasing membrane-water interaction, the osmotic pressure difference might be reduced. Finally, the osmotic force at the equilibrium state was balanced with an elasticity force. It should be noted that the elasticity force prevents the deformation of the onion membrane cells by the stretching balance of the cells.

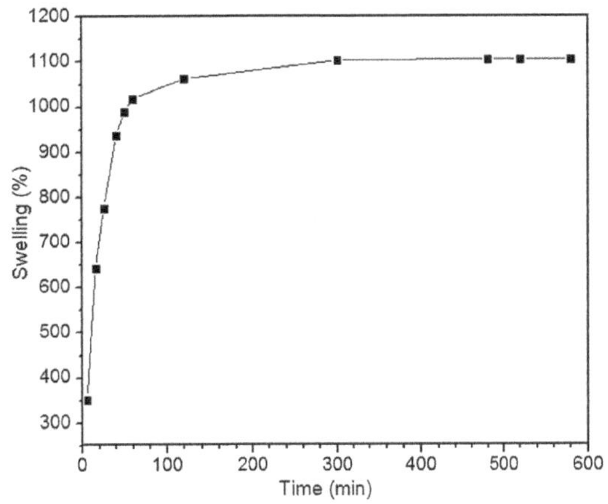

Figure 1 Swelling behavior of the onion membrane was plotted as a function of time. In this experiment, 0.06 g of membrane was immersed in 250 mL of water with a pH of 7.1 at 20°C.

Dye adsorption properties of onion membrane

The MB adsorption capacity of the onion membranes was examined. Figure 2 shows the preparation of the membranes for MB adsorption (Figure 2a) and color changes in the membrane and dye solutions before and after adsorption during the first and eight hours of contact time (Figure 2b-d). In addition, the scanning electron microscopy (SEM) images of the membranes before and after adsorption of MB reflect their surface morphology (Figure 2e and f). As can be seen, before adsorption the membrane has a smooth surface, whereas it exhibits a coarse surface due to the presence of MB molecules after adsorption. In addition to this distinctive change in the surface of the membrane, the optical microscope images of the membrane before and after MB adsorption (Figure 2g and h) also revealed the adsorption of MB by the onion membrane.

The FTIR spectrum of the onion membrane after adsorption of the dye was compared with the spectra of pure MB and dried onion membrane before adsorption in Figure 2i. The several peaks in the spectrum of dye-adsorbed membrane related to the MB and membrane are merged and slightly shifted. The peaks at 2,894 cm^{-1}, 2,900 cm^{-1}, and 1,744 cm^{-1} due to the C-H stretching in an aromatic methoxyl group and C = O stretching of carbonyl group of onion membrane, respectively, became stronger and were shifted to 2,916 cm^{-1}, 2,850 cm^{-1}, and 1,731 cm^{-1} in the dye adsorbed membrane [20]. The sharp and strong peak at 1,592 cm^{-1} of MB due to the presence of C = C vibration and N-H bending was merged with a peak at 1,599 cm^{-1} of membrane and showed a broader peak at 1,598 cm^{-1} in the spectrum of the dye-adsorbed membrane [21]. Like the two peaks at 1,443 cm^{-1} and 1,488 cm^{-1}, which indicates C = N stretching, the peaks at 1,220 cm^{-1} and 1,250 cm^{-1} of C = C stretching in aromatic rings of MB are merged and form broad peaks at 1,416 cm^{-1} and 1,232 cm^{-1}, respectively, in the spectrum of the dye-adsorbed membrane [18]. Finally, the peaks corresponding to the C-O stretching of the onion membrane and the C-S bending of the MB rings appeared at 1,008 cm^{-1} and 954 cm^{-1}, respectively [22]. The FTIR results accompanied with the supportive results of the SEM and the optical microscope confirmed the adsorption of MB by the onion membrane.

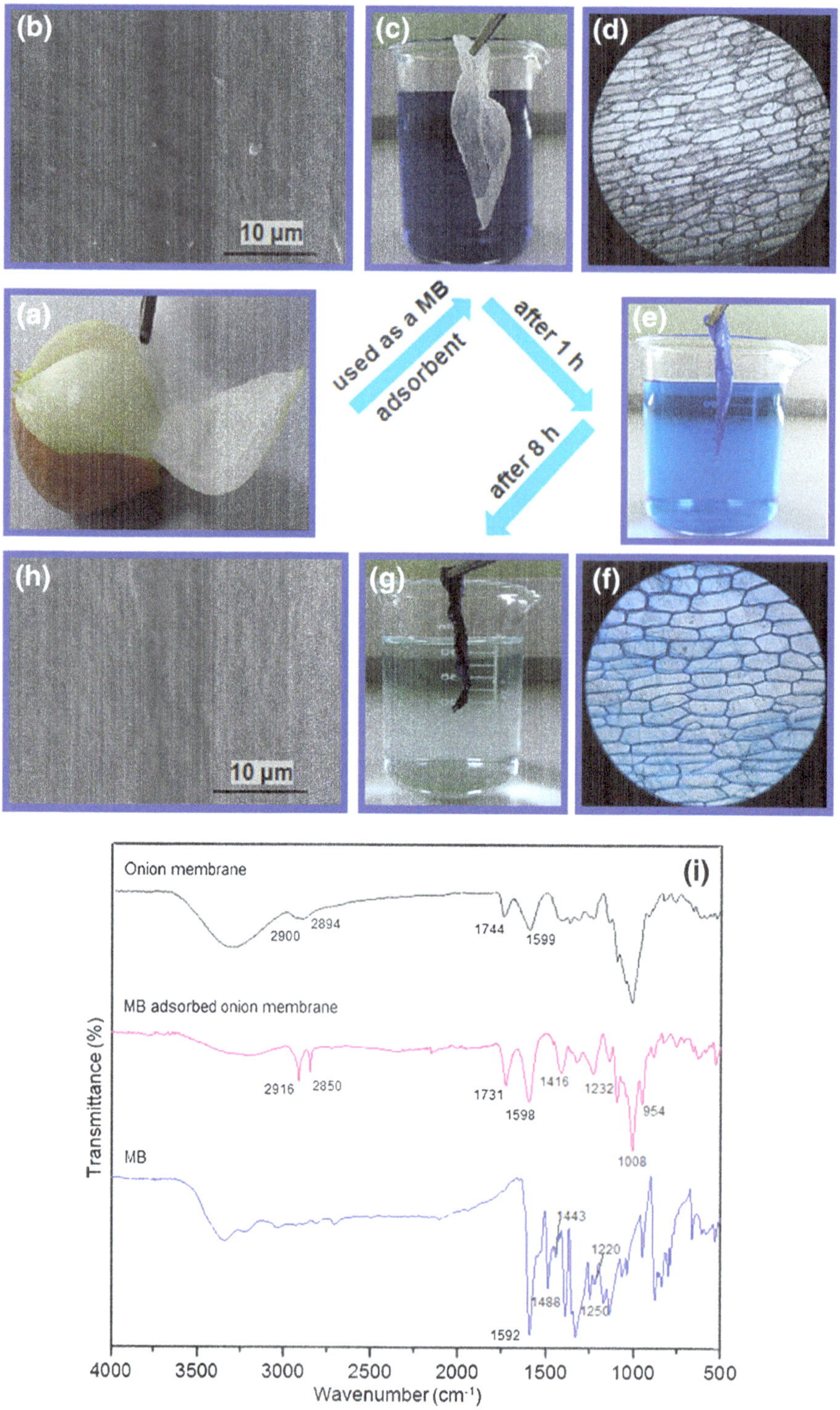

Figure 2 (a-d) Digital photographs, (e and f) SEM images, (g and h) optical microscope images, and (i) FTIR spectra of the onion membrane before and after dye adsorption are shown.

Onions contain protein (with –COOH and $-NH_2$ groups), sugars, carbohydrate, and vitamins A, B_6, and C (with –OH groups), minerals, and over 80% water [23]. As can be seen from Scheme 1, the onion membrane has several anionic groups such as –COOH and –OH. On the other hand, MB is a cationic dye consisting of = S– and $-N(CH_3)_2$ can become charged species and have ionic and dipole–dipole interactions with anionic groups in the surface of the onion membrane [24]. In addition, the = N– and $-N(CH_3)_2$ groups in the structure of MB can have hydrogen bonds with hydrogen atom of –COOH and –OH groups of the onion membrane. Therefore, the adsorbent can uptake MB very fast with high efficiency through the strong electrostatic attraction between the surface groups on the membrane and the cationic MB.

Effect of time on adsorption

The adsorption performance of the onion membrane was evaluated by a batch equilibration technique as a function of time. As shown in Figure 3, the adsorption capacity of MB ions on the membrane increased rapidly during the first hour of contact and then became slower until equilibrium was reached after eight hours (480 min). The maximum adsorption was 1.055 $g.g^{-1}$ with 84.45% efficiency after the first hour and 1.202 $g.g^{-1}$ with 96.20% efficiency after eight hours. This behavior can be attributed to the larger surface area of the onion membrane at the initial stage of the adsorption process. Subsequently, as the surface sites became saturated, adsorption did not increase significantly with further contact time.

Adsorption kinetics

In order to investigate the possibility of using an adsorbent for a particular separation task and to determine the adsorption efficiency as well as the adsorption rate, the kinetic mechanism of the adsorption process was considered. The adsorption kinetics of the MB ions with the onion membranes was investigated using three kinetic models: pseudo-first-order, pseudo-second-order, and intra-particle diffusion, which are given in the following equations, respectively.

$$\log(q_e - q_t) = \log q_e - \frac{k_1}{2.303} t \tag{5}$$

$$\frac{t}{q_t} = \frac{1}{k_2 q_e^2} + \frac{t}{q_e} \tag{6}$$

$$q_t = k_3 (t)^{\frac{1}{2}} + C_i \tag{7}$$

where t is the time (min) and q_e, q_t, ($g.g^{-1}$) and q_e^2 are the amounts of MB adsorbed by the onion membrane at

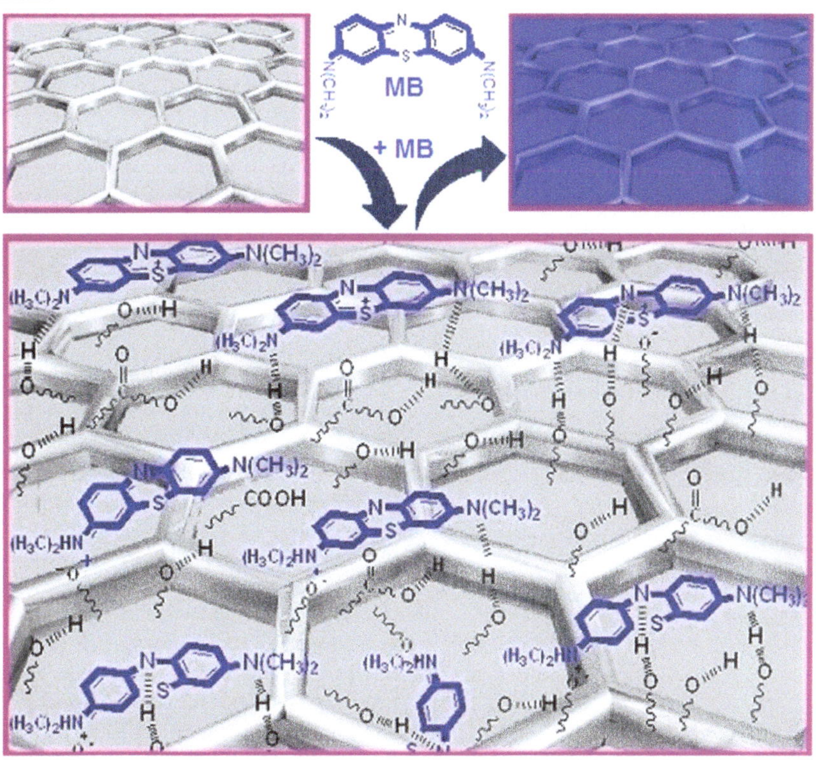

Scheme 1 Schematic illustration for the adsorption mechanism of MB by onion membrane.

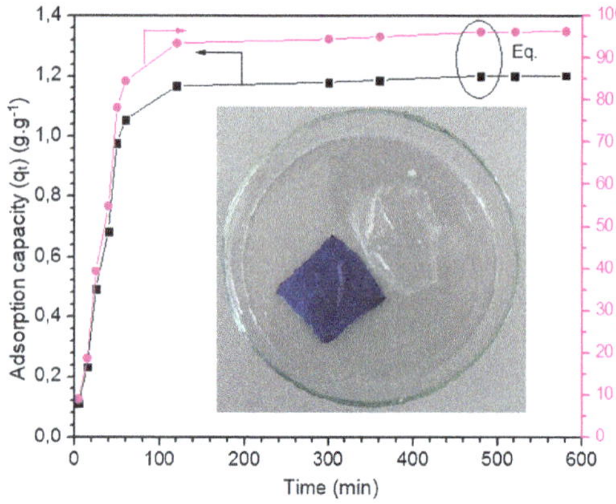

Figure 3 Effect of time on MB adsorption capacity ($g.g^{-1}$) and efficiency (%) of membrane was plotted. In this experiment, dye molecules from a 0.3 $g.L^{-1}$ dye solution (250 ml) with a pH of 7.1 at 20°C were taken up by 0.06 g of the membrane. Insert shows the onion membrane in swollen and dye-adsorbed state.

equilibrium, at time t, and at maximum adsorption capacity, respectively. k_1 (min^{-1}), k_2 ($g.g^{-1}.min^{-1}$), and k_3 ($g.g^{-1}.min^{-0.5}$) are the adsorption rate constants of the pseudo-first-order, pseudo-second order and the intra-particle diffusion models, respectively. In addition, C_i ($g.g^{-1}$) is the intra-particle diffusion constant, which is directly proportional to the boundary layer thickness. As shown in Table 1, the theoretical equilibrium adsorption capacity (1.3166 $g.g^{-1}$) using the pseudo-second-order model compared well with the experimental data (1.2025 $g.g^{-1}$), with a better R^2 value. Moreover, Figure 4a

Table 1 Comparison of kinetic models for adsorption of MB using onion membrane

Kinetic models and parameters	MB
q_e exp. ($g.g^{-1}$)	1.2025
Pseudo-first order	
K_1 (min^{-1})	0.0278
q_e cal. ($g.g^{-1}$)	0.6831
R^2	0.8255
Pseudo-second order	
$K_2 \times 10^{-4}$ ($g.g^{-1}.min^{-1}$)	0.0205
q_e cal. ($g.g^{-1}$)	1.3166
R^2	0.9893
Intraparticle diffusion	
$K_{3(1)}$ ($g.g^{-1}.min^{-1/2}$)	0.1747
C_1 ($g.g^{-1}$)	0.3567
R^2	0.9414
$K_{3(2)}$ ($g.g^{-1}.min^{-1/2}$)	0.0086
C_2 ($g.g^{-1}$)	1.0266
R^2	0.7264

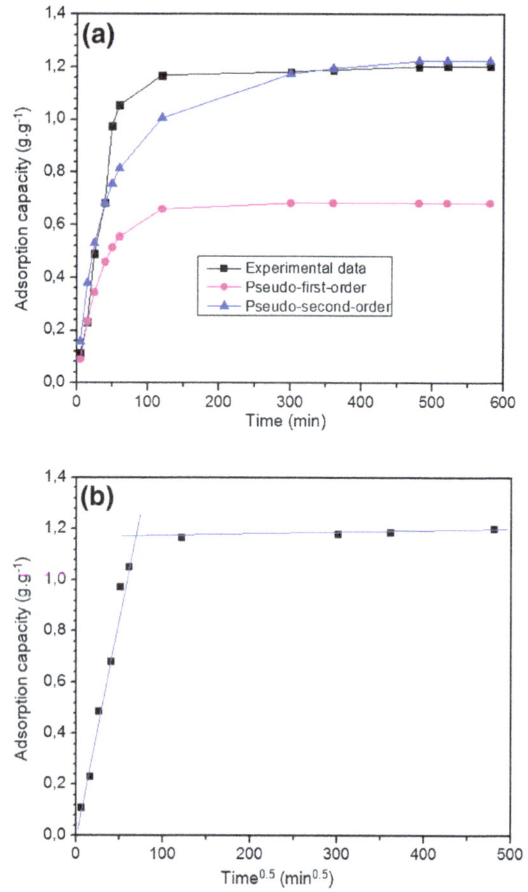

Figure 4 Adsorption kinetics of MB on membrane by (a) pseudo-first-order and pseudo-second-order, and (b) intra-particle models kinetic was plotted. In this experiment, dye molecules from a 0.3 $g.L^{-1}$ dye solution (250 ml) with a pH of 7.1 at 20°C were taken up by 0.06 g of the membrane.

shows the agreement between the experimental adsorption capacities with the calculated values of pseudo-second-order, which were obtained using the data in Table 1. Therefore, the agreement between experimental data and pseudo-second-order can prove the physical adsorption of MB on a highly heterogeneous onion membrane.

According to Equation 7, if the intra-particle diffusion is the main rate-controlling step, the plot of q_t versus $t^{0.5}$ should be linear and pass through the origin. However, the plot shown in Figure 4b did not pass through the origin and presented multilinearity, indicating the presence of two steps in the adsorption process. The intra-particle diffusion parameters for these steps are summarized in Table 1. The first linear segments can be attributed to the dye transfer from the solution onto the external surface or boundary layer of the onion membrane. The second step could be attributed to the final apparent equilibrium process, which reflects the intra-particle diffusion slowing down due to lowering the dye concentration in the solution [5]. As seen from the data in Table 1, the intra-particle diffusion constants of the two linear segments are not similar and the first step comprises the bigger $k_{3(1)}$ value ($0.1747\ g.g^{-1}.min^{-0.5}$) and the higher correlation coefficient 0.9414. This observation indicates that the adsorption of dye onto the onion membrane at the first section occurs more rapidly due to the availability of adsorption centers, then this is followed by the slow diffusion, which takes up to eight hours.

Effect of pH on adsorption

The pH value of the solution plays a significant role in the adsorption capacity of the adsorbate onto the adsorbent. As can be seen in Figure 5, with an increase in the initial pH of the MB solution from 3 to 8, adsorption capacity and efficiency increases rapidly and then increases slowly with a further increase in the pH. The maximum adsorption capacity was obtained at $1.245\ g.g^{-1}$, with 99.64% efficiency at pH 11. This result can be explained by the electrostatic interaction between the cationic MB species and the surface of the adsorbent, which should be a negatively charged species. The lower adsorption at acidic pH levels was probably due to the presence of an excess of H^+ ions competing with the dye cations for adsorption sites [19]. In order to confirm these results, the pHzpc of the onion membrane was determined. In this study, pHzpc value was 5.9, which at this pH the adsorbent surface has net electrical neutrality. At a pH below the pHzpc, the surface of the adsorbent is positive, and at a pH above the pHzpc, the surface of the adsorbent becomes more negatively charged by losing protons. Therefore, the adsorption of the MB reached its maximum value in the higher pH because of strong electrostatic attractions between the negatively charged surface of the onion membrane and the cationic MB.

Effect of adsorbent amount on adsorption

In order to find the influence of various onion membrane amounts on their dye uptake capacity, an adsorption of 250 mL MB solutions ($0.3\ g.L^{-1}$) was examined using five different membrane doses ranging from 0.015 to 0.12 g for eight hours in the atmospheric conditions. As shown in Figure 6, with an increase in the amount of membrane to 0.12 g, the adsorption amount and consequently the adsorption efficiency increases to 98.83%. This is most likely due to an increase in the numbers of adsorption sites at the adsorbent surface area, and as a result, increases the removal efficiency of MB. However, it is reasonable to observe a decrease in adsorption capacity to $0.617\ g.g^{-1}$ by increasing the adsorbent dose, which is a denominator of the fraction in Equation 3.

Effect of the initial concentration of dye solution on adsorption

Figure 7 shows the maximum capacity of an onion membrane in the adsorption of MB using adsorbent-adsorbate solutions with different initial dye concentrations (0.1-0.9 $g.L^{-1}$). It is clear that the MB adsorption capacity of an onion membrane increases with an increase in the initial concentration of the solution. This is most likely due to a greater availability of adsorbate ions in the vicinity of the onion membrane and a high driving force for mass transfer before the adsorption-desorption equilibrium was reached [25]. However, in this study, unlike the adsorption amount and capacity, the efficiency of the dye removal decreased,

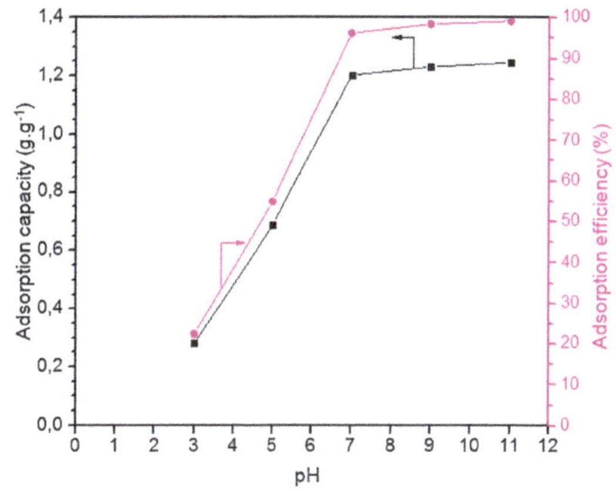

Figure 5 Effect of pH on the MB adsorption capacity ($g.g^{-1}$) and efficiency (%) of membrane was plotted. In these experiments, 0.06 g of membrane adsorbed dye molecules from a 0.3 $g.L^{-1}$ dye solution (250 ml) at 20°C for 8 hours.

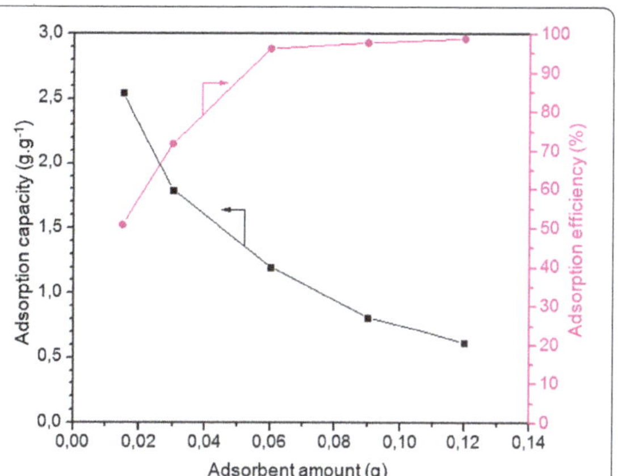

Figure 6 Effect of adsorbent amount on the MB adsorption capacity ($g.g^{-1}$) and efficiency (%) of membrane was plotted. In these experiments, the membrane adsorbed dye molecules from a 0.3 $g.L^{-1}$ dye solution (250 ml) with a pH of 7.1 at 20°C for 8 hours.

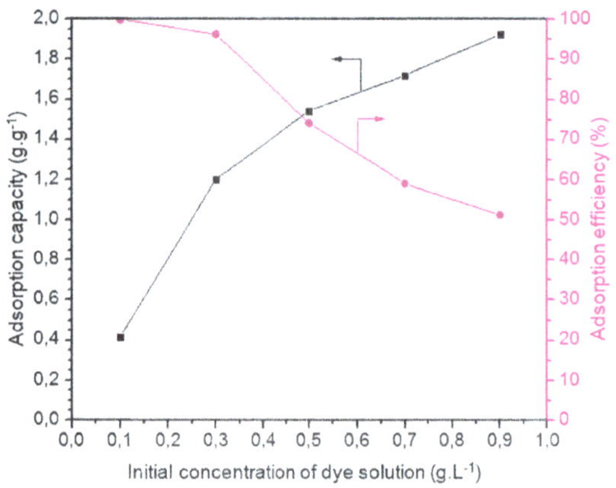

Figure 7 Effect of initial dyes concentration on the MB adsorption capacity (g.g^{-1}) and efficiency (%) of membrane was plotted. In these experiments, 0.06 g of the membrane adsorbed dye molecules from a dye solution (250 ml) with a pH of 7.1 at 20°C for 8 hours.

which may be attributed to the saturation of adsorption sites on the adsorbent surface [9]. The maximum MB adsorption capacity of an onion membrane is 1.9230 g.g^{-1} with the lowest efficiency at 51.28%, which is significantly higher than the other adsorbents [26-29] listed in Figure 8.

Isotherm of adsorption

The adsorption isotherm generally illustrates the interaction of an adsorbate with the adsorbent and also it can indicates the adsorption capacity of the adsorbent. Therefore, two isotherm models, Langmuir and Freundlich were investigated to find a more suitable model for the design process. The Langmuir model, the most popular, has been widely used to describe single-solute systems. The Langmuir model is based on the assumption that adsorbates produce monolayer coverage on the outer surface with uniform energies of adsorption, which is structurally homogeneous [30]. In the Freundlich model, the adsorption of an adsorbate occurs on a heterogeneous surface via multilayer adsorption with non-uniform distribution of heat of adsorption. The theoretical Langmuir and Freundlich isotherm models are represented by the following equations:

$$\frac{C_e}{q_e} = \frac{C_e}{q_m} + \frac{1}{q_m k_L} \tag{8}$$

$$\log q_e = \log k_F + \frac{1}{n}\log C_e \tag{9}$$

where q_e (g.g^{-1}) is the amount of dye adsorbed at equilibrium time, q_m (g.g^{-1}) is the maximum adsorption capacity, and C_e (g.L^{-1}) is the equilibrium dye concentration. k_L and k_F (L.g^{-1}) are the Langmuir and Freundlich adsorption equilibrium constant. 1/n is the empirical Freundlich constant. As it is clear from Figure 9, the calculated values of q_e belong to the Freundlich model is in agreement with the experimental value, which revealed that the Freundlich model is more suitable than the Langmuir model for describing the adsorption. This is confirmed by the correlation coefficient (R^2) of the Freundlich isotherm model (0.9922), which is greater than R^2 (0.9878) of the Langmuir model (Table 2). The empirical Freundlich constant (1/n) which can be obtained from the linear plot of $\log q_e$ versus $\log C_e$, is an indicator of the favorability and surface affinity for the solute. When the 1/n values are in the range 0.1-1,

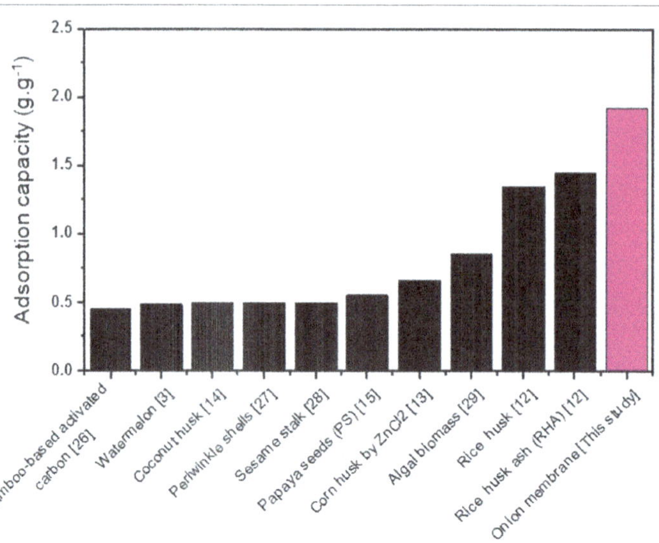

Figure 8 The maximum MB adsorption capacities of onion membrane were compared with several biomass adsorbents.

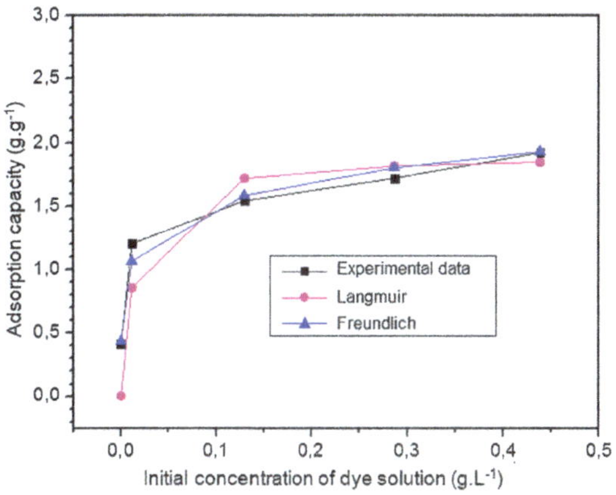

Figure 9 Adsorption isotherm of MB on onion membrane by Langmuir and Freundlich were plotted. In these experiments, 0.06 g of the membrane adsorbed dye molecules from a dye solution (250 ml) with a pH of 7.1 at 20°C for 8 hours.

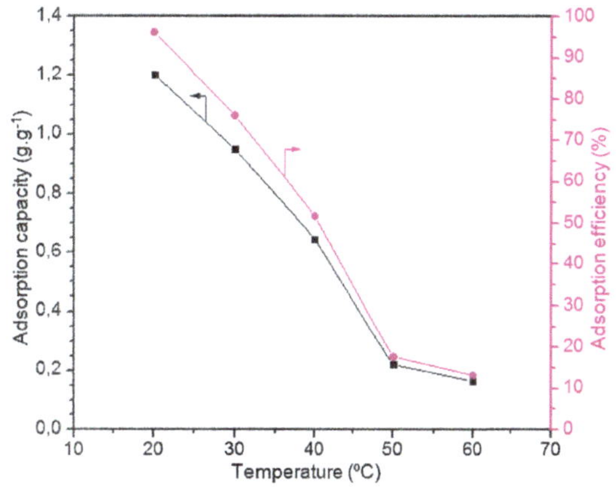

Figure 10 Effect of temperature on the MB adsorption capacity ($g.g^{-1}$) and efficiency (%) of membrane was plotted. In these experiments, 0.06 g of membrane adsorbed dye molecules from a 0.3 $g.L^{-1}$ dye solution (250 ml) with a pH of 7.1 for 8 hours.

the adsorption process is favorable. In addition, if the n is below one, then the adsorption is a chemical process; otherwise, the adsorption is a physical process. In this study, the value of 1/n is 0.24, lying between 0.1 and 1, indicating that adsorption of MB ions by an onion membrane is favorable with physisorption.

Effect of temperature on adsorption

The effect of temperature on the adsorption capacity of onion membrane (0.06 g) was studied using 250 mL of MB solution in different temperatures (20°C-60°C) for eight hours (480 min) in the atmospheric conditions. As shown in Figure 10, increasing the temperature leads to a decrease in the MB adsorption capacity of the membrane (0.164 $g.g^{-1}$, with 13.15% efficiency) after eight hours of contact time. This can be attributed to a weakening of the adsorptive forces between the active sites on the sorbent and the dye molecules due to the degradation of the onion membrane in the high temperature. The results suggest that a high temperature is not suitable for adsorbing MB when the onion membrane is adsorbent. Therefore, it is better to let the temperature of industrial outcome solutions decrease to 20°C to achieve maximum adsorption capacity.

Table 2 Comparison of isotherm models for adsorption of MB using onion membrane

Isotherm models and parameters	MB
Langmuir	
q_{max} ($g.g^{-1}$)	1.9054
q_e cal. ($g.g^{-1}$)	1.8471
K_L ($L.g^{-1}$)	72.387
R^2	0.9878
Fruendlich	
q_e cal. ($g.g^{-1}$)	1.9312
K_F ($L.g^{-1}$)	2.2074
n	6.1690
R^2	0.9922

Adsorption thermodynamics

The effect of temperature can be further investigated by calculating the thermodynamic parameters, including standard enthalpy change (ΔH°), the Gibbs free energy change (ΔG°), and standard entropy change (ΔS°). They have been determined using the following equations:

$$\Delta G^0 = -RT \ln K_d \tag{10}$$

The distribution ratio (K_d), can be calculated using the below equation:

$$K_d = \frac{q_e}{C_e} \tag{11}$$

Then, the relation between ΔG°, ΔH°, and ΔS° can be expressed by the following equations:

$$\Delta G^\circ = \Delta H^\circ - T\Delta S^\circ \tag{12}$$

Table 3 Thermodynamic parameters for adsorption of MB using onion membrane

Thermodynamic constant	Temperature (K)				
	293	303	313	323	333
ΔG° ($kJ.mol^{-1}$)	−10.79	−7.533	−4.273	−1.013	2.247
ΔH° ($kJ.mol^{-1}$)	−106.3				
ΔS° ($kJ.mol^{-1}.K^{-1}$)	−0.326				

Standard enthalpy (ΔH°) and entropy (ΔS°) were determined from the slope and intercept of the plot of $\ln K_d$ vs 1/T, which came from the Van's Hoff equation:

$$\ln K_d = \frac{\Delta S^{\circ}}{R} - \frac{\Delta H^{\circ}}{RT} \quad (13)$$

Table 3 presents the thermodynamic parameters of MB adsorption by the onion membrane in different contact temperatures. It is clear that the values of free energy (ΔG°) at all temperatures except 60°C were negative. This confirms that the adsorption of dye at these temperatures is spontaneous and thermodynamically favorable. The negative value of ΔH° confirms the exothermic nature of adsorption, which is supported by the decrease in the adsorption capacity of the onion membrane. Besides, the negative value of ΔS° resulted from the decreased randomness at the solid–liquid interface during the adsorption of MB ions onto the onion membrane.

Conclusion

The present study confirms the high potential of onion membranes with special physical and chemical characteristics for quick and efficient removal of MB from aqueous solutions. The amount of dye adsorbed varied with time, temperature, pH, adsorbent dosage, and initial dye concentration. The adsorption experiments indicated that onion membrane have a high MB adsorption capacity (1.9230 $g.g^{-1}$) when 0.06 g of adsorbent was immersed in 250 ml of dye solution (0.9 $g.L^{-1}$) with a pH of 7.1 at 20°C. The adsorption of MB by the onion membrane agreed with the pseudo-second-order model. Moreover, analysis of the equilibrium isotherms using the Langmuir and Freundlich isotherms showed that the Freundlich model fitted well with the experimental data. The thermodynamic studies suggested that the adsorption reaction was an exothermic and spontaneous process. Finally, the results suggest the synthesis of polymer-based membranes with similar physical and chemical properties of onion membrane as valuable and highly efficient adsorbents, which can be applied for dye removal in water treatment processes.

Competing interests

The authors declare that they have no competing interests.

Authors' contributions

SS-S as a first and corresponding author has contributed to performing the experiments, acquisition of data, analysis and interpretation of data, writing the manuscript. JH as a second author has contributed to performing the experiments, acquisition of data and preparing the tables and figures. All authors read and approved the final manuscript.

Acknowledgements

The authors thank Dr. Saeed Saber-Samandari of the Amirkabir University of Technology for his help with the SEM. The authors would like to acknowledge Mr. Ehsan Bahramzadeh (PhD student in Eastern Mediterranean University) for his help in preparing the manuscript.

References

1. Bayramoglu G, Adiguzel N, Ersoy G, Yilmaz M, Arica MY. Removal of textile dyes from aqueous solution using amine-modified plant biomass of a. caricum: equilibrium and kinetic studies. Water Air Soil Pollut. 2013;224:1.
2. Crini G. Recent developments in polysaccharide-based materials used as adsorbents in waste water treatment. Prog Polym Sci. 2005;30:38.
3. Lakshmipathy R, Sarada NC. Adsorptive removal of basic cationic dyes from aqueous solution by chemically protonated watermelon (Citrullus Lanatus) rind biomass. Desalin Water Treat. 2013;52:6175.
4. Santhi T, Manonmani S. Adsorption of methylene blue from aqueous solution onto a waste aquacultural shell powders (Prawn Waste). Sustain Environ Res. 2012;22:45.
5. Constantin M, Asmarandei I, Harabagiu V, Ghimici L, Ascenzi P, Fundueanu G. Removal of anionic dyes from aqueous solutions by an ion-exchanger based on pullulan microspheres. Carbohydr Polym. 2013;91:74.
6. Saber-Samandari S, Saber-Samandari S, Nezafati N, Yahya K. Efficient removal of lead (II) ions and methylene blue from aqueous solution using Chitosan/Fe-Hydroxyapatite nanocomposite beads. J Environ Manage. 2014;146:481.
7. Mishra G, Tripathy M. A critical review of the treatment for decolorization of textile effluent. Colourage. 1993;40:35.
8. Eren E. Investigation of a basic dye removal from aqueous solution onto chemically modified Unye Bentonite. J Hazard Mater. 2009;166:88.
9. Salleh MAM, Mahmoud DK, Karim WAWA, Idris A. Cationic and anionic dye adsorption by agricultural solid wastes: a comprehensive review. Desalination. 2011;280:1.
10. Saber-Samandari S, Gulcan HO, Saber-Samandari S, Gazi M. Efficient removal of anionic and cationic dyes from an aqueous solution using pullulan-graft-polyacrylamide porous hydrogel. Water Air Soil Pollut. 2014;225:2177.
11. Vadivelan V, Kumar KV. Equilibrium, kinetics, mechanism, and process design for the sorption of methylene blue onto rice husk. J Colloid Interface Sci. 2005;286:90.
12. Sharma P, Kaur R, Baskar C, Chung WJ. Removal of methylene blue from aqueous waste using rice husk and rice husk ash. Desalination. 2010;59:249.
13. Khodaie M, Ghasemi N, Moradi B, Rahimi M. Removal of Methylene Blue from Wastewater by Adsorption onto $ZnCl_2$ Activated Corn Husk Carbon Equilibrium Studies. J Chemistr. 2013;383985.
14. Khodaie M, Ghasemi N, Moradi B, Rahimi M. Removal of Methylene Blue from Wastewater by Adsorption onto $ZnCl_2$ Activated Corn Husk Carbon Equilibrium Studies. J Chemistr. 2013; Article ID 383985, 6 pages, http://dx.doi.org/10.1155/2013/383985.
15. Hameed BH. Evaluation of papaya seeds as a novel nonconventional low-cost adsorbent for removal of methylene blue. J Hazard Mater. 2009;162:939.
16. Saber-Samandari S, Gazi M, Yilmaz O. Synthesis and characterization of chitosan-graft-poly (N-Allyl Maleamic Acid) hydrogel membrane. Water Air Soil Pollut. 2013;224:1624.
17. Sharma K, Kaith BS, Kumar V, Kalia S, Kumar V, Swart HC. Water retention and dye adsorption behavior of Gg-Cl-Poly(Acrylic Acid-Aniline) based conductive hydrogels. Geoderma. 2014;232–234:45.
18. Sartape AS, Patil SA, Patil SK, Salunkhe ST, Kolekar SS. Mahogany fruit shell: a new low-cost adsorbent for removal of methylene blue dye from aqueous solutions. Desalin Water Treat. 2013;53:98.
19. Saka C, Sahin O, Celik MS. The removal of methylene blue from aqueous solutions by using microwave heating and pre-boiling treated onion skins as a new adsorbent. Energ Source Part A. 2012;34:1577.
20. Saka C, Sahin O. Removal of methylene blue from aqueous solutions by using cold plasma- and formaldehyde-treated onion skins. Color Technol. 2011;127:246.
21. Chowdhury A, Bhowal A, Datta S. Equilibrium, thermodynamic and kinetic studies for removal of copper (II) from aqueous solution by onion and garlic skin. Water. 2012;4:37.
22. Pathani D, Sharma S, Singh P. Removal of Methylene Blue by Adsorption onto Activated Carbon Developed from Ficus Carica Bast. Arab J Chem. 2013; Received 9 May 2012; accepted 17 April 2013. doi:10.1016/j.arabjc.2013.04.021.
23. Suleria HAR, Butt MS, Anjum FM, Saeed F, Khalid N. Onion: nature protection against physiological threats. Crit Rev Food Sci. 2015;55:50.

24. Al-Ghouti MA, Khraisheh MAM, Ahmad MNM, Allen S. Adsorption behaviour of methylene blue onto Jordanian diatomite: a kinetic study. J Hazard Mater. 2009;165:589.
25. Saber-Samandari S, Saber-Samandari S, Gazi M. Cellulose-Graft-Polyacrylamide/Hydroxyapatite composite hydrogel with possible application in removal of Cu(II) ions. React Funct Polym. 2013;73:1523.
26. Hameed BH, Din ATM, Ahmad AL. Adsorption of methylene blue onto bamboo-based activated carbon: kinetics and equilibrium studies. J Hazard Mater. 2007;141:819.
27. Bello OS, Adeogun IA, Ajaelu JC, Fehintola EO. Adsorption of methylene blue onto activated carbon derived from periwinkle shells: kinetics and equilibrium studies. Chem Ecol. 2008;24:285.
28. Maiti S, Purakayastha S, Ghosh B. Production of low-cost carbon adsorbents from agricultural wastes and their impact on dye adsorption. Chem Eng Comm. 2008;195:386.
29. Rubin E, Rodriguez P, Herrero R, Vicente MES. Adsorption of methylene blue on chemically modified algal biomass: equilibrium, dynamic and surface data. J Chem Eng Data. 2010;55:5707.
30. Mahmoodi NM, Arami M, Bahrami H, Khorramfar S. The effect of pH on the removal of anionic dyes from colored textile wastewater using a biosorbent. J Appl Polym Sci. 2011;120:2996.

Photocatalytic degradation of Metronidazole with illuminated TiO_2 nanoparticles

Mahdi Farzadkia[1], Edris Bazrafshan[2], Ali Esrafili[1], Jae-Kyu Yang[3] and Mehdi Shirzad-Siboni[1*]

Abstract

Metronidazole (MNZ) is a brand of nitroimidazole antibiotic, which is generally used in clinical applications and extensively used for the treatment of infectious diseases caused by anaerobic bacteria and protozoans. The aim of this investigation was to degrade MNZ with illuminated TiO_2 nanoparticles at different catalyst dosage, contact time, pH, initial MNZ concentration and lamp intensity. Maximum removal of MNZ was observed at near neutral pH. Removal efficiency was decreased by increasing dosage and initial MNZ concentration. The reaction rate constant (k_{obs}) was decreased from 0.0513 to 0.0072 min^{-1} and the value of electrical energy per order (E_{Eo}) was increased from 93.57 to 666.67 (kWh/m^3) with increasing initial MNZ concentration from 40 to 120 mg/L, respectively. The biodegradability estimated from the BOD5/COD ratio was increased from 0 to 0.098. The photocatalyst demonstrated proper photocatalytic activity even after five successive cycles. Finally, UV/TiO_2 is identified as a promising technique for the removal of antibiotic with high efficiency in a relatively short reaction time.

Keywords: Titanium dioxide, Metronidazole, Photocatalysis, Kinetics

Background

Recently, several different types of emerging contaminants in water systems are known as new environmental hazards those need to be treated with suitable methods [1]. As various pharmaceutical compounds have been used since the 1950s due to rapid population growth and development of medical science, several pharmaceutical compounds have been found in surface water, ground water and effluents from wastewater treatment plants. Metronidazole (2-methyl-5-nitroimidazole-1-ethanol) has been widely used to treat infections caused by anaerobic bacteria, bacteroides and protozoa [2-4]. Residual concentrations of metronidazole (MNZ) in surface waters and wastewater are $1 \sim 10$ ng/L [5,6]. As MNZ is non-biodegradable and highly soluble in water, it can be accumulated in the aquatic environment [7,8]. Elimination of MNZ from water system is an important issue considering its toxicity, potential mutagenicity and carcinogenity [7,8]. In order to remove MNZ, many techniques such as adsorption [9,10], reduction with nanoscale zero-valent iron particles [11], biological methods [12,13], ozonation technology [14], photolysis [15], Fenton and photo-Fenton processes [16], heterogeneous photocatalysis [15,17,18] and electro-Fenton process with a Ce/SnO_2–Sb coated titanium anode [1] have been applied.

Adsorption is widely used method for the treatment of wastewater containing toxic organic compounds. However, it just transfer contaminants from water to a solid phase without any degradation [9,10,19,20]. Biological method is also known as one of the suggested techniques. However this method generally requires long periods for treatment [12,21]. Oxidation is a promising process but sometimes it is regarded as a limited process due to the formation of intermediates with higher toxicity than the parent compound [5,8,22]. Therefore near complete mineralization of MNZ is the most relevant option. For this purpose, advanced oxidation process (AOP) is regarded as a promising option to treat wastewater containing MNZ due to a complete mineralization of parent material as well as lack of selectivity [7,23]. Generally AOPs involve generation of hydroxyl radicals through UV/photocatalyst, UV/H_2O_2 and UV/O_3 processes [24-26]. Among these methods, photocatalytic reaction using TiO_2/UV can treat non-biodegradable organic compounds to biodegradable species [23,24,27]. Considering characteristics of the AOP, it can be used as pre- or post-

* Correspondence: mshirzadsiboni@yahoo.com
[1]Department of Environmental Health Engineering, School of public Health, Iran University of Medical Sciences, Tehran, Iran
Full list of author information is available at the end of the article

treatment process in wastewater treatment because of its installation easiness in conventional wastewater treatment facilities [23,24,27].

Therefore, in the present work, P-25 TiO_2 was selected as a catalyst in the photocatalytic removal of MNZ. Effects of several operational parameters including pH, TiO_2 dosage and MNZ concentration on photocatalytic degradation of MNZ were investigated. Kinetic parameters for the photocatalytic degradation were obtained by application of the Langmuir–Hinshelwood (L–H) model. Finally, electrical energy per order (E_{Eo}) was obtained to evaluate cost-efficiency of the processes used in this research.

Material and methods

Chemicals

Analytical grade of MNZ ($C_6H_9N_3O_3$; 99% chemical reagent) was purchased from Merck (Darmesdat, Germany) and its physical and chemical characteristics are summarized in Table 1. Potassium dihydrogen phosphate (KH_2PO_4) and acetonitrile (99.7%, HPLC grade) were purchased from Merck. P-25 TiO_2 (80/20 mixture of anatase and rutile) was obtained from Degussa Corp. It has approximately spherical shape and has greater than 99.5% purity. The specific surface area of the TiO_2 particles was 50 ± 15 m^2/g according to Evonik-Industrial Co. The average size of the TiO_2 particles was 21 nm.

Table 1 Physical and chemical properties of MNZ

Characteristic	Metronidazole antibiotic (MNZ)
Molecular structure	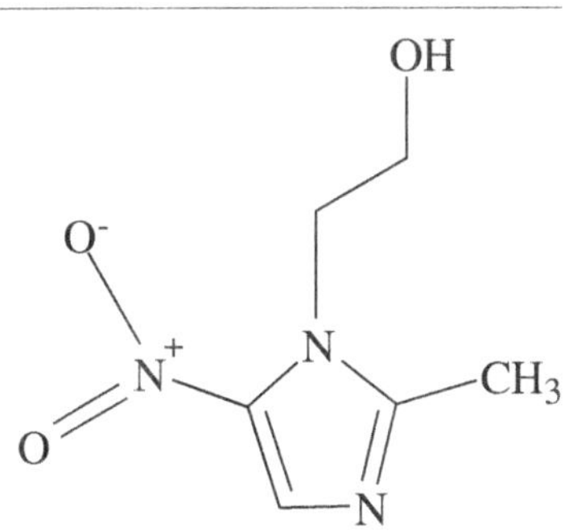
Molecular formula	$C_6H_9N_3O_3$
Molecular weight (g/mol)	171.2
Water solubility (g/L)	9.5
pK_a	2.55
Melting point (°C)	159-163
K_H (mol/dm^3.atm)	5.92×10^7
V_p (Pa)	4.07×10^{-7}

The antibiotic aqueous solution was prepared by dissolving 1 g of MNZ in 1 L distilled water. The antibiotic aqueous solution was prepared weekly and stored at 4°C. Initial COD and BOD_5/COD ratio of 1000 mg/L MNZ was 126 mg/L and approximately 0, respectively.

Figure 1a and b shows X-ray diffraction (XRD) and Fourier transform infrared spectroscopy (FT-IR) image of TiO_2, respectively. The main peaks at 2θ values of 25.367, 37.909, 38.667, 48.158, 54.051, 55.204, 62.817 and 68.976 were correspond to the (101), (004), (112), (200), (105), (211), (204) and (116) planes of P-25 TiO_2 (JCPDS card no. 36–1451). FT-IR analysis of TiO_2 was performed in the range of 400–4000 1/cm (Figure 1b). The absorption bands at 438 1/cm and 620 1/cm was attributed to the E_g and A_{2g} mode, respectively. The pH_{ZPC} of TiO_2 nanocatalyst was determined adopting the previously reported method.

Experimental set-up

The experimental reactor used for the photocatalytic degradation of MNZ is shown in Figure 2. The total volume of the reactor was 2 L with working volume of 1 L. The solution in the reactor was constantly stirred via a magnetic stirrer (170 rpm). A 125 W medium-pressure UVC lamp emitting maximum wavelength at 247.3 nm and a low-pressure UV lamp with irradiation intensity 8 W were applied as light sources. The light intensity of the UVC lamp was equal to 1020 μw/cm^2 measured by a Spectroline model DRC-100X digital radiometer combined with a DIX-365 radiation sensor (ShokofanTosee, Company, Iran).

Experimental procedure and analysis

In batch experiments, a selected dosage of TiO_2 (0.5-3 g/L) was added in 1000 mL of MNZ solution with a certain concentration (40–120 mg/L) at different solution pH ranging from 3 to 11. Initial pH of the solution was adjusted by adding NaOH and HCl (0.1 mol/L) and measured by pH meter (Metron, Switzerland). All runs were performed under ambient conditions for 3 h. During the experiments, the solution in the photoreactor was constantly stirred and kept at constant temperature (25 ± 1°C). The MNZ solutions loaded with TiO_2 were equilibrated in the dark for 30 min. After the equilibration period, the UV-lamp was switched on and 10 mL of the solution was taken at distinct time intervals. The aqueous samples were centrifuged (Sigma-301, Germany) at 4000 revolution per minute (rpm) for 10 min to eliminate TiO_2 and then measured concentration of residual MNZ. The concentration of residual MNZ was determined by high performance liquid chromatography (HPLC, Waters, USA) equipped with a UV detector at 348 nm. A Diamonsil (R) C18 column (5 μm, 250 mm long × 4.6 mm ID) was used. The data were recorded by a chemistation software.

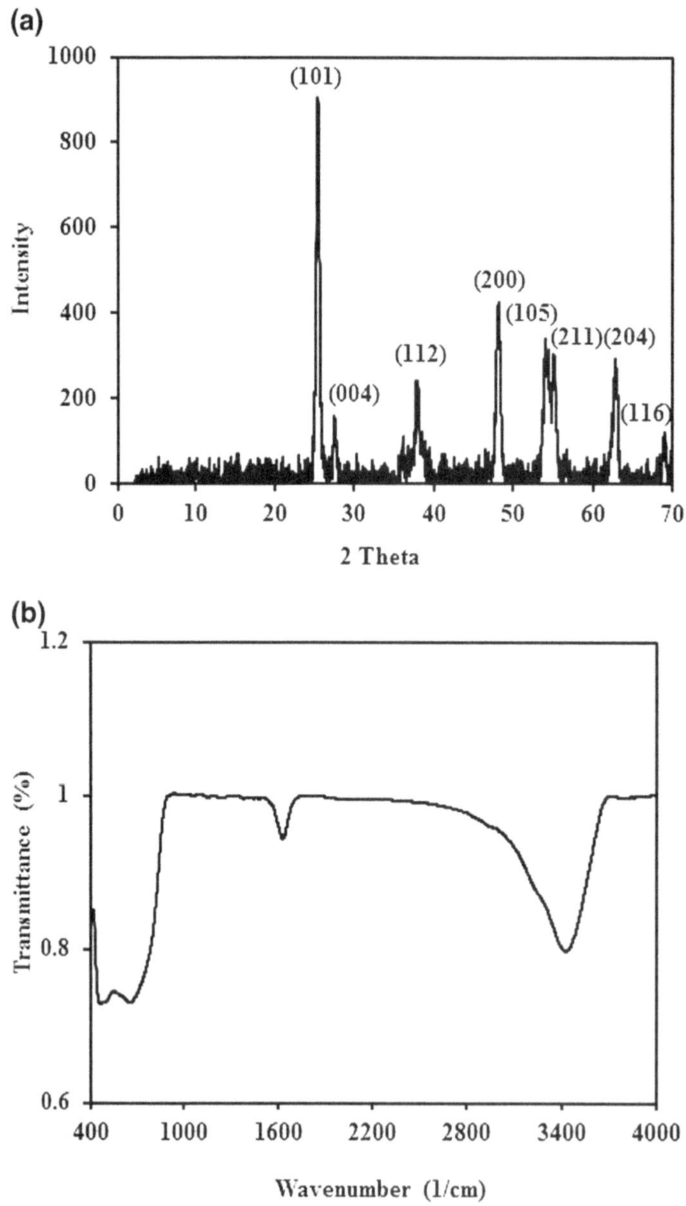

Figure 1 Characteristics of titanium dioxide: **(a)** XRD pattern **(b)** FT-IR pattern.

The mobile phase was composed of a mixture of acetonitrile and distilled water (30/70, v/v). The flow speed was set at 1.0 mL/min and 20 μL injections were used [4]. COD was determined by COD reactor model AR851 (HACH, USA) and biodegradability was measured by five-day biochemical oxygen demand (BOD5) according to the Standard Methods [28]. A typical HPLC chromatogram of MNZ is shown in Figure 3.

The removal efficiency (%) is calculated by Eq. (1).

$$\text{Removal efficiency } (\%) = \frac{C_0\text{-}C}{C_0} \times 100 \tag{1}$$

where C_0 and C are the concentrations of MNZ at initial and at time t (mg/L), respectively.

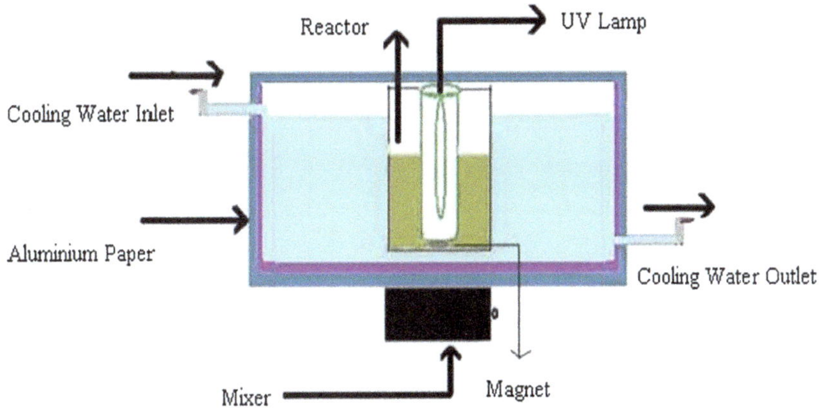

Figure 2 A schematic diagram of the experimental reactor.

All experiments were repeated three times and the average values with error percents were reported.

Results and discussion

Effect of TiO_2 dosage

Effect of TiO_2 dosage on the photocatalytic degradation of MNZ (80 mg/L) was investigated at pH 7. As shown in Figure 4, degradation efficiency of MNZ was increased from 64.28 to 97.61% by increasing irradiation time from 30 to 180 min at 0.5 g/L TiO_2. A greater degradation efficiency of MZN was observed over the entire reaction time at low TiO_2 dosage. This phenomena can be explained by the increased blockage of the incident UV light with increasing photocatalyst dosage [18,29]. Since the photocatalytic degradation of MNZ was not much increased over the 0.5 g/L of TiO_2, further experiments were performed with 0.5 g/L TiO_2. Similar results have been reported by other researchers [23,24,27].

Biodegradability of MNZ was evaluated in this work. To measure the biodegradability, BOD5 and COD values were measured before and after UV irradiation and the ratio of BOD5/COD was used as a biodegradability indicator. After 3 h reaction time, removal efficiency of COD was above 97.6% at all catalyst dosages and the ratio of BOD5/COD increased from 0 to 0.098 as the dosage increased from 0.5 to 3 g/L. This result indicates that MNZ can be changed to more biodegradable products.

Effect of pH

Effect of pH on the photocatalytic degradation of MNZ (80 mg/L) was investigated at constant TiO_2 dosage (0.5 g/L) by varying the initial pH of solution. Figure 5

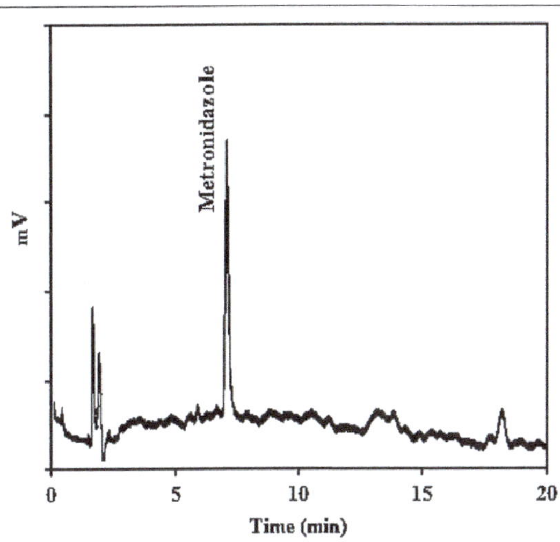

Figure 3 A typical HPLC chromatogram of Metronidazole.

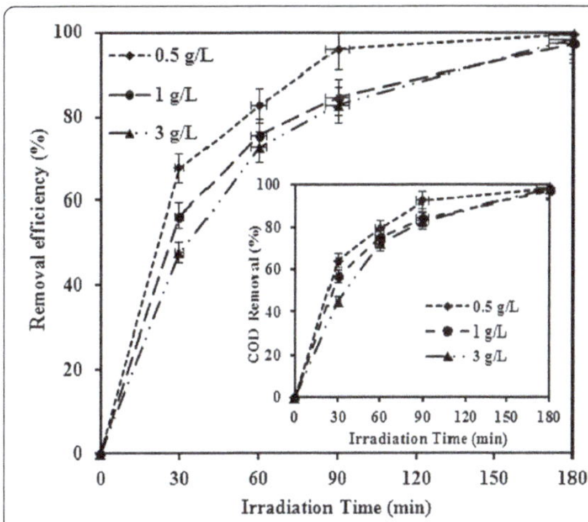

Figure 4 The effect of catalyst dosage on the photocatalytic degradation of MNZ and COD removal (pH = 7, MNZ =80 mg/L, BOD_5/COD ~ 0, COD = 126 mg/L).

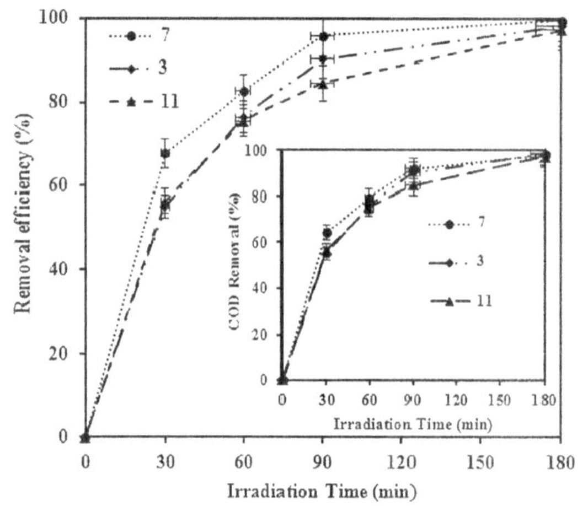

Figure 5 The effect of initial pH on the photocatalytic degradation of MNZ and COD removal (dosage = 0.5 g/L, MNZ =80 mg/L, $BOD_5/COD \sim 0$, COD = 126 mg/L).

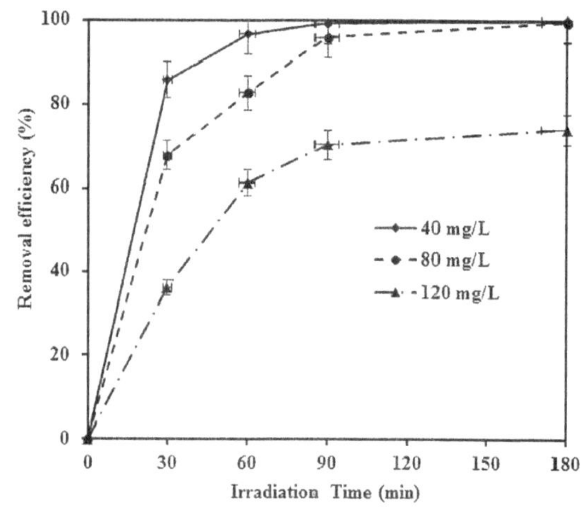

Figure 6 The effect of initial MNZ concentration on the photocatalytic degradation of MNZ (dosage = 0.5 g/L, pH = 7, $BOD_5/COD \sim 0$, COD = 126 mg/L).

shows that the greatest degradation efficiency was obtained at neutral pH over the entire reaction time. MNZ degradation after 180 min in pH 3, 7 and 11 was 98.2, 99.48 and 97.3%, respectively. Also, COD removal after 180 min in pH 3, 7 and 11 was 97.61, 98.02 and 96.82%, respectively. This trend can be explained by the variation of charges on MNZ as well as on the surface of TiO_2 at different solution pH. The pH_{zpc} of TiO_2 is determined as 6.52 and pK_a value of MNZ is 2.55. Therefore, at acidic pH, both TiO_2 and MNZ are positively charged, causing negative effect for the adsorption of MNZ on the surface of TiO_2. At neutral pH, no repulsive forces between the TiO_2 and MNZ might be developed. At basic pH, both TiO_2 and MNZ have negative charges, causing negative effect for the adsorption of MNZ on the surface of TiO_2. In this study, even though a distinct removal efficiency of MNZ was not observed at different solution pH, the most effective degradation of MNZ was observed at pH 7. Thus further experiments were performed at neutral pH [4,15,18].

Effect of initial MNZ concentration

Photocatalytic degradation of MNZ by TiO_2 was studied by varying the initial MNZ concentration at pH 7 and dosage equal to 0.5 g/L. Figure 6 shows that photocatalytic degradation efficiency decreased as the initial MNZ concentration increased. The presumed reason is that more surface of the TiO_2 surface may be occupied by MNZ as the initial MNZ concentration increased. In addition, more degradation intermediates can be accumulated on the TiO_2 surface, causing a negative effect in the utilization of hydroxyl radicals or positive holes in the valence band of the TiO_2 surface. Moreover, once the concentration of the MNZ increases, more absorption of UV light by MNZ molecules, known as inner filtration effect, can occur. This effect causes decrease of photons reaching to the TiO_2 surface [4]. Similar results have been reported by other researchers [15,18,23].

Kinetic study and electrical energy determination

In order to obtain kinetic information, experimental result in Figure 6 was fitted with a pseudo-first-order equation as expressed in Eq. (2).

$$\ln\left[(MNZ)_0/(MNZ)_t\right] = k_1 t \tag{2}$$

To calculate the rate constant from the plot $\ln[C_0/C]$ versus t, only initial data points were considered. Figure 7 shows the plot of $\ln[C_0/C]$ versus t for the degradation of MNZ. The first-order rate constants of photocatalytic process (k_{obs} (1/min)) at different initial concentrations of MNZ are summarized in Table 2. The relationship between the initial photocatalytic degradation rate (r) and the initial concentration of organic substrate for a heterogeneous photocatalytic process can be described by Langmuir–Hinshelwood (L-H) model (Eqs. 3 and 4) [30,31]:

$$r = \frac{k_c K_{MNZ}[MNZ]}{1 + K_{MNZ}[MNZ]_0} = k_{obs}[MNZ] \tag{3}$$

$$\frac{1}{k_{obs}} = \frac{1}{k_c\, K_{MNZ}} + \frac{[MNZ]_0}{k_c} \tag{4}$$

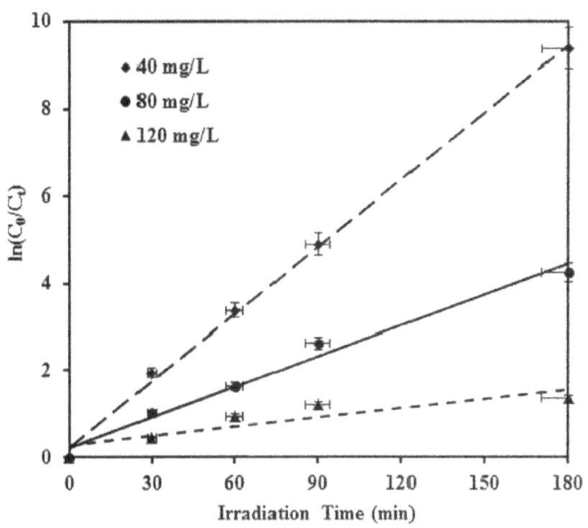

Figure 7 First-order kinetic model for the photocatalytic degradation of MNZ (dosage = 0.5 g/L, pH = 7, BOD_5/COD ~ 0, COD = 126 mg/L).

where $[MNZ]_0$ is the initial concentration of the antibiotic in mg/L, k_c (mg/L/min) is the kinetic rate constant of surface reaction and K_{MNZ} (L/mg) is the Langmuir adsorption constant. The values of K_{MNZ} and k_c were obtained as 0.0285 L/mg and 0.67 mg/L/min, respectively. This L–H kinetic model has been used by several authors to analyze heterogeneous photocatalytic reactions [30,31].

For the case of photocatalytic reaction, electrical energy is very important factor for the real application and evaluation for the electrical energy should be provided. Thus, in this work, electrical energy was evaluated by calculating electrical energy per order (E_{EO}). It is defined as the number of kWh of electrical energy required to reduce concentration of a pollutant by 1 order of magnitude (90%) in 1 m^3 of contaminated water. The E_{EO} (kWh/m^3) can be calculated from the following equation:

$$E_{EO} = \frac{p \times t \times 1000}{V \times 60 \times \log(C_I/C_f)} \tag{5}$$

Table 2 Pseudo-first order kinetic parameters and E_{Eo} values for the photocatalytic degradation of MNZ at different initial MNZ concentrations (catalyst dose = 0.5 g/L and pH =7)

E_{Eo} (kWh/m^3)	R^2	$1/k_{obs}$(min)	k_{obs} (1/min)	$[MNZ]_0$ (mg/L)
93.57	0.998	19.493	0.0513	40
206.01	0.9828	42.918	0.0233	80
666.67	0.7874	138.888	0.0072	120

Table 3 The E_{Eo} values for the removal of MNZ ($[MNZ]_0$ = 80 mg/L, catalyst dose = 0.5 g/L and pH =7)

Process	E_{Eo} (kWh/m^3)
UV 8 W-alone	290.11
UV125W-alone	245.17
UV 8 W/TiO_2	230.04
UV 125 W/TiO_2	197.95

$$E_{EO} = \frac{38.4 \times P}{V \times k_{obs}} \tag{6}$$

where P is the rated power (kW) of the AOP system, t is the irradiation time (min), k_{obs} is the pseudo-first order rate constant (1/min), V is the volume (L) of the wastewater in the reactor, C_i and C_f is the initial and final MNZ concentrations, respectively. The E_{EO} value for UV-alone and UV/TiO_2 processes are reported in Table 3. E_{EO} value for UV/TiO_2 process was lower than UV-alone process.

Comparison of different MNZ removal processes and reusability test

MNZ removal by TiO_2-alone, UV 8 W-alone, UV 125 W-alone, UV 8 W/TiO_2 and UV 125 W/TiO_2 processes are shown in Figure 8. Removal efficiency of MNZ through adsorption process (TiO_2-alone) was low. Overall removal efficiency of MNZ by TiO_2-alone, UV 8 W-alone, UV 125 W-alone and UV 8 W/TiO_2 process was 9.63%, 24.52, 42.32% and 53.53%, respectively. But 99.48% of

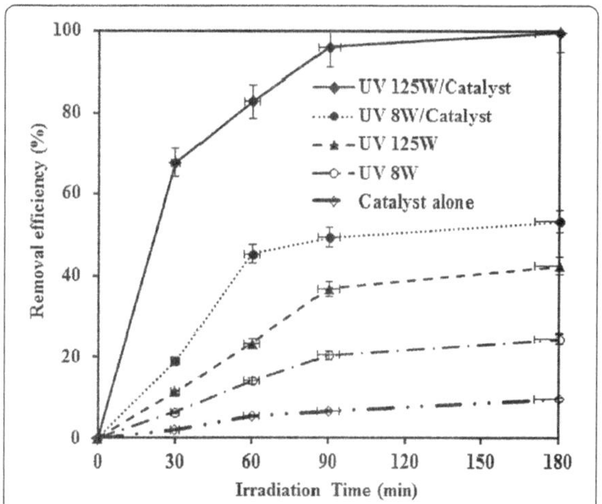

Figure 8 The contribution of each process involved in the photocatalytic degradation of MNZ (dosage = 0.5 g/L, pH = 7, MNZ = 80 mg/L, BOD_5/COD ~ 0, COD = 126 mg/L).

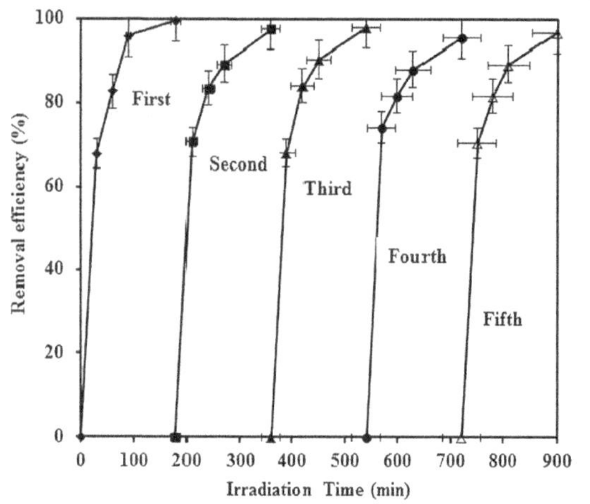

Figure 9 Reusability test of UV/TiO_2 for the photocatalytic degradation of MNZ over five consecutive runs (dosage = 0.5 g/L, pH = 7, MNZ =80 mg/L, BOD_5/COD ~ 0, COD = 126 mg/L).

MNZ was removed with UV 125 W/TiO_2. These experiments demonstrate that both UV light and TiO_2 are necessary for the effective degradation of MNZ.

Based on the above experiments and analysis, mechanism of the photocatalysis could be proposed as following:

An electron excites from the valence band to the conduction band of TiO_2, generating electron–hole pair, with UV light ($\lambda < 390$ nm) (Eq. 7) [24,27]:

$$\mathrm{TiO2} + h\upsilon \rightarrow \mathrm{TiO2}\left(e^-_{CB} + h^+_{VB}\right) \tag{7}$$

Then, the generated electron–hole pairs can participate in the reactions with electron acceptors like O_2 and donors like H_2O or OH^- to generate highly reactive radical species particularly hydroxyl radicals ($E^0 = +3.06$ V), which can oxidize organic contaminants and their degradation intermediates unselectively. Furthermore, positive holes can oxidize pollutants directly, too (Eqs. 8–11) [24,27]. Also Homem and Santos [32] reviewed degradation and removal methods of antibiotics from aqueous matrices and suggested removal mechanisms.

$$h^+_{VB} + \mathrm{MNZ} \rightarrow \text{intermediates or products} \tag{8}$$

$$h^+_{VB} + H_2O \rightarrow H^+ + \cdot\cdot OH \tag{9}$$

$$h^+_{VB} + OH^- \rightarrow \cdot\cdot\cdot OH \tag{10}$$

$$\cdot\cdot OH + \mathrm{MNZ} \rightarrow \text{intermediates or products} \tag{11}$$

The reusability of a photocatalyst is an important factor for real application. Hence, five consecutive photocatalytic experiments were performed by UV/TiO_2 process. As can be seen in Figure 9, quite similar photocatalytic activity was maintained over five consecutive runs. Photocatalytic degradation of MNZ with illuminated TiO_2 was compared with other reported data. Removal efficiency and reaction rate constant were compared and summarized in Table 4.

Conclusions

From the application of TiO_2 for the photocatalytic degradation of MNZ in aqueous solutions, a maximum removal of MNZ was observed at neutral pH. Removal efficiency was decreased by increasing TiO_2 dosage and initial MNZ concentration. Electrical energy per order was increased and reaction rate constant was decreased with increasing initial MNZ concentration. Photocatalytic activity was maintained even after five consecutive runs. Finally, UV/TiO_2 is identified as a promising technique for the removal of MNZ with high efficiency in a relatively short reaction time.

Table 4 Comparison of photocatalytic degradation of MNZ

Systems	pH	Catalyst dosage (g/L)	$[MNZ]_0$ (mg/L)	Lamp (W)	Time (min)	Removal efficiency (%)	k_{obs} (min^{-1})	Reference
Visible/ZnO	-	1.0	5	300	160	16.9	-	[3]
Visible/ZnO-RGO	-	1.0	5	300	160	49.3	-	[3]
Visible	-	-	5	300	160	5.5	-	[3]
UV/ZnO	10	1.5	80	125	180	96.55	-	[4]
UV	6	-	0.006	Lp Mp	5 5	6 12	0.005616 0.02304	[16]
UV/Niobate $K_6Nb_{10.8}O_{30}$	-	1.5	10	18	180	57	0.00449	[18]
UV/TiO_2	7	0.5	80	125	120	99.48	0.0233	Present study

Competing interests
The authors declare that they have no competing interests.

Authors' contribution
MF carried out the degradation studies of Metronidazole. EB contributed in writing of the manuscript and analyzing of data. AE involved in design of removal experiments, analyzing of data. J-KY discussed XRD and FT-IR data of titanium dioxide and participated in the sequence alignment of the manuscript. MS-S involved in design of removal experiments, analyzing of data, writing of the manuscript and reviewing of the manuscript. All authors read and approved the final manuscript.

Acknowledgment
The authors thank the Iran and Zahedan Universities of Medical Sciences, Iran for all of the support provided. Also, authors would like to thank Mr. Bonyani for the HPLC analysis in the laboratory of nutrition department.

Author details
[1]Department of Environmental Health Engineering, School of public Health, Iran University of Medical Sciences, Tehran, Iran. [2]Health Promotion Research Center, Zahedan University of Medical Sciences, Zahedan, Iran. [3]Divisions of General Education, Kwangwoon University, Seoul 139-701, South Korea.

References

1. Cheng W, Yang M, Xie Y, Liang B, Fang Z, Tsang EP. Enhancement of mineralization of metronidazole by the electro-Fenton process with a Ce/SnO_2–Sb coated titanium anode. Chem Eng J. 2013;220:214–20.
2. Chatzitakis A, Berberidou C, Paspaltsis I, Kyriakou G, Sklaviadis T, Poulios I. Photocatalytic degradation and drug activity reduction of chloramphenicol. Water Res. 2008;42:386–94.
3. Dong S, Li Y, Sun J, Yu C, Li Y, Sun J. Facile synthesis of novel ZnO/RGO hybrid nanocomposites with enhanced catalytic performance for visible-light-driven photodegradation of metronidazole. MCP. 2014;145:357–65.
4. Farzadkia M, Esrafili A, Baghapour MA, Shahamat YD, Okhovat N. Degradation of metronidazole in aqueous solution by nano-ZnO/UV photocatalytic process. Desalin Water Treat. 2013;52:4947–52.
5. Dantas RF, Rossiter O, Teixeira AKR, Simões AS, da Silva VL. Direct UV photolysis of propranolol and metronidazole in aqueous solution. Chem Eng J. 2010;158:143–7.
6. Vulliet E, Cren-Olivé C. Screening of pharmaceuticals and hormones at the regional scale, in surface and groundwaters intended to human consumption. Environ Pollut. 2011;159:2929–34.
7. Zhenhu X, Zaixu C, Jianming L. Comparison of metronidazole degradation by different advanced oxidation processes in low concentration aqueous solutions. Chin J Environ Eng. 2009;3:465–9.
8. Johnson MB, Mehrvar M. Aqueous metronidazole degradation by UV/H_2O_2 process in single-and multi-lamp tubular photoreactors: kinetics and reactor design. Ind Eng Chem Res. 2008;47:6525–37.
9. Méndez-Díaz J, Prados-Joya G, Rivera-Utrilla J, Leyva-Ramos R, Sánchez-Polo M, Ferro-García MA, et al. Kinetic study of the adsorption of nitroimidazole antibiotics on activated carbons in aqueous phase. JCIS. 2010;345:481–90.
10. Rivera-Utrilla J, Prados-Joya G, Sánchez-Polo M, Ferro-García M, Bautista-Toledo I. Removal of nitroimidazole antibiotics from aqueous solution by adsorption/bioadsorption on activated carbon. J Hazard Mater. 2009;170:298–305.
11. Fang Z, Chen J, Qiu X, Qiu X, Cheng W, Zhu L. Effective removal of antibiotic metronidazole from water by nanoscale zero-valent iron particles. Desalination. 2011;268:60–7.
12. Ingerslev F, Halling-Sørensen B. Biodegradability of metronidazole, olaquindox, and tylosin and formation of tylosin degradation products in aerobic soil–manure slurries. Ecotoxicol Environ Saf. 2001;48:311–20.
13. Ingerslev F, Toräng L, Loke M-L, Halling-Sørensen B, Nyholm N. Primary biodegradation of veterinary antibiotics in aerobic and anaerobic surface water simulation systems. Chemosphere. 2001;44:865–72.
14. Sánchez-Polo M, Rivera-Utrilla J, Prados-Joya G, Ferro-García M, Bautista-Toledo I. Removal of pharmaceutical compounds, nitroimidazoles, from waters by using the ozone/carbon system. Water Res. 2008;42:4163–71.
15. Prados-Joya G, Sánchez-Polo M, Rivera-Utrilla J, Ferro-Garcia M. Photodegradation of the antibiotics nitroimidazoles in aqueous solution by ultraviolet radiation. Water Res. 2011;45:393–403.
16. Shemer H, Kunukcu YK, Linden KG. Degradation of the pharmaceutical metronidazole via UV, Fenton and photo-Fenton processes. Chemosphere. 2006;63:269–76.
17. Gao J, Liu B, Wang J, Jin X, Jiang R, Liu L, et al. Spectroscopic investigation on assisted sonocatalytic damage of bovine serum albumin (BSA) by metronidazole (MTZ) under ultrasonic irradiation combined with nano-sized ZnO. Spectrochim Acta A Mol Biomol Spectrosc. 2010;77:895–901.
18. Wang H, Zhang G, Gao Y. Photocatalytic degradation of metronidazole in aqueous solution by niobate $K_6Nb_{10.8}O_{30}$. Wuhan Univ J Nat Sci. 2010;15:345–9.
19. Ahmed MJ, Theydan SK. Microporous activated carbon from Siris seed pods by microwave-induced KOH activation for metronidazole adsorption. J Anal Appl Pyrolysis. 2013;99:101–9.
20. Çalışkan E, Göktürk S. Adsorption characteristics of sulfamethoxazole and metronidazole on activated carbon. SS&T. 2010;45:244–55.
21. Saidi I, Soutrel I, Floner D, Fourcade F, Bellakhal N, Amrane A, et al. Indirect electroreduction as pretreatment to enhance biodegradability of metronidazole. J Hazard Mater. 2014;278:172–9.
22. Jimmy C. In situ synthesis of Zn_2GeO_4 hollow spheres and their enhanced photocatalytic activity for the degradation of antibiotic metronidazole. DTr. 2013;42:5092–9.
23. Palominos RA, Mondaca MA, Giraldo A, Peñuela G, Pérez-Moya M, Mansilla HD. Photocatalytic oxidation of the antibiotic tetracycline on TiO_2 and ZnO suspensions. Catal Today. 2009;144:100–5.
24. Elmolla ES, Chaudhuri M. Photocatalytic degradation of amoxicillin, ampicillin and cloxacillin antibiotics in aqueous solution using UV/TiO_2 and UV/H_2O_2/TiO_2 photocatalysis. Desalination. 2010;252:46–52.
25. Giraldo AL, Penuela GA, Torres-Palma RA, Pino NJ, Palominos RA, Mansilla HD. Degradation of the antibiotic oxolinic acid by photocatalysis with TiO_2 in suspension. Water Res. 2010;44:5158–67.
26. Farrokhi M, Yang J-K, Lee S-M, Shirzad-Siboni M. Effect of organic matter on cyanide removal by illuminated titanium dioxide or zinc oxide nanoparticles. J Environ Health Sci Eng. 2013;11:23.
27. Dimitrakopoulou D, Rethemiotaki I, Frontistis Z, Xekoukoulotakis NP, Venieri D, Mantzavinos D. Degradation, mineralization and antibiotic inactivation of amoxicillin by UV-A/TiO_2 photocatalysis. J Environ Manage. 2012;98:168–74.
28. Federation WE, Association APH. Standard methods for the examination of water and wastewater. Washington, DC, USA: American Public Health Association (APHA); 2005.
29. Wang J, Wang Z, Jin X, Guo Y, Gao J, Li K, et al. Catalytic damage of bovine serum albumin by metronidazole under ultrasonic irradiation in the presence of nano-sized TiO_2 powder. Rus J Physic Chem A. 2012;86:867–74.
30. Daneshvar N, Salari D, Khataee AR. Photocatalytic degradation of azo dye acid red 14 in water: investigation of the effect of operational parameters. J Photochem Photobiol A Chem. 2003;157:111–6.
31. Daneshvar N, Salari D, Khataee AR. Photocatalytic degradation of azo dye acid red 14 in water on ZnO as an alternative catalyst to TiO_2. J Photochem Photobiol A Chem. 2004;162:317–22.
32. Homem V, Santos L. Degradation and removal methods of antibiotics from aqueous matrices - A review. J Environ Manage. 2011;92:2304–47.

Application of Reverse Transcriptase –PCR (RT-PCR) for rapid detection of viable *Escherichia coli* in drinking water samples

Neda Molaee[1], Hamid Abtahi[2], Mohammad Javad Ghannadzadeh[3], Masoude Karimi[4] and Ehsanollah Ghaznavi-Rad[2,5*]

Abstract

Background: Polymerase chain reaction (PCR) is preferred to other methods for detecting *Escherichia coli (E. coli)* in water in terms of speed, accuracy and efficiency. False positive result is considered as the major disadvantages of PCR. For this reason, reverse transcriptase-polymerase chain reaction (RT-PCR) can be used to solve this problem. The aim of present study was to determine the efficiency of RT-PCR for rapid detection of viable *Escherichia coli* in drinking water samples and enhance its sensitivity through application of different filter membranes.

Materials and methods: Specific primers were designed for *16S rRNA* and elongation Factor II genes. Different concentrations of bacteria were passed through FHLP and HAWP filters. Then, RT-PCR was performed using 16srRNA and *EF –Tu* primers. Contamination of 10 wells was determined by RT-PCR in Arak city. To evaluate RT-PCR efficiency, the results were compared with most probable number (MPN) method.

Results: RT-PCR is able to detect bacteria in different concentrations. Application of EF II primers reduced false positive results compared to *16S rRNA* primers. The FHLP hydrophobic filters have higher ability to absorb bacteria compared with HAWB hydrophilic filters. So the use of hydrophobic filters will increase the sensitivity of RT-PCR.

Conclusion: RT-PCR shows a higher sensitivity compared to conventional water contamination detection method. Unlike PCR, RT-PCR does not lead to false positive results. The use of *EF-Tu* primers can reduce the incidence of false positive results. Furthermore, hydrophobic filters have a higher ability to absorb bacteria compared to hydrophilic filters.

Keyword: Coliforms, Reverse transcriptase, Drinking water

Background

The presence of pathogens in drinking water is a major health problem. Therefore, detection and removal of pathogens are considered as main health issues for drinking water. In diagnostic workup, presence of *E.coli* is considered as an indicator of water pollution by wastewater. The conventional methods for detecting pathogens in water such as (most probable number) MPN and water culture are usually costly and time consuming and presumably lack of sufficient accuracy. This is why new methods are expected to detect pathogens in drinking water [1].

* Correspondence: e.ghaznavirad@arakmu.ac.ir
[2]Molecular and Medicine Research Center, Arak University of Medical Sciences, Arak, Iran
[5]Department of Medical Microbiology and Immunology, Faculty of Medicine, Arak University of Medical Sciences, Arak, Iran
Full list of author information is available at the end of the article

Polymerase chain reaction (PCR) could be a good alternative to conventional assays. PCR is a sensitive, accurate and rapid method that its effectiveness has been demonstrated in numerous studies [2]. PCR is able to detect even one bacterium per 100 ml of water [3]. Polymerase chain reaction is a sensitive and accurate method that not only detects pollution, but determines the type of bacteria [4]. However, due to relatively high stability of DNA in the culture medium, presence of dead cells will produce positive result. Some studies showed that the PCR result for bacteria killed by boiling or UV radiation becomes positive. Studies on *E. coli* and *Listeria monocyte genes* showed that the PCR result for autoclaved bacteria is still positive [5].

Due to incidence of false positive results in DNA-based detection procedures, other methods such as initial

Table 1 The sequence and position of the oligonucleotide primers used in the study

Gene	Forward	Reverse	Size (bp)	Access number
16S rRNA	5'CGA GTG GCG GAC GGG TGA GT3' (FROM 81)	5' TCG ACA TCG TTT ACG GCG TGG A3' (FROM 786)	723	EF620925
EF-Tu	5'CGCTGGAAGGCGACGCAGAG 3' (FROM 1253)	5'CGGAAGTAGAACTGCGGACGGTAG3' (FROM 1698)	470	X57091

enrichment before PCR testing are recommended. Although this method increases the detection efficiency of the test for live and dead samples, the duration of the assay will be increased. In addition, in the case where the number of dead bacteria is high, it may lead to false positive results [6].

Due to the low stability of RNA outside the cell, the use of reverse transcriptase polymerase chain reaction (RT-PCR) for detecting RNA is considered as a suitable marker for tracking the living cells. At the same time, the stability of different RNAs varies outside the cell. Davis *et al.*, found that of the four species of nucleic acid, mRNA is the most promising candidate as an indicator of viability in bacteria [7]. Klein and Juneja showed a good correlation between the presence of mRNA and the viability of *L. monocytogenes* when comparing growing cells with those killed by autoclaving [8]. Therefore, this study designed to examine the efficiency of RT-PCR by preparing various concentrations of *E. coli* in water. In addition, the impact of bacterial filters (hydrophilic and hydrophobic) on concentrated water samples and RT-PCR results are studied.

Materials and methods

PCR primers targeting *16S rRNA* and *EF-Tu* regions of the *E. coli* genome were designed using Primer Select (DNAstar, Inc., Madison, WI) software package. Two sets of primer pairs were designed and tested. The nucleotide sequences of the primers have been shown in Table 1.

Water dilutions

To prepare water dilutions, sequential dilutions of *E. coli* bacteria were prepared in 100 ml of sterile water. The McFarland Solution No.1 was used to prepare different bacterial concentrations. For this purpose, the bacterial suspension is adjusted to match the one McFarland turbidity standard.

Then, the suspension was used to prepare sequential dilutions of 8/100 to 1/1600 as listed in Table 2 (two samples for each dilution). To verify the number of bacteria in various concentrations, the bacterial sediment was obtained by centrifuging the whole water at 5000 rpm for 5 min and cultured by pour plate method in nutrient agar medium. Two concentrations were prepared in two series.

After preparing water samples with various bacterial concentrations, a series of dilutions were passed through FHLP filter (Millipore, pore diameter of 0.5 microns) and the second series were passed through HAWP filter (Millipore, pore diameter of 0.45 microns). Then, the filters were placed inside sterile micro tubes and 50 ml water containing 0.1% diethylpyrocarbonate (DEPC water) was added. The micro tubes were vortexed vigorously to release bacteria from the filter surface to the fluid.

RT-PCR

The bacterial RNA was extracted and purified using the RNX-plus kit (Sinagene, Iran). Deoxyribonuclease I enzyme was used to remove DNA contamination of the purified RNA. To remove the enzyme, 1 µl ethylene diamine tetraacetic acid (EDTA, 25 Mm) was added for 10 min at 65°C. RT-PCR was performed for *16 s rRNA* and *EF-Tu* under the circumstances described elsewhere [9]. The method is described briefly in Figure 1.

The first phase of PCR is composed of 35 cycles, each consists of three steps including 1-denaturation (at 94°C for 1 min), 2 binding the primers to the DNA template (at 59°C, 1 min for EF-Tu and 1 min for 16SrRNA) and 3- target gene amplification (at 72° for 1 min). After the end of the cycles, the final extension was performed for one cycle at 72 ° C for 5 min.

To evaluate the PCR products, the products were electrophoresed on 1% agarose gel in Tris base- boric acid-EDTA (TBE, pH = 8) buffer solution. To analyze the electrophoresis results, the samples were stained with ethidium bromide solution and visualized by an UV transilluminator apparatus.

To confirm the difference between PCR and RT-PCR in diagnosis of live and death bacteria, control for living and dead bacteria through RT-PCR method and a control of PCR for dead bacteria have been performed in this experiment (Figures 2).

Table 2 Coliforms serial dilutions prepared in laboratory

Dilutions	1600/1	1/800	1/400	1/200	1/100	2/100	4/100	8/100
Number of bacteria	1	1	1	1	1	2	4	8
The volume of water(ml)	1600	800	400	200	100	100	100	100

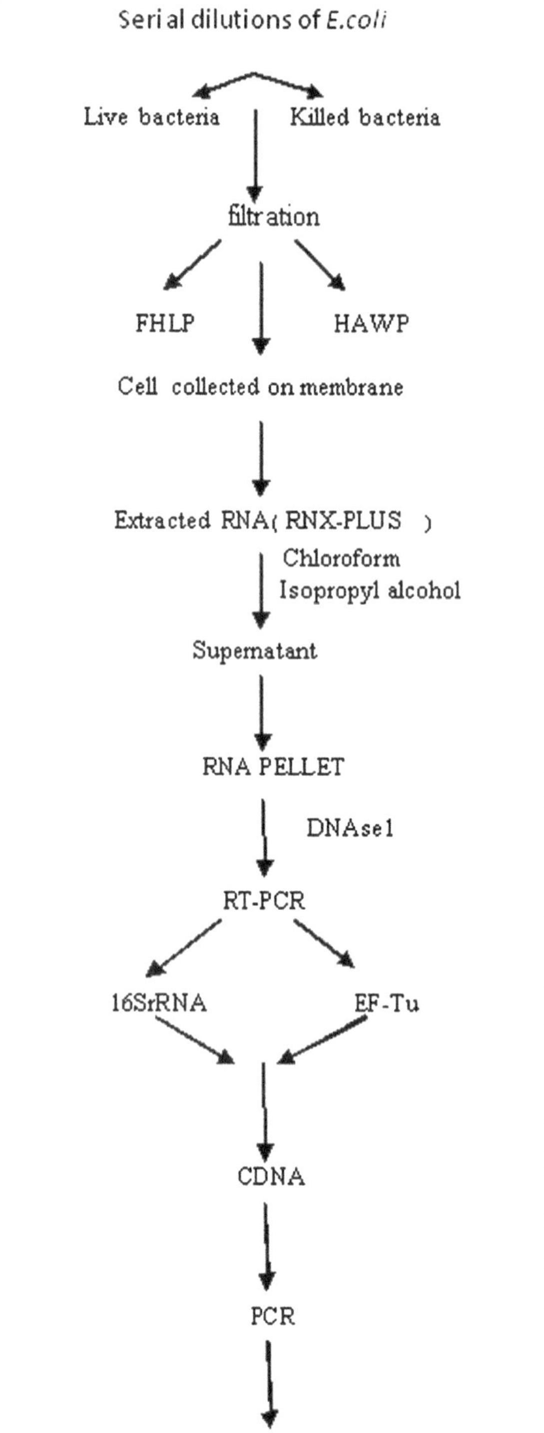

Figure 1 Flow chart illustrates the RT-PCR procedure for detecting *16S rRNA* and *EF-Tu* mRNA of *E.coli*.

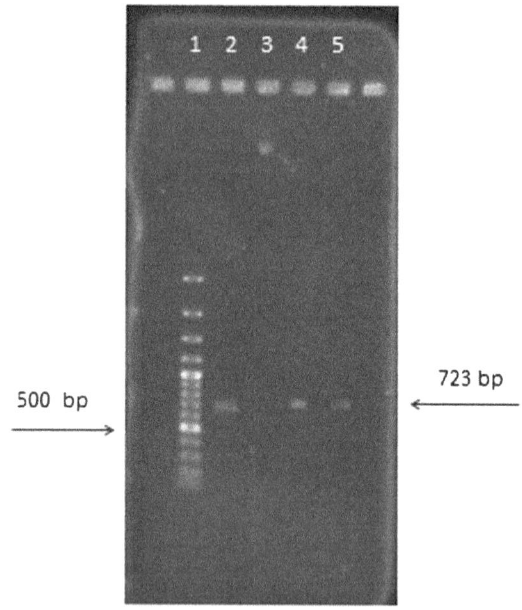

Figure 2 16SrRNA gene RT-PCR and PCR results : Lane 1: Marker 100 bp, Lane2, a live bacteria RT-PCR, Lane3, death bacteria RT-PCR, Lane 4, a live bacteria PCR, Lane 5, death bacteria PCR.

The stability of *EF-Tu* and *16S rRNA*: mRNA detection in live bacteria

To investigate the stability of RNA in the medium, the bacterial dilutions were killed by chlorine. Then, RNA was extracted and purified at different times (0, 0.5, 1, 2, 3, 4, 6, 10 and 16 h after bacterial death).

To prepare the chlorine solution, 0.1 g of the powdered calcium hypochlorite granules 70% was dissolved in 100 ml water. Then, 30 ml chlorine solution was added to the bacterial dilutions so that the concentration of the residual chlorine was 0.2 to 0.4 mg/l after 30 minutes. After chlorination, the water dilutions were cultured in nutrient agar medium by pour plate method to ensure the death of all bacteria.

After chlorination, series of bacterial dilutions passed through both filters. RT-PCR was performed for genes, *EF-Tu* and *16srRNA* as described before.

Examination of well water samples by RT-PCR and MPN

To achieve this purpose of the study 10 wells were selected and 250 ml water was collected in sterile containers from each well in Arak city according to standard procedure.

The MPN method was used to examine the consistency of RT-PCR results. The presence of coliform in the samples was evaluated using both methods. In the RT-PCR method, 100 ml water was filtered using HAWP and FHLP filters and then checked for *Escherichia coli*. The MPN test was performed by three-tube method and the

Table 3 The number of colony obtained on in agar nutrient medium by pour plate method

Dilution	1/1600	1/800	1/400	1/200	1/100	2/100	4/100	8/100
Colony number	1	1	1	1	1	2	4	8

number of *E. coli* bacteria was determined based on gas production.

Results

Water dilutions

The number of bacteria was confirmed by culturing the water dilutions in agar nutrient medium by pour plate method. The result has been shown in Table 3.

Water dilutions filtration and RT-PCR

The result of RT-PCR on water dilutions showed that the RT-PCR results become positive only after filtration with hydrophobic filters (FHLP). When FHLP filters were used, the presence of even one bacterium in 1600 ml water can be detected by RT-PCR. The RT-PCR results for the genes *16S rRNA* (Figures 3 and 4) and *EF-Tu* (Figures 5 and 6) demonstrate the role of FHLP and HAWP filters in the detection of low numbers of bacteria in water samples. The RT-PCR results for all dilutions passed through FHLP showed a band as observed by UV transilluminator.

The stability of *16SrRNA* and *EF-Tu* after chlorination

No bacteria were found in cultures after chlorination of water dilution samples. Therefore, it was confirmed that bacteria were killed.

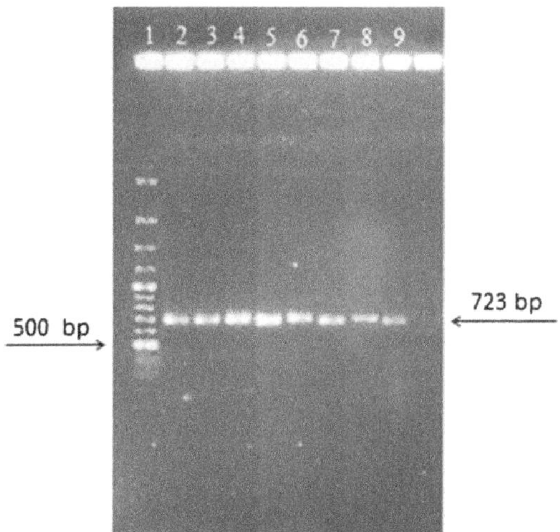

Figure 3 Dilution of bacterial *16SrRNA* gene RT-PCR results filtered with FHLP, Lane1, Marker 100 bp, Lane2, 1/1600Dilution, Lane3, 1/800Dilution, Lane 4, 1/400Dilution, Lane 5, 1/200Dilution, Lane 6, 1/100Dilution, Lane 7, 2/100Dilution, Lane 8, 4/100Dilution, Lane 9, 8/100Dilution.

Table 4 shows the stability of *16SrRNA* and *EF-Tu* RNAs after the death of bacteria by chlorine. As shown, *EF-Tu* and 16S rRNA remained stable up to 4 h and over 16 h, respectively.

Comparison of molecular and MPN methods

Table 5 shows the results of MPN and RT-PCR tests for 10 drinking water wells. Comparison of RT-PCR results demonstrates the higher efficiency of RT-PCR method for bacteria detection compared to MPN method. The results of this comparison are given in Table 5.

Discussion

Due to the importance of water borne diseases, in particular those transmitted by drinking water, the evaluation of water quality in terms of pathogenic microorganisms has a major influence on public health program. The presence of coliforms (especially *E. coli*) in water should be considered as a pollution indicator. Various methods have been designed to detect pathogens in water samples. To approve the water quality in terms of pathogens, the water samples should be exactly checked for the presence of coliforms, especially *Escherichia coli*. Therefore, the presence of coliforms after treatment indicate the water pollution, needs further action. In the case of water contamination with coliforms, the water samples may be contaminated with other pathogens, parasites, viruses, and etc. [10].

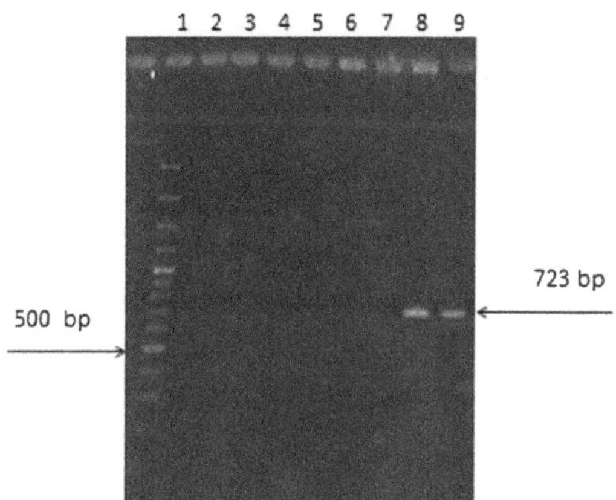

Figure 4 Dilution of bacterial *16SrRNA* gene RT-PCR results filtered with HAWP, Lane 1, Marker 100 bp, Lane2,1/1600Dilution, Lane3, 1/800Dilution, Lane 4, 1/400Dilution, Lane 5, 1/200Dilution, Lane 6, 1/100Dilution, Lane 7, 2/100 Dilution, Lane 8, 4/100Dilution, Lane 9, 8/100Dilution.

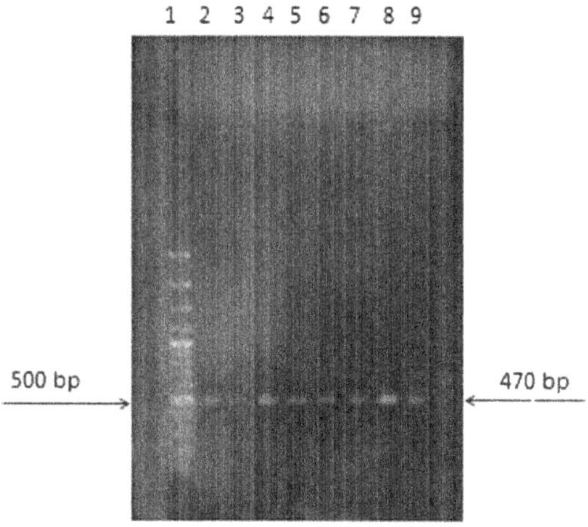

Figure 5 Dilution of bacterial *EF-Tu* gene RT-PCR results filtered with FHLP, Lane 1, Marker 100 bp, Lane2, 1/1600 dilution, Lane3, 1/800 dilution, Lane 4, 1/400 dilution, Lane 5, 1/200 dilution, Lane 6, 1/100 dilution, Lane 7, 2/100 Dilution, Lane 8, 4/100 dilution, Lane 9, 8/100 dilution.

There are several problems with viable culture methods (MPN) used for routine monitoring of the bacteriological safety of water supplies, including maintaining the viability of bacteria between the time of collection and enumeration, lack of growth of viable but nonculturable bacteria. Therefore, the use of an ideal method with advantages such as high speed, sensitivity and accuracy, ease of doing and low cost to evaluate a high volume of water samples can be effective in preventing the spread of infectious diseases through water. In addition, detection, separation of most pathogens in contaminated water is difficult, time consuming and often associated with high costs [11]. Although the use of molecular techniques for detecting pathogens is preferred in terms of speed and accuracy, techniques like PCR have some drawbacks. The major disadvantages is that this method is not able to discriminate dead and living bacteria, hence presence of dead bacteria leading to false positive result [6].

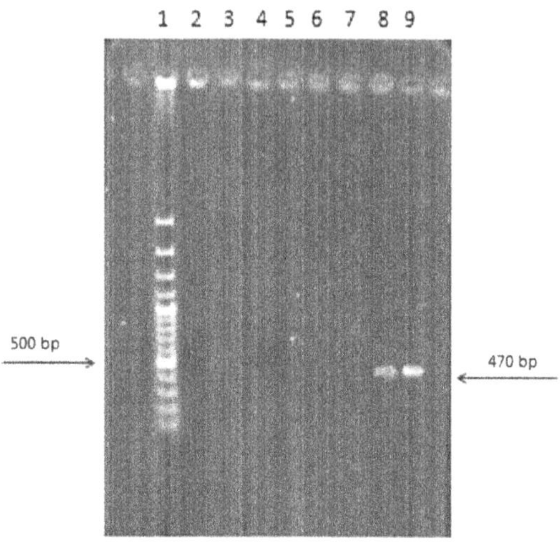

Figure 6 Dilution of bacterial *EF-Tu* gene RT-PCR results filtered with HAWP, Lane 1,100 bp ladder, Lane2, 1/1600Dilution, Lane3, 1/800Dilution, Lane 4, 1/400Dilution, Lane 5, 1/200Dilution,Lane 6, 1/100Dilution,Lane 7, 2/100Dilution, Lane 8, 4/100Dilution, Lane 9, 8/100Dilution.

Table 4 Stability of the mRNA (*EF-Tu* and *16S rRNA*) in different times was shown

Target	0 min	30 min	1 h	2 h	3 h	4 h	6 h	10 h	16 h
16SrRNA	Y	Y	Y	Y	Y	Y	Y	Y	Y
EF-Tu	Y	Y	Y	Y	Y	Y	N	N	N

Y, Positive RT-PCR. N, négative RT-PCR.NP not performed.

Methods that only detect live bacteria must be used to fix this problem. Techniques like RT-PCR can be used to detect live bacteria. In general, RNA-based techniques can prove the presence of living cells only when the target molecule has little stability after cell death. In fact, mRNA molecules are constantly reproduced and increased inside live cells. However, RNA unlike the DNA has a very short half-life, so that RNA content decreases rapidly after the cell death. Therefore, the presence of RNA molecules is a good marker to prove the existence of living cells. Vaitilingom *et al.*, used RT-PCR method and found RNA molecules only in living cells [3]. However, some types of RNA molecules are more stable. For instance, the results of study conducted by Sheridan *et al.*, showed that *16S rRNA* genes remain stable for about 16 h. Therefore, less stable RNA molecules should be sought [12].

The results of the present study showed that the molecular RT-PCR method is more efficient for detecting less stable *EF-Tu*, can reduce the detection time to 4 hours.

Another important point is the higher efficiency of methods like RT-PCR. Various studies suggest the lower sensitivity of RT-PCR than PCR. In this regard, Liu et al. indicated that RT-PCR is not capable of detecting bacteria in suspension with 1 CFU/ml [13]. Thus, hydrophobic filters can be used to concentrate bacteria and increase the sensitivity of RT-PCR to prevent loss of RNA molecules. Bej *et al.*, found that hydrophobic filters have a higher ability to absorb bacteria and DNA

Table 5 Comparison of RT-PCR result for *EF-Tu* and *16S rRNA* gene with the MPN method of 10 wells

Number of wells	1	2	3	4	5	6	7	8	9	10
RT-PCR(*16S rRNA*)	-	+	+	+	-	+	+	+	+	+
RT-PCR(*EF-Tu*)	-	+	+	+		+	+	+	+	+
MPN	-	-	+	-	-	-	-	+	+	-

particles than hydrophilic filters [11]. Our results indicating that the RT-PCR efficiency increases using hydrophobic filter even at low bacterial concentrations. The enhanced efficiency can be attributed to the lack of bacteria loss and thus the presence of bacteria nucleic acids. Although the pore diameter of hydrophilic filter (e.g. HAWP) is less than FHLP filters, the hydrophilic filters are less able to absorb bacteria. HAWP filters only able to isolate the bacteria at dilutions of 4 bacteria in 100 ml water. In other words, RT-PCR is not able to detect bacteria at dilutions less than 4 bacteria using hydrophilic filters.

Beside the ability to detect one bacterium in 100 ml water, the results also indicating that RT-PCR is able to detect a bacterium in higher volumes (up to 1600 ml water) using hydrophobic filters. In addition to the high accuracy and efficiency of the RT-PCR method in water pollution detection, it reduces the time of bacterial detection. The routine MPN test lasts at least 24 h, while this time is reduced to 6 to 7 h using RT-PCR method. Therefore, the test could be started within four hours after sampling to avoid detection of possible contamination with dead bacteria.

The results of polymerase chain reaction (PCR) test in water purification and disinfection systems become false positive due to the stability of DNA molecule. Accordingly, molecular methods like PCR cannot reflect the impact of disinfectants on water pollution index. To resolve this problem, other cell molecules (e.g. RNAs) with relatively low stability such as *EF-Tu* with the stability period of 4 h can be used. Reverse transcriptase polymerase chain reaction (RT-PCR) must be used to determine the presence of RNA in the medium. The detection performance can be enhanced using hydrophobic filters for relatively high volumes of water with low bacterial concentrations.

Conclusions

Reverse transcriptase polymerase chain reaction (RT-PCR) is an efficient method for detecting the bacterial contamination of water. The detection performance can be enhanced using hydrophobic filters. The detection time is significantly reduced using less stable ribonucleic acids such as *EF-Tu*.

Competing interests
The authors declare that they have no competing interests.

Authors' contribution
All authors have equal contribution. All authors read and approved the final manuscript.

Acknowledgement
This project was supported by Arak University of Medical Sciences, Arak, Iran.

Author details
[1]Department of Microbiology and Immunology, Arak University of Medical sciences, Arak, Iran. [2]Molecular and Medicine Research Center, Arak University of Medical Sciences, Arak, Iran. [3]Department of Environmental Health, Faculty of Health, Arak University of Medical Sciences, Arak, Iran. [4]Department of Medical Microbiology and Immunology, Arak University of Medical sciences, Arak, Iran. [5]Department of Medical Microbiology and Immunology, Faculty of Medicine, Arak University of Medical Sciences, Arak, Iran.

References
1. Toze S. PCR and the detection of microbial pathogens in water and waste water. Wat Res. 1999;33(17):3545–56.
2. Procop GW. Molecular diagnostics for the detection and characterization of microbial pathogens. Clin Infect Dis. 2007;45 Suppl 2:S99–111.
3. Vaitilingom M, Gendre F, Brignon P. Direct detection of viable bacteria, molds, and yeasts by reverse transcriptase PCR in contaminated milk samples after heat treatment. Appl Environ Microbiol. 1998;64(3):1157–60.
4. Horakova K, Mlejnkova H, Mlejnek P. Direct detection of bacterial faecal indicators in water samples using PCR. Water Sci Technol J Int Assoc Water Pollut Res. 2006;54(3):135–40.
5. Kobayashi H, Oethinger M, Tuohy MJ, Procop GW, Hall GS, Bauer TW. Limiting false-positive polymerase chain reaction results: detection of DNA and mRNA to differentiate viable from dead bacteria. Diagn Microbiol Infect Dis. 2009;64(4):445–7.
6. Sabat G, Rose P, Hickey WJ, Harkin JM. Selective and sensitive method for PCR amplification of Escherichia coli 16S rRNA genes in soil. Appl Environ Microbiol. 2000;66(2):844–9.
7. Davis BD, Luger SM, Tai PC. Role of ribosome degradation in the death of starved Escherichia coli cells. J Bacteriol. 1986;166(2):439–45.
8. Klein PG, Juneja VK. Sensitive detection of viable Listeria monocytogenes by reverse transcription-PCR. Appl Environ Microbiol. 1997;63(11):4441–8.
9. Morin NJ, Gong Z, Li XF. Reverse transcription-multiplex PCR assay for simultaneous detection of Escherichia coli O157:H7, Vibrio cholerae O1, and Salmonella Typhi. Clin Chem. 2004;50(11):2037–44.
10. Pommepuy M, Le Guyader F. Molecular approaches to measuring microbial marine pollution. Curr Opin Biotechnol. 1998;9(3):292–9.
11. Bej AK, Mahbubani MH, Dicesare JL, Atlas RM. Polymerase chain reaction-gene probe detection of microorganisms by using filter-concentrated samples. Appl Environ Microbiol. 1991;57(12):3529–34.
12. Sheridan GF, Masters CI, Shallcross JA, MacKey BM. Detection of mRNA by reverse transcription-PCR as an indicator of viability in Escherichia coli cells. Appl Environ Microbiol. 1998;64(4):1313–8.
13. Liu Y, Gilchrist A, Zhang J, Li XF. Detection of viable but nonculturable Escherichia coli O157:H7 bacteria in drinking water and river water. Appl Environ Microbiol. 2008;74(5):1502–7.

Evaluation of chromosomal aberrations caused by air pollutants in some taxi drivers from two polluted districts of urban Tehran and its comparison with drivers from rural areas of Lahijan

Sara Taghizadeh[1], Hossein Najmabadi[1], Koorosh Kamali[2] and Farkhondeh Behjati[1*]

Abstract

Background: Chromosome instability is the most common form of genomic instability. Genomic instability can lead to tumorogenesis. High level of chromosomal aberrations in peripheral blood lymphocytes can be used as a biomarker for cancer. Air pollution is one of the most important factors that cause chromosomal instability (CIN). In this comparative study we used classic Cytogenetic technique to analyze the effects of air pollutants on chromosome stability. We collected peripheral blood from 30 taxi drivers of two polluted districts (districts 6 and 7) in Tehran and 30 taxi drivers from rural areas of Lahijan, north of Iran.

Results: Comparison of the level of chromosome breakage in the two groups showed an increased level of chromosome breakage in the drivers from polluted districts of Tehran, although not significant, using Fisher exact test (p-value = 0.300). However, the overall chromosome aberration rate (including both chromosome and chromatid gaps), the difference was significant using Chi-square test (p-value = 0.012).

Conclusion: An increased level of chromosome aberration was present in the drivers from polluted districts of Tehran compared to drivers from non-polluted areas in Lahijan.

Keywords: Air pollution, Chromosome aberration, Taxi drivers, Tehran, Lahijan

Introduction

Air pollution is concerned with many ill effects on health including pulmonary and cardiovascular diseases, cancer as well as increased mortality [1]. Additionally, a relationship between intrauterine growth retardation and high exposure to air pollutants during pregnancy has been reported [2]. This has been demonstrated in children and pregnant mothers living in industrial regions. Chromosomal aberrations and gene mutations lead to different kinds of diseases including cancer, particularly Leukemia [3]. The damaging pollutants include poly aromatic hydrocarbons (PAH), methylbenzene, inhaled Ozone, stress oxidative damage of oxygen (ROS), nitrogen (RNS), and persistent particulate matter with size less than 2.5 micron [4].

PAHs are widespread environmental toxicants in ambient air produced from the partial combustion of fossil fuels. Different studies have evaluated the genetic damage in residents in polluted cities and compared them with those living in rural areas. They have shown that air pollution can have carcinogenic effect causing chromosomal aberrations in adults [5].

Adverse health effects are inflicted through physical and chemical properties of air born particulate matter (PM). These pollutants may induce either direct or indirect damage to biological macromolecules, including DNA. Several studies have indicated that pollutants have destructive effect on chromosomes and other important

* Correspondence: f_behjati@uswr.ac.ir
[1]Genetics Research Center, University of Social Welfare and Rehabilitation Sciences, Tehran, Iran
Full list of author information is available at the end of the article

biomolecules [6]. There are both exogenous physical agents and endogenous chemical genotoxic agents, both of which cause DNA damage including double strand and single strand breaks. Besides, ultraviolet can induce both interstrand and intrastrand crosslinks. They can all contribute towards formation of DNA adducts. Defect in repair and replication mechanisms are two outcomes of DNA damage. Such DNA defects can cause mutation or chromosomal aberrations leading to genomic instability [7]. The common damages on chromosomes are breaks, gaps, translocations and acentric fragments [8].

Genomic instability is recognized as a major stimulating force of tumorogenesis [9]. The final goal of cell division for most non-cancerous somatic cells is to accurately duplicate the genome and then evenly divide into the two daughter cells. However any deregulation of cell cycle can lead to aberrant cells. Accumulation of these genetic alterations due to failure in regulation of cell division, the imbalance between cell growth and death can eventually lead to cancer [10]. There are different forms of genomic instability. The most common form is called chromosomal instability (CIN), leading to high rate of changes in chromosome structure and number, which were first observed more than a hundred years ago [11].

The accepted technique for biological monitoring of genetic damage to somatic cells is conventional cytogenetic analysis of peripheral blood lymphocytes, which has been adapted internationally since 1970. It has the advantage of determining the DNA damage by physical and chemical clastogenic agents in the occupational situation. Today, chromosomal aberration in human peripheral lymphocytes is recognized as a valuable biomarker of effect. It is generally accepted that a high frequency of chromosomal aberrations in peripheral lymphocytes is predictive of an increased risk of cancer [12].

The air pollution in Tehran

The world Health organization (WHO) was warned about air pollution as a serious problem in developing countries [13]. According to particle matter index (PMI); there are pollutants such as HC,Pb,No2,Co2,Co,O3 and particles with PM of less than 2.5 all having genotoxic and carcinogenic effects on the genome. If the pollutants concentration increased up to 100 we have air pollution; however, the level lower of 100 indicates healthy air. The quality control center of air pollution in Tehran has announced that the quality of air in Tehran is in a critical situation. Also this center determined four districts as the most pollutant districts: 6, 7, 11, and 12. As a result, we selected districts 6 and 7 to collect our samples. The quality control center of air pollution in Tehran has compared the level of air pollution. The comparison of the level of air pollution from March to October of the three successive years in Tehran is presented in Figure 1 [14]. Meantime, the quality control center of air pollution in Guilan has not reported any air pollution in the rural areas in Lahijan [15]. In this study we used classic cytogenetic methods for the investigation of chromosome aberration to detect the effect of air pollution on chromosomes and genomic stability.

Materials and method

Sampling

The study population consisted of 30 taxi drivers (exposed group) from two polluted districts in Tehran and 30 taxi drivers from Lahijan (North of Iran) (the control

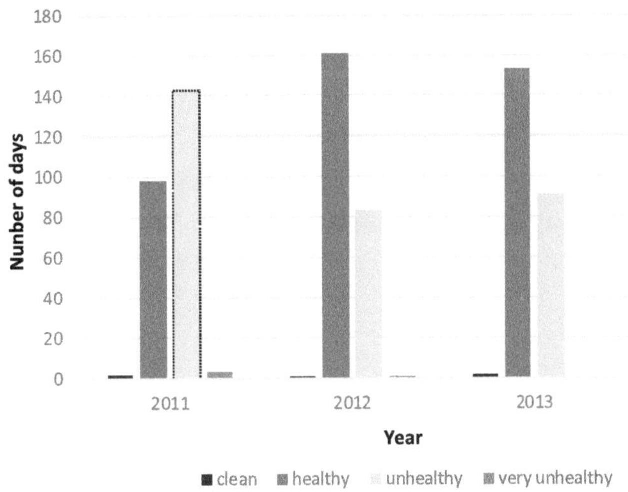

Figure 1 Comparison of the level of air pollution from March to October [14].

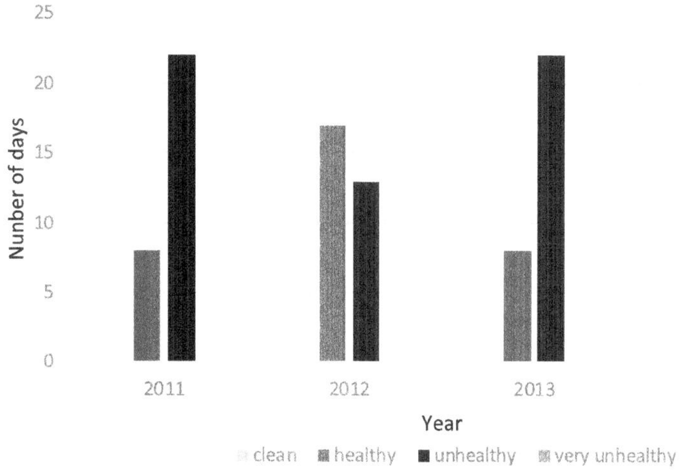

Figure 2 Comparison of air quality index in October [14].

group). The drivers' working hours outdoor were eight hours daily. The exposed group consisted of 30 individuals, median age 35 years and the control group was 30 individuals, median age 33 years. All participating subjects were healthy volunteers who were recruited in convenience way (non-random sampling) and all completed a questionnaire. The inclusion criteria in this study were non smoker, no intake of alcohol, no family history of genetic disorder, non-exposure to chemical reagents and radiation. Any individual with medical treatment, radiation exposure or vaccination up to three months before sampling was not included in the study. The participants signed a consent form. The ethical code of practice of the University of Social welfare and Rehabilitation Sciences was observed. The sampling was performed during October and November 2013 for the case group and May to June for the control. The clean air was constant throughout the year for the control group. The level of air pollution during October and November in three successive years in Tehran is presented in Figures 2 and 3 [14].

Cytogenetic technique

Heparinized blood was collected from the divers. Blood cultures were established within 24 h of specimen collection. Cell cultures were cultivated for 48 h at 37°C in RPMI 1640 with 0.5 cc Of PBS and 1% phytohemagglutinin. Two duplicate cultures were set up from each sample. After 24 h we added 50 λ Colcemid to each tube and then after 1 h incubation both cultures were harvested

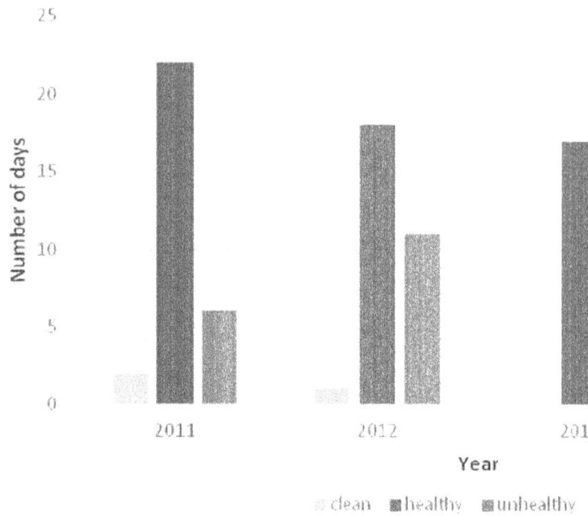

Figure 3 Comparison of air quality index in November [14].

Table 1 Frequency of different types of chromosome aberration in case and control groups with aberrant cells (X^2-test, P-value = 0.012)

abnormalities group	R	Dic	F	Ctg	Ctb	Csg	Csb	tr	qr	Rea
Case	No	No	14 (26.7%)	15 (23.3%)	7 (20%)	1 (3.3%)	2 (6.7%)	No	No	No
control	NO	No	1 (3.3%)	4 (10%)	0 (0%)	1 (3.3%)	1 (3.3%)	No	No	No

R (Ring), Dic (Dicentric), F (Fragment), Ctg (Chromatid gap), Ctb (Chromatid break), Csg (Chromosome gap), Csb (Chromosome break), tr (triradial), qr (quadriradial), Rea(rearrangement).

using a classic technique that include centrifugation, treatment with hypotonic solution of KCL for 20 min followed by repeated fixation with methanol/acetic acid(3/1) [16].

Microscopic analysis

After processing the cultures and preparation of slides, the slides were stained by Giemsa. The slides were examined with light microscope. A total of 100 chromosome spreads were examined for chromosome aberrations. The chromosome aberrations included chromatid gap, chromatid break, chromosome gap, chromosome break, chromosome rearrangements, ring, fragment, and dicentric chromosome. Gaps were scored as chromosome aberration. Dicentric and rearrangements were scored as two breaks. Ring, fragment, chromatid break, and chromosome break were scored as one break (Table 1). Chromosome breakage per cell was calculated for both the case and control groups.

Statistical analysis

Data were analyzed using SPSS 11.5 software. Data are shown as frequency and percentage in study groups. X^2test was carried out. P value of less than 0.05 was considered as statistically significant.

Results

In this study, we have discovered an increased level of chromosome aberration in the drivers from polluted districts of Tehran. The difference was significant, using Chi-square test (p-value = 0.012) (Table 1). Based on the comparison of the level of chromosome breakage in case and control groups, there was an increased level of chromosome breakage (fragment, chromatid break, and chromosome break) in the drivers from polluted districts of Tehran, although not significant, using Fisher exact test (p-value = 0.300). The number of aberrant cells with chromosome aberration in 1000 scored cells showed a significant difference between the case and control groups, using X^2-test (P-Value = 0.001)(Table 2). Also there is no significant difference between the average age of two groups using t-test (p-value = 0.191).

Discussion

The air quality of Tehran has deteriorated in recent years. In particular during autumn and winter seasons the concentration of pollutants increase because of the inverted air phenomenon [14]. The effect of air pollution on morbidity and mortality has become a public health concern [17]. Numerous studies have related high levels of air pollutants to chromosome instability. Genomic instability is a principal agent that can lead to cancer [18]. Some studies have indicated that air pollution causes epigenetic alterations, mitochondrial and nuclear damage. Such genetic alterations can account for behavior disorder in Autistic children. These genetic changes are both microscopic and submicroscopic that can be detected using micro array analyses and DNA sequencing [19]. Similar studies have shown different panel of methylation in DNA in industrial residents exposed to pollutants in comparison with rural residents. They used polymerase chain reaction (PCR) and pyrosequencing to investigate these changes on template of DNA methylation with biomarkers such as LINE-1, P53, IL-6, and P16. Several of these methylation markers showed differences between industrial workers and rural controls [20]. Harmful effects of air pollution on health have been demonstrated in several investigations. It can lead to several diseases such as cancer, especially lung cancer. Stress oxidative damage results in inflammation and increasing coagulopathy activities in blood [21]. Several studies have used cytogenetic parameters including chromatid and chromosome aberrations to demonstrate the adverse effect of air pollutants on genomic stability. Both classic and molecular cytogenetic techniques have been used [22]. Few studies have compared conventional cytogenetic method with FISH and Micronucleus (MN) techniques and found noticeable differences between conventional cytogenetic

Table 2 Frequency of aberrant cells with breaks

Group	Aberrant No. of cells with breaks	Total No. of cells scored	Rate of aberrant cells/1000 (CI95%)	OR (CI95%)	P-Value
Case	35	3000	1.17 (0.83-1.61)	5 (2.2-11.3)	0.001*
Control	7	3000	2.3 (7.02-1.62)		

OR: Odd Ratio, (X^2-test).

and the latter techniques [23]. The FISH technique using whole chromosome painting probes is as a rapid and sensitive method for detecting structural rearrangements, in particular reciprocal translocations. Such rearrangements can be inherited and passed on to the next generation if affecting the germ cells. The micronucleus technique is also an efficient method for the detection of aneuploidies and large number of cells can be screened [24]. Using of FISH and Micronucleus (MN) can be useful to detect translocations and aneuploidies in the nuclei [25]. In some studies focusing on the different seasons, significant differences in chromosome aberrations have been found during summer and winter [26]. In a study by Rossner et al. using classic Cytogenetic technique, they determined the level of vitamins A, C, E, and folate in both case and control groups and did not find any significant difference between the two groups [27]. The level of chromosome aberration was not significant either.

In this study using classic Cytogenetic technique we demonstrated a significantly increased level of chromosome aberration (gaps and breaks) in the drivers from polluted districts of Tehran compared to drivers from non-polluted areas in North of Iran. However this is a preliminary study and such an investigation should be carried out on a larger sample size.

Conclusion

An increased level of chromosome breakage was present in the drivers from polluted districts of Tehran compared to drivers from non-polluted areas in Lahijan. Based on these results and the importance of air pollution on morbidity and mortality, it is highly recommended that further similar studies on a larger sample size from other polluted areas of Tehran should be carried out for more conclusive results. Use of FISH and Micronucleus techniques are also highly recommended.

Competing interests

The authors declare that they have no competing interests.

Authors' contributions

ST coordinated the sampling, carried out the Cytogenetics work, and drafted the manuscript; HN helped with the design of the study and its follow ups; KK carried out the statistical analysis; FB did the design of the study, supervision of the project, editing and finalising the paper. All authors read and approved the final manuscript.

Acknowledgements

The authors gratefully acknowledge all the participants who took part in this study. We thank the Student's Research Committee of the University of Social Welfare and Rehabilitation Sciences for funding this project. Our special thanks to the Center of quality control of air in Tehran and Guilan state for providing the data on level of pollutions in the studied areas. We are grateful to Mr. Hajipour from Tehran taxi bus services, Mr. Ali Taghizadeh from Guilan province, and Mrs Fatemeh Ostaresh for helping with collecting blood samples from the individuals. We are thankful to Miss Susan Banihashemi and Mr. Eiman Bagheizadeh for their assistance in the laboratory work.

Author details

[1]Genetics Research Center, University of Social Welfare and Rehabilitation Sciences, Tehran, Iran. [2]Department of Public Health, School of Public Health, Zanjan University of Medical Sciences, Zanjan, Iran.

References

1. Yang W, Omaye ST: **Air pollutants, oxidative stress and human health.** *Mutat Res* 2009, **647**:45–54.
2. Novotna B, Topinka J, Solansky I, Chvatalova I, Lnenickova Z, Sram RJ: **Impact of air pollution and genotype variability on DNA damage in prague policeman.** *Toxicol Lett* 2007, **172**:37–47.
3. Domenico Franco M, Silvia A, Livia A, Harrie Besse L, Maria B, Nigel B: **Micronulei in cord blood lymphocytes and associations with biomarkers of exposure to carcinogens and hormonally active factors, gene polymorphisms and gene expression: The newgeneris cohort.** *ehp* 2013, **122**:1–38.
4. Valavanidis A, Vlachogianni T, Fiotakis K, Loridas S: **Pulmonary Oxidative Stress, Inflammation and Cancer: Respirable Particulate Matter, Fibrous Dusts and Ozone as Major Causes of Lung Carcinogenesis through Reactive Oxygen species mechanisms.** *Int J Environ Res Public Health* 2013, **10**:3886–3907.
5. Bocskay KA, Tang D, Orjuela MA, Liu X, Warburton DP, Perera FP: **Chromosomal aberrations in cord blood Are associated with prenatal exposure to carcinogenic polycyclic aromatic hydrocarbons.** *Cancer Epidemiol Biomarkers Prev* 2005, **14**:506–511.
6. Moller P, Loft S: **Oxidative damage to DNA and lipids as biomarkers of exposure to air pollution.** *Environ Health Prospect* 2010, **118**:1126–1136.
7. Hoeijmakers JHJ: **DNA damage, aging, and cancer.** *N Engl J Med* 2009, **361**:1475–1485.
8. Rossner P Jr, Rossnerova A, Spatova M, Beskid O, Uhlirova K: **Analysis of biomarkers in a Czech population part II: chromosomal aberrations and oxidative stress.** *Mutagenesis* 2012, **28**:97–106.
9. **Julio Cesar Nepomuceno:** Nutrigenomics and cancer prevention. **2013, chapter 17, 1–26.**
10. **Zhiyuan Shen, Robert Wood Johnson:** Genomic instability and cancer: an introduction. **2011, 3:1–3.**
11. Negrini S, Gorgoulis VG, Halazonetis TD: **Genomic instability an evolving hallmark of cancer.** *Nature* 2010, **11**:220–228.
12. Sram RJ, Beskid O, Binkova B, Rossner P, Smerhovsky Z: **Cytogenetic analysis using fluorescence in situ hybridization to evaluate occupational exposure carcinogens.** *Elsevier* 2004, **149**:335–344.
13. Word Health Organization. Outdoor air quality database. Geneva: WHO;2011. available at: http://www.who.int/phe/health_topics/outdoorair.
14. Air pollution data [http://air.tehran.ir] March 2013.
15. Air pollution data [http://gilan.doe.air.ir] March 2013.
16. Human Cytogenetics: In *A practical Approach Volume I.* Edited by Roony D, Czepulkowski BH. Oxford University press; 2001.
17. Kleeberger SR: **Genetic aspects of susceptibility to air pollution.** *Eur Respir J* 2003, **21**(Suppl. 40):52–56.
18. Demetrioul CA, Ole Raaschou N, Peter M, Roel V, Domenico P, Marc Chadeau H: **Biomarkers of ambient air pollution and lung cancer: a systematic review.** *Occup Environ Med* 2011, **69**:619–627.
19. Moyra S: **Nuclear and Mitochondrial Genome defects in Autism.** In *Genomic instability and Impact of epigenetic and environmental factors, Comprehensive Guide to Autism.* Irvine, CA, USA: Springer, College of Health Sciences; 2014:1679–1698.
20. Marco P, Valentina B, Armelle M, Petcharin S, Adisorn J, Suleeporn S: **DNA methylation differences in exposed workers and nearby residents of the Ma Ta Phut industrial estate, Rayong, Thailand.** *IJe* 2012:1–8.
21. Pedersen M, Vinzents P, Petersen JH, Kleinjans JCS, Plas G, Kirsch-Volders M, Dostál M, Rössner P: **Cytogenetic effects in children and mothers exposed to air pollution assessed by the frequency of micronuclei and fluorescence in situ hybridization (FISH): A family pilot study in the Czech Republic.** *Mutat Res* 2006, **608**:112–120.
22. Xiangy M, Aoy L, Yang H, Liu W, Sun L, Han X, Liu J, Cao J: **Chromosomal damage and polymorphisms of metabolic genes among 1, 3-butadiene-exposed workers in a matched study in China.** *Mutagenesis* 2012, **27**(4):415–421.

23. Kim Vande L, Eleni F, Ilse D, Georgia C, Maria K, Gina P: **Maternal and Gestational Factors and Micronucleus Frequencies in Umbilical Blood: The NewGeneris Rhea Cohort in Crete.** *Children's Health* 2011, **119**:1460–1465.
24. Sram RJ, Beskid O, Rössnerova A, Rössner P, Lnenickova Z, Milcova A, Solansky I, Binkova B: **Environmental exposure to carcinogenic polycyclic aromatic hydrocarbons; the interpretation of cytogenetic analysis by FISH.** *Toxicol Lett* 2007, **172**:12–20.
25. Holland NT, Luoping Z, Smith MT: **Cytogenetic markers and air pollution, In relationship between acute and chronic effects of air pollution.** 2000:65–78.
26. Demirgil GC, Erdem O, Gaga EO, Altug H, Van Doorn W, Burgaz S: **Cytogenetic biomonitoring of primery school children exposed to air pollutants:micronuclei analysis of buccal epithelial cells.** *Environ Sci Pollut Res* 2013, **21**:1197–1207.
27. Rossner P, Bavorova H, Ocadlikova D, Svandova E, Sram RJ: **Chromosomal aberrations in peripheral lymphocytes of children as biomarkers of environmental exposure and life style.** *Toxicol Lett* 2002, **134**:79–85.

12

Fabrication and characterization of a polysulfone-graphene oxide nanocomposite membrane for arsenate rejection from water

Reza Rezaee[1], Simin Nasseri[2,1*], Amir Hossein Mahvi[1,3,4], Ramin Nabizadeh[1], Seyyed Abbas Mousavi[5], Alimorad Rashidi[6], Ali Jafari[7] and Shahrokh Nazmara[1]

Abstract

Background: Nowadays, study and application of modified membranes for water treatment have been considered significantly. The aim of this study was to prepare and characterize a polysulfone (PSF)/graphene oxide (GO) nanocomposite membrane and to evaluate for arsenate rejection from water.

Materials and methods: The nanocomposite PSF/GO membrane was fabricated using wet phase inversion method. The effect of GO on the synthesized membrane morphology and hydrophilicity was studied by using FE-SEM, AFM, contact angle, zeta potential, porosity and pore size tests. The membrane performance was also evaluated in terms of pure water flux and arsenate rejection.

Results: ATR-FTIR confirmed the presence of hydrophilic functional groups on the surface of the prepared GO. FE-SEM micrographs showed that with increasing GO content in the casting solution, the sub-layer structure was enhanced and the drop like voids in the pure PSF membrane changed to macrovoids in PSF/GO membrane along with increase in porosity. AFM images indicated lower roughness of modified membrane compared to pure PSF membrane. Furthermore, contact angle measurement and permeation experiment showed that by increasing GO up to 1 wt%, membrane hydrophilicity and pure water flux were increased. For PSF/GO-1, pure water flux was calculated about 50 L/m^2h at 4 bar. The maximum rejection was obtained by PSF/GO-2 about 83.65 % at 4 bar. Moreover, it was revealed that arsenate rejection depended on solution pH values. It was showed that with increasing pH, the rejection increased.

Conclusions: This study showed that application of GO as an additive to PSF casting solution could enhance the membrane hydrophilicity, porosity, flux and arsenate rejection.

Keywords: Mixed matrix membrane, Polysulfone, Graphene oxide, Hydrophilicity, Arsenate

Background

In recent years, a growing public concern has arisen over release of toxic pollutants such as inorganic ions, metals and synthetic organic matters into the water due to increasingly industrial and agricultural activities. Among these toxicants, arsenic is a serious threat in water resources of some regions [1, 2]. Toxicological and epidemiological studies proven that inorganic arsenic could cause carcinogenic and non-carcinogenic effects in human [3]. World health organization (WHO) and united state protection agency (USEPA) had classified arsenic as class A carcinogens list [4]. International agency for research on cancer (IARC) also classified inorganic form of arsenic in class I carcinogens list [5]. With regard to strict regulations for control and removal of arsenic in drinking water, and limitations of conventional water treatment processes (e.g. generation of toxic intermediates and low efficiencies) looking for new technologies is of great interest [3, 6]. Membrane process can be considered as a promising technology for arsenic removal due to its several advantages such as no need to add

* Correspondence: naserise@tums.ac.ir
[2]Center for Water Quality Research, Institute for Environmental Research, Tehran University of Medical Sciences, Tehran, Iran
[1]Department of Environmental Health Engineering, School of Public Health, Tehran University of Medical Sciences, Tehran, Iran
Full list of author information is available at the end of the article

chemicals, no generation of sludge, ease of system capacity development, separation in continuous mode, ease of integration with other processes, minimum dependency to environmental conditions and capable of microorganisms and solutes removal [7, 8]. However, certain drawbacks associated with common membranes are low water recovery, fouling problem and high-energy consumption [9, 10]. In recent years to overcome these drawbacks, different studies have been conducted in order to modify polymeric membranes to enhance the permeability, rejection and decreasing fouling problem and reduce the investment and operational costs [11]. Accordingly, various works such as physical blending, plasma treatment, polymer grafting and chemical reactions have been carried out to modify the membranes [12, 13]. Among these methods physical blending is preferred due to the simplicity procedure using phase inversion technique [14]. Physical blending consist of mixing of polymeric materials with inorganic nanoparticles (e.g. TiO_2 [15], ZnO [16], silica [17]) and recently carbon allotropes [11, 18, 19]. Adding inorganic nanoparticles to membrane matrix can enhance the membrane hydrophilicity, strength, permeability and antifouling characteristics [18, 20]. Graphene and its derivatives due to unique two-dimensional structure, one-atom-layer-thick, high theoretical surface area (2630 m^2/g), good mechanical properties, non-harmful effects, low cost production have attracted interest for different application especially polymeric membrane modification [21, 22]. Graphene oxide (GO) is also highly hydrophilic due to presence of oxygen containing functional groups (e.g. hydroxyl, carboxyl, carbonyl and epoxy) [12, 23]. When thin sheets of carbon atoms (GO) are added to a polymer matrix at low content and proper procedure, it could significantly improve the physical properties of the base polymer [21, 24]. Among different synthetic polymers, polysulfone (PSF) is the one that is widely used for various membranes fabrication such as filtration, ultrafiltration, hemodialysis and bioreactor technologies [13, 25]. The reasons for wide use of this type of polymer are good characteristics such as desire mechanical and thermal properties, high chemical stability, high resistance in a wide range of pH and high solubility in a broad range of polar solvents (dimethylformamide, dimethylacetamide, dimethylsulfoxide) [13, 21, 25]. One of the main drawbacks of PSF membrane is fouling problem and consequently reduction of the membrane lifetime. Actually, this type of membrane is influenced by fouling problem more than other membrane materials because of the hydrophobic nature of the membrane and interactions between the membrane surface charges and the foulants [13, 21]. A few studies have used GO in casting solution to improve the water permeability, antifouling properties and mechanical strength characteristics of the mixed matrix membrane. Zhao et,al showed that synthesized PVDF/GO ultrafiltration membrane had higher pure water flux compared to PVDF due to improvement of the surface hydrophilicity [12]. Wang et, al also reported that GO nanosheet as a hydrophilic modifier could enhance the water flux of the fabricated ultrafiltration membrane with an improvement in the antifouling property [14]. In another study, Zinadini et.al showed that water permeability, hydrophilicity and antifouling properties of the PES/GO membrane were enhanced compared to pure PES membrane [26]. Xia et, al also revealed that employment of a certain amount of GO in the matrix could improve the water flux, hydrophilicity and antifouling characteristics of a type of synthesized PVDF/GO membrane used for natural organic matter removal [27]. The aim of this study is to synthesis and characterizes a PSF/GO nanocomposite membrane in order to reject arsenic from water. In this work, GO was applied to PSF matrix as a hydrophilic agent. The performance of the synthesized membranes was evaluated by pure water flux measurement and arsenate rejection.

Materials and methods

Materials

All chemicals used in the experiments were of reagent grade. Graphite fine powder extra pure (with a mean particle size of <50 μm) was purchased from Merck-Germany. PSF (with average $M_w = 22{,}000$ g/mol) was obtained from Sigma-Aldrich Co-Germany. N,N-Dimethylformamide >(DMF) was purchased from Sigma-Aldrich and used without purification as a solvent to prepare cast solution. Analytical grade H_2SO_4 (98 %-Merck), $NaNO_3$ (99 %, Sigma–Aldrich), $KMnO_4$ (99 %, Sigma–Aldrich) and H_2O_2 (30 % solution, stabilized Merck) were used as received. Sodium arsenate dibasic heptahydrate (Na_2HAsO_4-$7H_2O$) was obtained from Sigma-Aldrich. The deionized (DI) water was used in the sample preparation and for pure water flux measurements.

Preparation and characterization of graphene oxide (GO)

In this study GO was prepared using modified Hummer's method [28]. Firstly, 5 g graphite powder and 2.5 g sodium nitrate were added to a 500-ml neck flask containing 120 ml concentrated sulfuric acid in ice bath and thoroughly mixed for 30 min. Then under vigorous mixing, 15 g $KMnO_4$ was slowly added to the suspension and mixing was continued for 30 min. The rate of adding was controlled to maintain temperature of the reaction below 20 °C. After that, ice bath was removed and the mixture was stirred overnight at room temperature. By elapsing the time, the mixture changed in to sticky and the color changed to brown. Then under mixing condition, 150 ml distilled water was slowly added to the mixture. The temperature was rapidly increased to 98 °C and the color turned to yellow. This aqueous suspension was stirred at 98 °C for 24 h. In order to remove $KMnO_4$, 50 ml H_2O_2 (30 %) was added to the liquid mixture. For more purification, the liquid mixture of GO was washed by HCL (5 %) and DI water and centrifuged for several times to reach the pH to natural range. Finally, for exfoliating the product, sonication was conducted for 1 h. Then it was filtered and dried in a vacuum oven (at 40 °C for 24 h) to obtain a grey color GO nanoplate powder. Raman spectra of the GO was obtained in the spectral range of 100-4200 cm^{-1} and with 532 nm wavelength incident laser light (Almega Thermo Nicolet Dispersive Raman Spectrometer, Germany). The measurements of the attenuated total reflectance fourier transform infrared spectroscopy (ATR-FTIR) of the GO was performed using a ATR-FTIR spectroscopy in the range between 600 cm − 1 and 4000 cm^{-1} (Tensor 27, Bruker Inc., Germany).

Fabrication of PSF/GO nanocomposite membrane

In present work, PSF/GO nanocomposite membrane was fabricated via common phase inversion method [14, 29]. For this purpose, PSF was used as bulk material, DMF as solvent, GO nanoplate as the additive and hydrophilic modifier, DMF as the solvent and DI water as the nonsolvent in coagulation bath. The casting solution consist of PSF = 15 %wt, DMF = 85 wt% and GO = (0-0.5-1-2 wt% PSF). PSF and GO powder were dried in vacuum oven at 60 °C for 4 h. At first, four different amounts of GO were dispersed in DMF and was sonicated for 1 h to obtain a homogenous casting solution. Then, under continuous stirring condition, PSF was added to GO/DMF mixture and was allowed to stir for 24 h. Then the casting solution was maintained in room temperature for 24 h without stirring. Finally, casting solution was sonicated to remove remaining air bubbles. The prepared casting solution was casted uniformly onto a smooth and clean glass plate using a casting knife at a thickness of 200 μm. The casted film on the glass was left for air exposure (20 s) followed by immersing into the nonsolvent coagulation bath (DI water at 25 °C). The glass plate was kept in the coagulation bath for 10 min to guarantee complete phase inversion process. Finally the peeled off synthesized membrane was washed with DI water for several times until all the residual solvent removed. The membranes were kept in DI water for characterization and experiments. The synthesized membrane based on GO content named pure PSF, PSF/GO-0.5, PSF/GO-1 and PSF/GO-2.

Characterization of the prepared membranes

The structure and surface morphology of the membranes were evaluated using a field-emission scanning electron microscope (FE-SEM, S-4160, Hitachi, Japan). For sample preparation, membrane were cut into small pieces and washed with distilled water. For obtaining a good cross section image, the wet pieces were immersed in liquid nitrogen for 1 min to freeze. The frozen pieces of the membranes were fractured and kept in air to dry. The dried samples were coated with a thin layer of gold to increase the electric conductivity before FE-SEM imaging. Atomic force microscopy (AFM) was applied for top surface morphology and roughness analysis. Thermo microscopes Auto probe CP Research (Veeco Instruments, Sunnyvale, CA, USA) was used for AFM analysis. The samples were cut into small pieces (1 cm × 1 cm), washed with distilled water and dried in room temperature. In this study, surface hydrophilicity changes of different fabricated membranes were determined via the contact angle and Zeta potential. The contact angle was analyzed using a water contact angle measurement (OCA 15 Plus, Dataphsycs, Germany). Before contact angle measurement, the samples were dried in oven at 50 °C for 4 h. For more accuracy in the determination of contact angle, 5 different top surface points were measured and the average was reported. The zeta potentials of fabricated membrane were measured by streaming potential method using Electro kinetic Analyzer (EKA, Anton Paar GmbH, Austria) equipped with plated sample cell. For this purpose membrane were cut in 5 cm × 5 cm pieces and zeta potentials were measured at 26 °C and pH of 7. In this measurement method, 0.001 M KCl solution was applied as electrolyte and zeta potential were measured in triplicate for each membrane.

Membrane porosity and pore size

To evaluate the effect of GO on the membrane structure, the porosity, as the ratio of the volume of voids to the total volume of membrane, was measured using a gravimetry method. For this, the membranes were dried in an air-circulating oven at 50 °C for 24 h. Then the samples were cut into small pieces (1 cm × 1 cm) (5 pieces for each membrane) and weighted. The pieces were immersed in distilled water for 24 h at 25 °C. After removing the droplets on the surface of membrane by a paper filter, the membrane was weighted again. The average of dry and wet weights for each membrane was recorded and the porosity (ε) was calculated using the gravimetry equation 1 [18, 30, 31].

$$\varepsilon = \frac{\frac{W_1 - W_2}{\rho_w}}{\frac{W_1 - W_2}{\rho_w} + \frac{W_2}{\rho_m}} \times 100\% \qquad (1)$$

Where, W_1 and W_2 are wet and dry weights of membrane respectively (g), ρ_w is the density of distilled water (0.998 g/mL) and ρ_m is the density of polymer (PSF = 1.24 g/mL at 25 °C). The average pore radius (r_m) of the membranes was calculated by following equation known as Guerout–Elford–Ferry equation (Eq. 2) [18, 32].

$$rm = \sqrt{\frac{(2.9-1.75\varepsilon) \times 8\eta l Q}{\varepsilon \times A \times \Delta P}} \quad (2)$$

where rm is the mean pore radius (m), η is the water viscosity (8.9×10^{-4} Pa · s), l is the membrane thickness (m), Q is the volume of the permeate water per unit time (m^3/s), A is the effective area of the membrane (m^2) and ΔP is the operational pressure (Pa).

Permeation tests and arsenate rejection experiments

In this study, to evaluate the permeation flux and arsenate rejection by fabricated nanocomposite membrane, a lab-scale filtration system was used at dead end mode operation. The main components of the filtration system include a 2-L feed tank (equipped with mixer and temperature control), low and high pressure feed pumps (1 to 15 bar), stainless steel flat membrane module (effective area of 9.6 cm^2), valves and pressure gauges (Fig. 1). For flux measurements, the membranes were first immersed in distilled water for 24 h. Then the membranes were compacted under 7 bar of distilled water at 25 ± 0.5 °C for 30 min until a constant flux was achieved. Immediately the pressure was reduced to 4 bar and pure water flux test was conducted for 1 h with collecting and measuring the filtrate volume at 5 min intervals. Finally, the flux was calculated using equation 3 [11, 33].

$$J_w = \frac{V}{A\Delta t} \quad (3)$$

Where J_w is the pure water flux (L/m^2h), V is the volume of permeated pure water (L), A is the effective area of membrane (m^2) and Δt is the sampling time (h).

after measuring the pure water flux, arsenate sodium solution with initial concentration of 300 ± 10 µg/L was prepared based on a standard procedure [34]. The rejection of arsenate was evaluated at 4 bar. The permeate was collected each 20 min for arsenate analysis, finally the average was reported. Arsenic concentrations was measured by inductively coupled plasma optical emission spectroscopy (HG-ICP/OES) (Model Spectro arcos, Specro Inc, Germany) connected to a hydride generator. The percentage of rejection was calculated using equation 4 [26].

$$\%R = \left(1-\frac{C_p}{C_f}\right) * 100 \quad (4)$$

Where R is the rejection of arsenate (%), and C_p and C_f are the concentrations of arsenate in the permeation and feed solution, respectively (µg/L). All pure water flux and rejection experiments were performed in triplicate.

Results and discussion

Characterization of graphene oxide

Figure 2 depicts the Raman spectrum of synthesized GO. From the Figures D, G and 2D appeared at 1348, 1585 and 2700 cm^{-1} as GO known peaks [35]. Generally, in graphene Raman spectrum, D band indicates the disordered and defect in graphene structure, G band shows that normal structure of graphene and 2D band is related to number of layers. Graphene Raman spectrum from a single layer and a few layer graphene consist of peak G at around 1580 cm^{-1} and peak 2D at around 2700 cm^{-1}. In GO Raman spectrum, as well as G and 2D peaks, typical D band is obvious which appears at around 1350 cm^{-1}. This peak (D) is absent in ordered graphene, while in GO, presence of D band is assigned to the developed defect structure in due to oxygen containing functional groups(e.g. hydroxyl) at the edge of

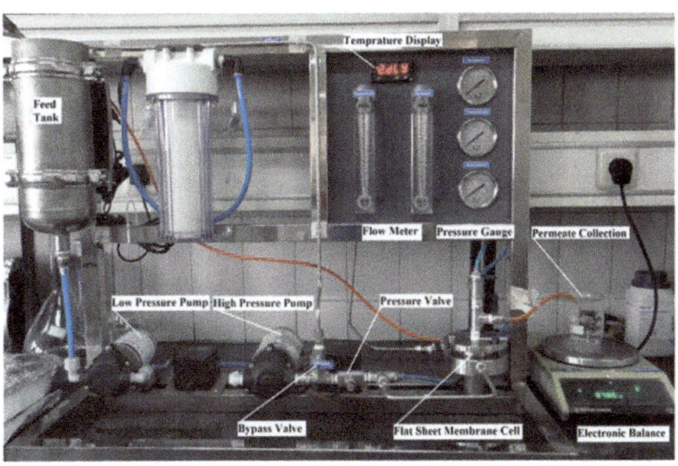

Fig. 1 Membrane filtration system used in experiment

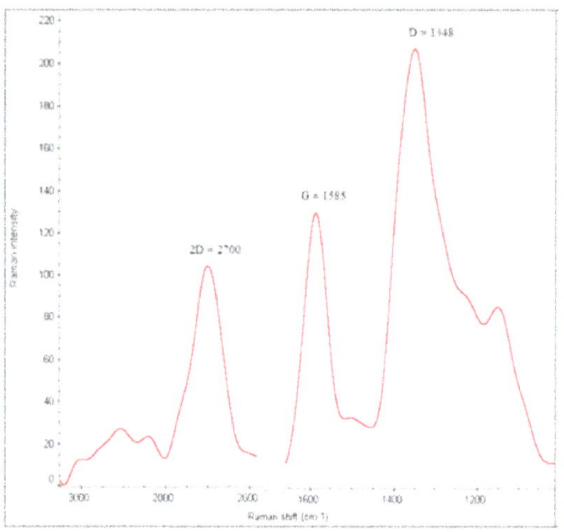

Fig. 2 Raman spectrum of synthesized GO

graphene plates. As the intensity of peak D is higher, the sample has higher disordered structure. In addition, Raman spectrum can be used for analysis of graphene quality and determination of the layers (up to 5 layers) through the 2D peak shape, width and position. With increase in number of the layers, 2D peak shifts to higher wavelengths and will broaden [36, 37]. In this study based on appeared peaks from Raman spectrum analysis confirmed a few-layer structure of GO.

In addition to Raman spectra, IR spectrum is also used for GO characterization. Figure 3 shows the GO ATR-FTIR spectrum. From the figure, a prominent adsorption peak appeared at 3411.94 cm^{-1} that reveals the typical GO characteristics. This strong peak assigns to stretching vibration O-H bond and indicates the presence of hydroxyl groups. O-H bond may exist in forms of alcoholic, phenolic, carboxylic and so on. This peak also confirms the hydrophilic properties of GO. The band 1395.86 cm^{-1} can be attributed to O-H deformation vibration [21]. The absorption peak in the 1713.63 cm^{-1} shows the carbonyl stretching vibration (C = O) and indicate the presence of carboxyl functional group. In addition, appearance of an adsorption peak at 1110.65 cm^{-1} could be assigned to the C-O bond stretching vibration [38]. With regard to presence of oxygen containing functional groups it is proved that the synthesized GO is highly hydrophilic. These observations are consistent with the results reported in other works [12, 14].

Characterization of the PSF/GO membrane

Effect of GO addition on membrane morphology

In next stage of the study, the effect of loaded GO on the micro-structure of the PSF membrane was analyzed. Cross-sectional FE-SEM micrographs of the prepared membranes are presented in Fig. 4. General structure of the membrane consists of a dense skin layer on the top and a porous support sub layer. Pure PSF membrane with mainly sponge structure and few separated closed end drop-like pores shown in Fig. 4a. With the addition of GO, the main characteristics of a asymmetric structure appears composing of a dense skin layer on top and a thick porous layer with finger like pores in the bottom (Fig. 4b-d). From Fig. 4b, in membrane with 0.5 wt% GO, drop like pores have been replaced by finger-like pores in the pure PSF membrane but the walls of the pores are thick and with closed ends, and the sponge parts are still exist as a significant part of the membrane. With further increase in loaded GO, finger like channels turned into a large, open-end macrovoids and the spongy portion decreased significantly. Furthermore, from the figure, the

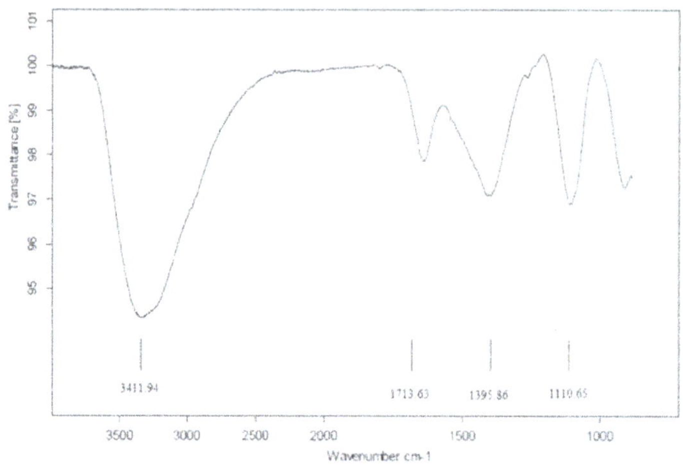

Fig. 3 ATR-FTIR spectrum of synthesized GO

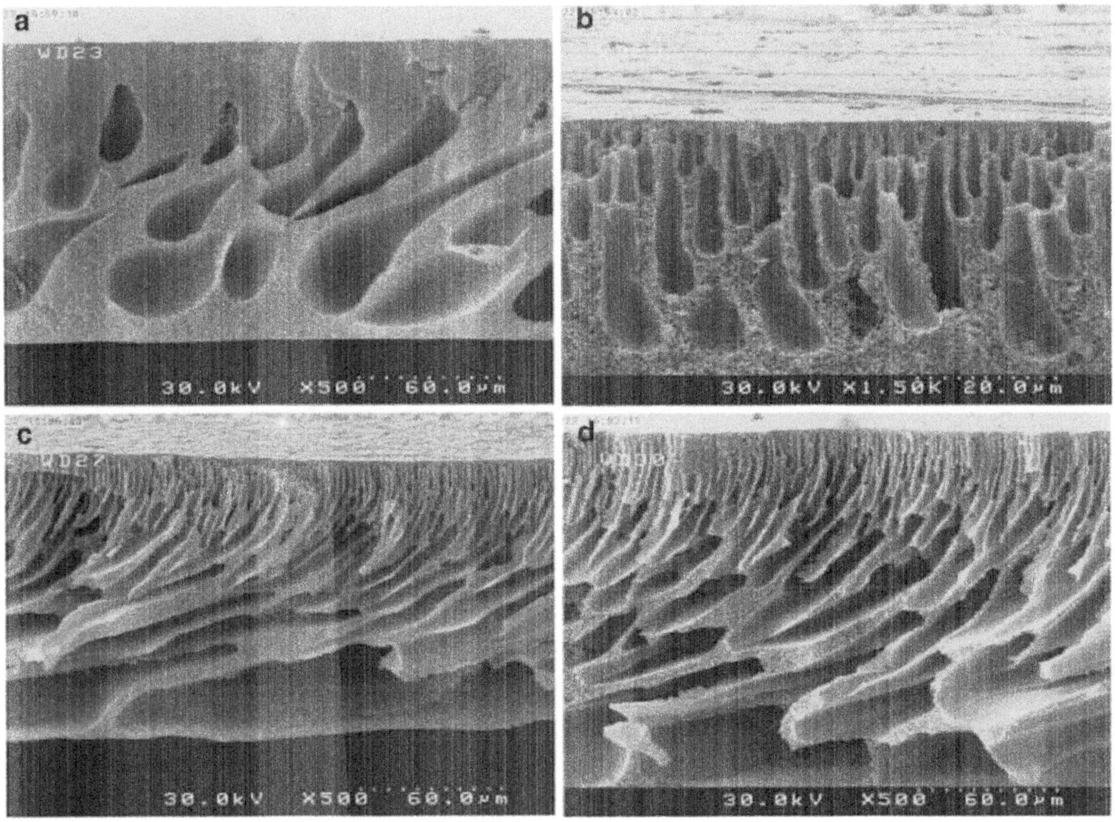

Fig. 4 Cross-section morphologies FE-SEM images of the prepared membranes. **a** Pure PSF, **b** PSF/GO-0.5, **c** PSF/GO-1 and **d** PSF/GO-2 membranes

number of their pores increased and walls thickness decreased compare to pristine PSF membrane (Fig. 4c-d). Generally, these structures have a low resistance to water permeation [39]. In addition, in the membranes with 1 and 2 wt% GO, horizontal channels appeared that can improve the water permeability. This issue is confirmed by other similar studies [14, 26]. The rate of pores production is the directly related to the exchange rate of solvent and non-solvent in the coagulation bath of phase inversion process. However, the faster the exchange rate of solvent and non-solvent in the coagulation process, the larger pores, more finger like pores and more channels. In contrast, the slower the exchange rate of solvent and non-solvent in the coagulation process, the smaller pores, more drop like pores and a spongy or non-void structure is resulted which finally alter the membrane permeability [40, 41]. By adding GO to the matrix of membrane the sub layer is effectively modified. This capability is attributed to GO hydrophilicity which results in thermodynamic instability in the casting solution, consequently rapid mass transfer between the solvent and nonsolvent is occurred. As a result, large pores are formed in the sub layer of membrane [5]. In this study, to evaluate the surface morphology of the synthesized membranes, AFM was used. In Fig. 5, three-dimensional images of the four types of synthesized membranes are illustrated. As it is obvious, the bright areas exhibit the highest points and dark areas depict the valleys or pores of the fabricated membranes. It seems that the direction of the dents is pointed to direction of applied coagulation bath. In addition, Table 1 presents the different roughness parameters of the membranes. From the Table, surface roughness of pure PSF membrane is greater than the modified membrane with 0.5 and 1 wt% GO, but it is less than membrane with 2 wt% GO. Adding a certain amount of GO changes the large peaks and valleys of the membrane to a large number of small peaks and valleys [26]. Actually, in low loading of carbon modifiers such as carbon nanotube and grapheme oxide, due to low electrostatic interaction and good compatibility with the membrane matrix, these nanomaterials could develop a suitable structure in the membrane, reducing the membrane roughness and thus create a smooth surface [42]. Similar behavior has been reported in previous studies [11, 43].

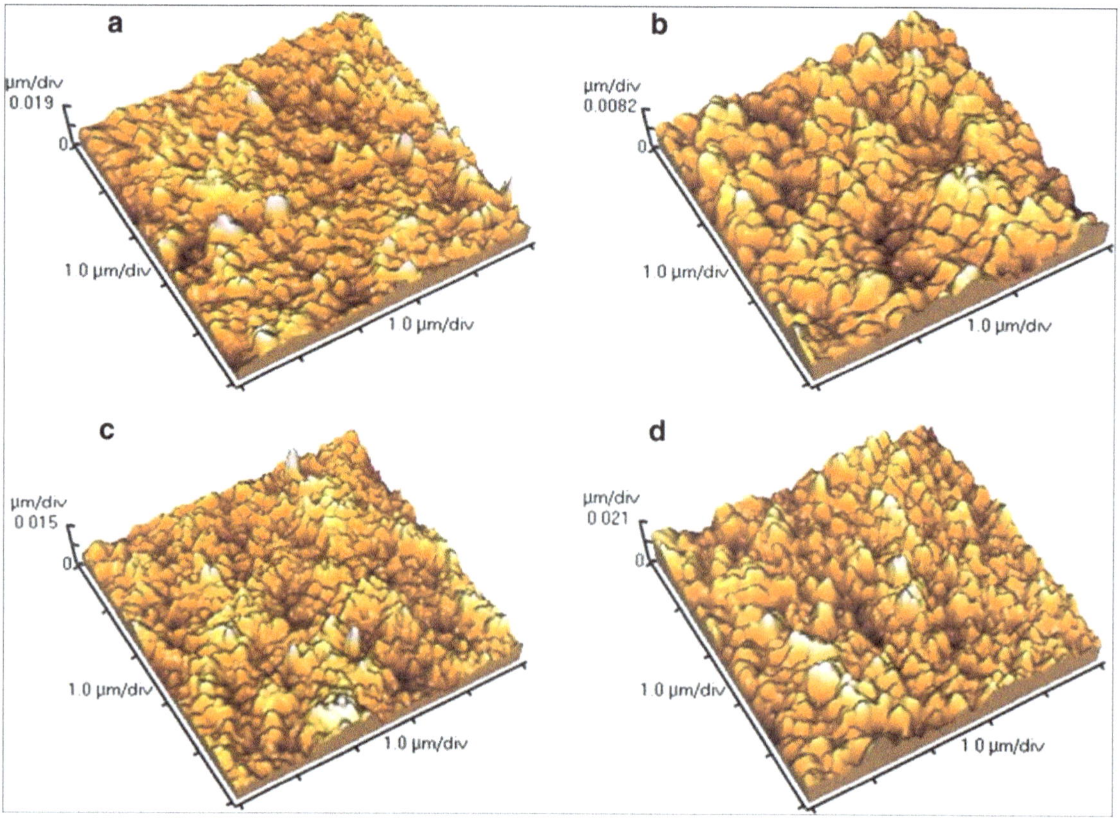

Fig. 5 AFM three-dimensional surface morphology of the prepared membranes. **a** pure PSF, **b** PSF/GO-0.5, **c** PSF/GO-1 and **d** PSF/GO-2 membranes

Membrane hydrophobicity, Water permeation flux and pore structure parameters

Zeta potential values for synthesized membranes are presented in Fig. 6. As shown, all given values are negative. With increasing the amount of GO to 1 wt%, negatively charge and zeta potential increased. The results of contact angle measurements, porosity, pore size and water flux are given in Table 2. As shown in the table with an increase of 1 % GO nanoparticles to the polymer matrix, water contact angle decreased, in contrast the porosity, pore size and water flux increased. Accordingly, net PSF membrane has the highest contact angle, lowest values of porosity, pore size and flux. Among the membranes, PSF/GO-1 has the lowest contact angle and maximum porosity, pore size and water flux. From the table, PSF/GO-2 has slightly higher contact angle and lower pure water flux compare to PSF/GO-1 membrane. Generally, zeta potential plays an important role in flux and anti-fouling properties of membranes [44]. The surface charge is an indication of presence of charged functional groups on the membrane surface. Inducing of hydroxylic and carboxylic functional groups can produce negative charges on the membrane surface [20]. During the phase inversion process hydrophilic functional groups in GO migrate to the surface resulting in negatively charged surface. Blended nano particles in the membrane casting solution migrate to the top of the membrane that is initially exposed to the non-solvent (water) liquid. Increase of hydrophilic groups density on the membrane surface results in decrease of intermediate energy (interface energy) with water. As a result, with increasing the surface hydrophilicity, contact angle decreased [12]. The hydrophilic nature of GO speed up the exchange process of solvent and non solvent in the phase inversion method which increases the

Table 1 Surface roughness parameters of the prepared membranes obtained from analyzing six randomly chosen surface AFM images

Membranes	Roughness parameters	
	Mean surface roughness (Ra-nm)	Root mean square roughness (Rq-nm)
Pure PSF	2.9 ± 0.23	3.9 ± 0.47
PSF/GO-0.5	2 ± 0.14	2.5 ± 0.15
PSF/GO-1	2.5 ± 0.30	3.4 ± 0.36
PSF/GO-2	4.4 ± 0.32	5.8 ± 0.50

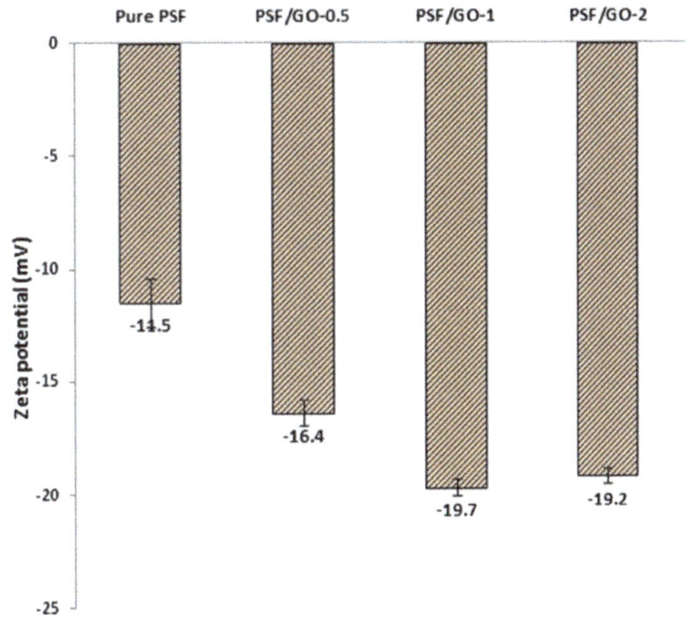

Fig. 6 Surface zeta potential of the prepared membranes with various GO contents

porosity and pore size of the membrane as clearly seen in FE-SEM micrographs (Fig. 4). These changes in the membrane properties enhance the membrane permeability [14, 45]. At GO contents of more than 1 wt%, (namely PSF/GO-2), the hydrophilicity of the membrane relatively reduced. This phenomenon may be due to accumulation and irregular positioning of GO nanoplates and decrease of the functional groups on the membrane surface. In addition, the reduction of water flux through membrane with GO content more than 1 wt%, is attributed to decrease of membrane porosity and pore size due to high viscosity of casting solution and delay of solvent and non-solvent exchange. In this situation, the pores are blocked by high concentrations of GO, resulting in flux reduction [11, 14]. The results of GO effects on the membrane characteristics are consistent with the similar works [12, 13, 21, 26].

Arsenate rejection performance evaluation

The results of arsenate rejection and membrane flux for different fabricated membranes are presented in Fig. 7. In the mentioned operating condition arsenate rejection for the pure PSF membrane and the modified membrane with 0.5, 1 and 2 wt% GO were 25.87 %, 65.80 %, 82.30 %, and 83.65 % respectively. The rejection by modified membranes are substantially higher than that of the pure PSF membrane. Moreover, by increasing the weight of GO in the casting solution the arsenate ions rejection increased. The reasons for this increase are described below. Negative hydrophilic functional groups such as hydroxyl and carboxyl groups on surface of GO can build up a high zeta potential by inducing negative charges on surface of the membrane. Negative charge of arsenate and negative charge on the membrane surface result in increase of Donnan repulsion, resulting in an increase in the arsenate rejection [46]. This feature does not exist in pure PSF membrane. Fundamentally, the charge repulsion of ions depends on the membrane charge, ionic strength and ions capacity [11]. Lohokare et al. reported that dominant removal mechanism of arsenate was Donnan exclusion using a modified hydrophilic UF membrane [46]. Moreover some researchers have previously proposed that modified hydrophilic membranes due to strong bonds with water can

Table 2 Effect of GO content on water contact angle, pure water flux and pore structure parameters of the prepared membranes

Membranes	Contact angle (deg)	Porosity (%)	Mean pore radius (nm)	Pure water flux (L/m^{2}h)
Pure PSF	73.5 ± 2.1	48.3 ± 2.6	6.9 ± 0.56	19.7 ± 3.2
PSF/GO-0.5	66.7 ± 1.6	77.9 ± 2.2	8.3 ± 0.31	32.3 ± 3.5
PSF/GO-1	51.3 ± 1.2	86.5 ± 1.8	9.1 ± 0.63	49.9 ± 2.6
PSF/GO-2	54.8 ± 1.4	82.1 ± 1.3	8.7 ± 0.42	46.4 ± 2.0

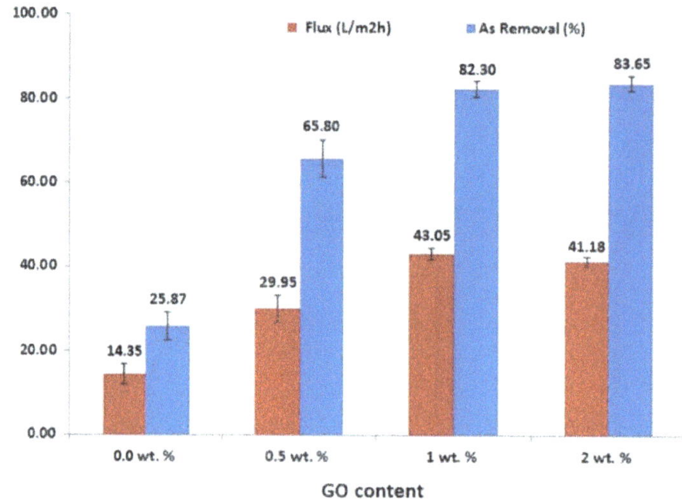

Fig. 7 As(V) rejection and flux of the prepared membranes with various GO contents. (Operating pressure =4 bar, pH = 8.5 ± 0.2, Initial As(V) concentration = 300 ± 10 μg/L, feed temperature =25 ± 0.5 °C)

effectively prevent the passage of molecules [27]. However, it has been expressed that carbon nano-materials, could absorb foulants by surface reactions and consequently increase the rejection rate [32]. From Fig. 7, with increase in GO to 1 wt%, the increase in arsenate rejection is obvious, which is justified by the previously mentioned reasons. However, with increase to more than 1 wt% GO (PSF/GO-2) the removal efficiency is not very significant compared to the PSF/GO-1 membrane. This could be because of high density of irregular GO on membrane structure, reducing the functional groups on the membrane surface, resulting in decrease in membrane hydrophilicity [26]. Consequently with reduction of functional groups, negatively charged on membrane surface is reduced, thus the removal of arsenate does not increase proportion to loaded GO [11, 14]. In addition, a slight increase of arsenate rejection in PSF/GO-2 compare to PSF/GO-1 can be assigned to lower flux and pore size value. From Fig. 7, the results of flux of arsenate solution filtration for modified membranes showed an approximate 10 % reduction compared to pure water flux (Table 2), while the flux reduction is more in pure PSF membrane (about 27 %). This difference can be attributed to the nature of the hydrophilic and anti-fouling properties of the modified membranes. The rejection of arsenic by membrane could be affected by various

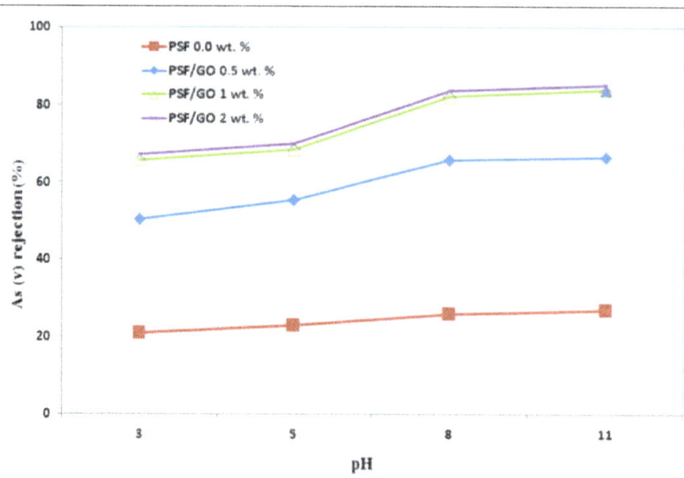

Figure 8 Percentage rejection of As (V) at different pH by prepared membranes with various GO contents. (Operating pressure =4 bar, Initial As (V) concentration = 300 ± 10 μg/L, feed temperature =25 ± 0.5 °C)

parameters such as operating pressure, initial concentration, pH, ionic strength [46]. However, one of the most influential parameters is solution pH, which plays a major role in the rejection of arsenic by membrane systems [21, 47]. The effect of pH on the rate of arsenate rejection by synthesized membranes has been presented in Fig. 8. With increasing pH, the rejection increased due to some reasons. First, by increasing the pH, zeta potential of membrane increases and membrane surface charge becomes more negative [46, 48]. Moreover, arsenic charge which is controlled by pH, becomes more negative with increasing the pH [49]. Second, changing the pH values will change the predominant species of arsenic in the environment. So that at pH <6.9 monovalent ions ($H_2AsO_4^-$) are dominant, while at pH > 6.9 divalent ions ($HAsO_4^{2-}$) are dominant. Therefore, with increasing pH, monovalent ions converted into divalent ions. Since the repulsive effect of Donnan is more dominant for divalent ions than monovalant ions, thus the rejection increased in higher pH values [47, 49, 50]. Accordingly Seidel et al. showed that the removal of arsenic by nanofiltration membranes was reduced from 85 % at pH = 8.5 to 8 % in pH = 4.5 [50]. Based on the good results of As (v) rejection obtained from the synthesized membrane, it seems that with determining the optimum operating parameters, the proposed standards for arsenic, especially in surface waters with the dominant species of arsenate, is achievable.

Conclusion

In present study, GO nanoplate were directly added to PSF casting solution to fabricate a mixed matrix membrane via phase inversion method. The results showed that presence of abundant containing hydrophilic functional groups on GO, strongly enhance the hydrophilicity and permeability of the synthesized membrane. Graphene oxide also could modify the morphology of the membrane so that the spongy structure and closed-end drop like pores of the pure PSF membrane could change to finger like pores and larger open-end channels in PSF/GO membrane. Adding GO up to 1 wt% in casting solution resulted in enhancement of membrane morphology so that the contact angle reduced and the porosity and pure water flux increased due to the improvement of the membrane surface hydrophilicity. The results also showed that the rejection of arsenic in the PSF/GO membranes has substantially increased compared to pure PSF membrane. In addition, with increase in GO weight in the casting solution the rejection of arsenate ions increased. The experiments also showed that the predominant mechanism of arsenate rejection is, Donnan repulsion due to the negative charges induced by GO on the membrane surface. The results of this study revealed that due to unique properties of GO especially hydrophilicity, it can be considered as a promising nanomaterial for membrane fabrication and modification.

Competing interests
The authors declare that they have no competing interests.

Authors' contributions
RR and SN has participated in all stages of the study (design of the study, conducting the experiment, analyzing of data and manuscript preparation). AHM and RN participated in the design of the study, final revised of manuscript and intellectual helping for analyzing of data. SAM and AMR carried out statistical and technical analysis of data and intellectual helping for analyzing of data. AJ carried out statistical and technical analysis of data, participated in design of study and manuscript preparation. SN performed data collection and carried out technical analysis. All authors read and approved the final manuscript.

Acknowledgements
This research was part of a PhD dissertation of the first author and has been financially supported by a grant (NO, 22716-46-02-92) from Center for Water Quality Research, Institute for Environmental Research, Tehran University of Medical Sciences, Tehran, Iran. The authors would like to express their thanks to the Department of Environmental Health Engineering, School of Public Health, Tehran University of Medical Sciences for their collaboration.

Author details
[1]Department of Environmental Health Engineering, School of Public Health, Tehran University of Medical Sciences, Tehran, Iran. [2]Center for Water Quality Research, Institute for Environmental Research, Tehran University of Medical Sciences, Tehran, Iran. [3]Center for Solid Waste Research, Institute for Environmental Research, Tehran University of Medical Sciences, Tehran, Iran. [4]National Institute of Health Research, Tehran University of Medical Sciences, Tehran, Iran. [5]Department of Chemical and Petroleum Engineering, Sharif University of Technology, Tehran, Iran. [6]Nanotechnology Research Center, Research Institute of Petroleum Industry (RIPI), Tehran, Iran. [7]Department of Environmental Health Engineering, School of Public Health, Lorestan University of Medical Sciences, Khorramabad, Iran.

References
1. Bhatnagar A, Sillanpää M. A review of emerging adsorbents for nitrate removal from water. Chem Eng J. 2011;168:493–504.
2. Maleki A, Amini H, Nazmara S, Zandi S, Mahvi AH. Spatial distribution of heavy metals in soil, water, and vegetables of farms in Sanandaj, Kurdistan, Iran. J Environ Health Sci Eng. 2014;29:33.
3. Jain CK, Singh RD. Technological options for the removal of arsenic with special reference to South East Asia. J Environ Manage. 2012;107:1–18.
4. Saitua H, Gil R, Padilla AP. Experimental investigation on arsenic removal with a nanofiltration pilot plant from naturally contaminated groundwater. Desalination. 2011;274:1–6.
5. Addo Ntim S, Mitra S. Adsorption of arsenic on multiwall carbon nanotube–zirconia nanohybrid for potential drinking water purification. J Colloid Interface Sci. 2012;375:154–9.
6. Ebrahimi R, Maleki A, Shahmoradi B, Daraei H, Mahvi AH, Barati AH, et al. Elimination of arsenic contamination from water using chemically modified wheat straw. Desalination Water Treat. 2013;51:2306–16.
7. Dutta T, Bhattacherjee C, Bhattacherjee S. Removal Of Arsenic Using Membrane Technology–A Review. International Journal of Engineering Research and Technology. 2012;1:1-23.
8. Jafari A, Mahvi AH, Nasseri S, Rashidi A, Nabizadeh R, Rezaee R, et al. Ultrafiltration of natural organic matter from water by vertically aligned carbon nanotube membrane. J Environ Health Sci Eng. 2015;13:51.
9. Shi X, Tal G, Hankins NP, Gitis V. Fouling and cleaning of ultrafiltration membranes: a review. J Water Process Eng. 2014;1:121–38.
10. Zazouli M, Nasseri S, Mahvi A, Gholami M, Mesdaghinia A, Younesian M. Retention of humic acid from water by nanofiltration membrane and influence of solution chemistry on membrane performance. Iran J Environ Health Sci Eng. 2008;5:11–8.
11. Vatanpour V, Madaeni SS, Moradian R, Zinadini S, Astinchap B. Fabrication and characterization of novel antifouling nanofiltration membrane prepared from oxidized multiwalled carbon nanotube/polyethersulfone nanocomposite. J Membr Sci. 2011;375:284–94.

12. Zhao C, Xu X, Chen J, Yang F. Effect of graphene oxide concentration on the morphologies and antifouling properties of PVDF ultrafiltration membranes. J Environ Chem Eng. 2013;1:349–54.
13. Lee J, Chae H-R, Won YJ, Lee K, Lee C-H, Lee HH, et al. Graphene oxide nanoplatelets composite membrane with hydrophilic and antifouling properties for wastewater treatment. J Membr Sci. 2013;448:223–30.
14. Wang Z, Yu H, Xia J, Zhang F, Li F, Xia Y, et al. Novel GO-blended PVDF ultrafiltration membranes. Desalination. 2012;299:50–4.
15. Rajaeian B, Heitz A, Tade MO, Liu S. Improved separation and antifouling performance of PVA thin film nanocomposite membranes incorporated with carboxylated TiO 2 nanoparticles. J Membr Sci. 2015;485:48–59.
16. Liang S, Xiao K, Mo Y, Huang X. A novel ZnO nanoparticle blended polyvinylidene fluoride membrane for anti-irreversible fouling. J Membr Sci. 2012;394:184–92.
17. Hassanajili S, Khademi M, Keshavarz P. Influence of various types of silica nanoparticles on permeation properties of polyurethane/silica mixed matrix membranes. J Membr Sci. 2014;453:369–83.
18. Zhao C, Xu X, Chen J, Yang F. Optimization of preparation conditions of poly(vinylidene fluoride)/graphene oxide microfiltration membranes by the Taguchi experimental design. Desalination. 2014;334:17–22.
19. Crock CA, Rogensues AR, Shan W, Tarabara VV. Polymer nanocomposites with graphene-based hierarchical fillers as materials for multifunctional water treatment membranes. Water Res. 2013;47:3984–96.
20. Yin J, Deng B. Polymer-matrix nanocomposite membranes for water treatment. J Membr Sci. 2015;479:256–75.
21. Ganesh BM, Isloor AM, Ismail AF. Enhanced hydrophilicity and salt rejection study of graphene oxide-polysulfone mixed matrix membrane. Desalination. 2013;313:199–207.
22. Yari M, Norouzi M, Mahvi AH, Rajabi M, Yari A, Moradi O, et al. Removal of Pb (II) ion from aqueous solution by graphene oxide and functionalized graphene oxide-thiol: effect of cysteamine concentration on the bonding constant. Desalination Water Treat. 2015; In press, doi: 10.1080/19443994.2015.1043953.
23. Hegab HM, Zou L. Graphene oxide-assisted membranes: fabrication and potential applications in desalination and water purification. J Membr Sci. 2015;484:95–106.
24. Hu K, Kulkarni DD, Choi I, Tsukruk VV. Graphene-polymer nanocomposites for structural and functional applications. Prog Polym Sci. 2014;39:1934–72.
25. Shah P, Murthy CN. Studies on the porosity control of MWCNT/polysulfone composite membrane and its effect on metal removal. J Membr Sci. 2013;437:90–8.
26. Zinadini S, Zinatizadeh AA, Rahimi M, Vatanpour V, Zangeneh H. Preparation of a novel antifouling mixed matrix PES membrane by embedding graphene oxide nanoplates. J Membr Sci. 2014;453:292–301.
27. Xia S, Ni M. Preparation of poly (vinylidene fluoride) membranes with graphene oxide addition for natural organic matter removal. J Membr Sci. 2014;473:54-62.
28. Hummers Jr WS, Offeman RE. Preparation of graphitic oxide. J Am Chem Soc. 1958;80:1339–9.
29. Blanco J-F, Sublet J, Nguyen QT, Schaetzel P. Formation and morphology studies of different polysulfones-based membranes made by wet phase inversion process. J Membr Sci. 2006;283:27–37.
30. Dong C, He G, Li H, Zhao R, Han Y, Deng Y. Antifouling enhancement of poly(vinylidene fluoride) microfiltration membrane by adding Mg(OH)2 nanoparticles. J Membr Sci. 2012;387–388:40–7.
31. Wang Y, Ou R, Ge Q, Wang H, Xu T. Preparation of polyethersulfone/carbon nanotube substrate for high-performance forward osmosis membrane. Desalination. 2013;330:70–8.
32. Xu Z, Zhang J, Shan M, Li Y, Li B, Niu J, et al. Organosilane-functionalized graphene oxide for enhanced antifouling and mechanical properties of polyvinylidene fluoride ultrafiltration membranes. J Membr Sci. 2014;458:1–13.
33. Zhao S, Wang Z, Wang J, Wang S. The effect of pH of coagulation bath on tailoring the morphology and separation performance of polysulfone/polyaniline ultrafiltration membrane. J Membr Sci. 2014;469:316–25.
34. APHA, AWWA, WEF. Standard methods for the examination of water and wastewater. 21st ed. Washington DC: APHA, AWWA, WEF; 2005.
35. Wu J, Tang Q, Sun H, Lin J, Ao H, Huang M, et al. Conducting film from graphite oxide nanoplatelets and poly (acrylic acid) by layer-by-layer self-assembly. Langmuir. 2008;24:4800–5.
36. Zhu Y, Murali S, Cai W, Li X, Suk JW, Potts JR, et al. Graphene and graphene oxide: synthesis, properties, and applications. Adv Mater. 2010;22:3906–24.
37. Yang D, Velamakanni A, Bozoklu G, Park S, Stoller M, Piner RD, et al. Chemical analysis of graphene oxide films after heat and chemical treatments by X-ray photoelectron and Micro-Raman spectroscopy. Carbon. 2009;47:145–52.
38. Lin Y, Jin J, Song M. Preparation and characterisation of covalent polymer functionalized graphene oxide. J Mater Chem. 2011;21:3455–61.
39. Lin D-J, Chang C-L, Huang F-M, Cheng L-P. Effect of salt additive on the formation of microporous poly(vinylidene fluoride) membranes by phase inversion from LiClO4/Water/DMF/PVDF system. Polymer. 2003;44:413–22.
40. Li YQ, Xi DL, Fan SL. Preparation and characterization of novel hollow fiber membrane with multicomponent polymeric materials. Adv Mater Res. 2012;534:8–12.
41. Kuilla T, Bhadra S, Yao D, Kim NH, Bose S, Lee JH. Recent advances in graphene based polymer composites. Prog Polym Sci. 2010;35:1350–75.
42. Qiu S, Wu L, Pan X, Zhang L, Chen H, Gao C. Preparation and properties of functionalized carbon nanotube/PSF blend ultrafiltration membranes. J Membr Sci. 2009;342:165–72.
43. Zhao H, Wu L, Zhou Z, Zhang L, Chen H. Improving the antifouling property of polysulfone ultrafiltration membrane by incorporation of isocyanate-treated graphene oxide. Phys Chem Chem Phys. 2013;15:9084–92.
44. Zazouli MA, Nasseri S, Ulbricht M. Fouling effects of humic and alginic acids in nanofiltration and influence of solution composition. Desalination. 2010;250:688–92.
45. Sun M, Su Y, Mu C, Jiang Z. Improved antifouling property of PES ultrafiltration membranes using additive of silica – PVP nanocomposite. Ind Eng Chem Res. 2009;49:790–6.
46. Lohokare H, Muthu M, Agarwal G, Kharul U. Effective arsenic removal using polyacrylonitrile-based ultrafiltration (UF) membrane. J Membr Sci. 2008;320:159–66.
47. Fang J, Deng B. Rejection and modeling of arsenate by nanofiltration: contributions of convection, zdiffusion and electromigration to arsenic transport. J Membr Sci. 2014;453:42–51.
48. Zhao G, Li J, Ren X, Chen C, Wang X. Few-layered graphene oxide nanosheets as superior sorbents for heavy metal ion pollution management. Environ Sci Technol. 2011;45:10454–62.
49. Akbari H, Mehrabadi AR, Torabian A. Determination of nanofiltration efficency in arsenic removal from drinking water. Iran J Environ Health Sci Eng. 2010;7:273–8.
50. Seidel A, Waypa JJ, Elimelech M. Role of charge (Donnan) exclusion in removal of arsenic from water by a negatively charged porous nanofiltration membrane. Environ Eng Sci. 2001;18:105–13.

Optimizing photo-mineralization of aqueous methyl orange by nano-ZnO catalyst under simulated natural conditions

Ahed Zyoud[1*], Amani Zu'bi[1], Muath H. S. Helal[2], DaeHoon Park[3], Guy Campet[4] and Hikmat S. Hilal[1]

Abstract

Background: Photo-degradation of organic contaminants into non-hazardous mineral compounds is emerging as a strategy to purify water and environment. Tremendous research is being done using direct solar light for these purposes. In this paper we report on optimum conditions for complete mineralization of aqueous methyl orange using lab-prepared ZnO nanopowder catalyst under simulated solar light.

Results: Nano-scale ZnO powder was prepared in the lab by standard methods, and then characterized using electronic absorption spectra, photolumenscence emission (PL) spectra, XRD, and SEM. The powder involved a wurtzite structure with ~19 nm particles living in agglomerates. Photo-degradation progressed faster under neutral or slightly acidic conditions which resemble natural waters. Increasing catalyst concentration increased photodegradation rate to a certain limit. Values of catalyst turn over number and degradation percentage increased under higher light intensity, whereas the quantum yield values decreased. The photocatalytic efficiency of nano-ZnO powders in methyl orange photodegradation in water with solar light has been affected by changing the working conditions. More importantly, the process may be used under natural water conditions with pH normally less than 7, with no need to use high concentrations of catalyst or contaminant. The results also highlight the negative impact of possible high concentrations of CO_2 on water purification processes. Effects of other added gaseous flows to the reaction mixture are also discussed.

Conclusion: ZnO nano-particles are useful catalyst for complete mineralization of organic contaminants in water. Photo-degradation of organic contaminants with ZnO nano-particles, methyl orange being an example, should be considered for future large scale water purification processes under natural conditions.

Keywords: Methyl orange, Contaminant mineralization, Solar simulated light, ZnO nanopowder

Introduction

Purification of water from hazardous chemicals is an important research area. Organic contaminants, such as industrial dyes, halocarbons and phenol derivatives, are among the main contaminants that demand complete safe removal [1]. Different strategies are being investigated for water remediation, including biological treatment [2, 3], ultra-filtration [4], adsorption methods [5] and others. Such methods may not be favored as they may not cause complete mineralization of the organic contaminant. They simply transfer the pollutant from one phase to another [6]. Advanced Oxidation Processes (AOP) have been proposed as alternative routes for water purification. Among those, oxidation via ozone or hydrogen peroxide has been reported as an effective technique [7–11]. Unfortunately, such methods may be costly, as ozonation demands artificial UV radiations, and hydrogen peroxide is not available free of charge. Contaminant complete mineralization with natural solar light seems to be the most practical process for future water purification. A semiconductor photo-catalyst speeds up the action of light by first absorbing photon and producing electrons and holes [12]. With the abundance of costless solar radiations, a low cost catalyst may thus be useful. Different semiconducting materials, in the powder form, have been assessed as photo-catalysts [13, 14]. TiO_2 in its anataze form is the most widely used effective photo-catalyst for its high efficiency, photochemical

* Correspondence: ahedzyoud@najah.edu
[1]SSERL, Department of Chemistry, An-Najah National University, Nablus, Palestine
Full list of author information is available at the end of the article

stability, non-toxic nature and low cost. It has been described for degradation of a wide range of organic contaminants [15–22]. Zinc oxide ZnO is a semiconductor with a comparable band gap ~3.2 eV (with wavelength shorter than 400 nm), but has been investigated to a lesser extent in water purification. ZnO is evaluated in many advanced applications such as field-effect transistors, lasers, photodiodes, chemical and biological sensors and solar cells, but to a lesser extent in photo-degradation catalysis [23–26]. One main advantage for ZnO is that it absorbs a larger fraction of solar spectrum, than TiO_2 does [27]. The performance of ZnO in degrading a number of organic contaminants has been reported [28, 29]. The quantum efficiency of ZnO nano-particles in photo-degrading organic contaminants process is higher than that of TiO_2 [30, 31], due to its higher absorptivity in waves shorter than 400 nm, which accounts to about 5 % of the reaching solar light.

In this communication the photo-catalytic activity of ZnO powder in complete mineralization of organic contaminants is revisited, focusing on finding optimum conditions that yield highest contaminant removal, for the first time. For application purposes, it is necessary to emulate natural conditions of contaminated waters in terms of pH, low contaminant concentration, low allowable catalyst amount and moderate water temperatures. Influence of CO_2 and other gas flows on methyl orange photo-degradation process will also be assessed here for the first time. All such reaction parameters will be studied in order to assess feasibility of using ZnO activated photo-degradation of methyl orange in water under simulated natural conditions. To assess feasibility of ZnO catalyst to function on its own in simulated natural waters, multiple use of the added ZnO to photo-degrade fresh methyl orange samples will also be investigated. All such studies are being investigated for the first time.

Methyl orange, with molecular structure shown in Fig. 1, is a dye that is believed to be mutagenic [32]. It slightly dissolves in water. Its color changes with pH, from yellow (at pH higher than 4.4) to red (at lower pH values), and therefore it is used as an indicator [33]. Methyl orange is also used as a dye in textile industry [34]. It is an example of the widely spread azo dies [35], which are resistant to complete biodegradation [36]. For these reasons, methyl orange is commonly used as a model dye to study in environmental cleanup, and this work is no exception.

In earlier study [37, 38], we reported on using commercial ZnO powders as catalysts in photo-degradation of methyl orange. As mentioned above, this work is intended to find optimum conditions for using ZnO nano-particles in methyl orange photo-degradation under natural water conditions, where ZnO is added to contaminated waters and allowed to function on its own under direct solar light.

Experimental

Chemicals

Hydrochloric acid, sodium hydroxide, and methyl orange were purchased from Merck. ZnO powder was prepared in the lab to obtain small particle sizes, as described earlier [39, 40]. A $ZnCl_2$ solution (250 mL, 0.25 M) was drop-wise added (within 40 min) to NaOH solution (200 mL, 0.90 M) with continuous stirring. The system was then left to settle, and the supernatant was decanted. The resulting precipitate was washed with water many times to remove any remaining ions. Enough amount of distilled water was added to convert the precipitate into slurry. The slurry was centrifuged at 6000 rpm for 10 min, and the supernatant was carefully decanted leaving the solid catalyst which was dried at 120 °C.

The CO_2 gas was prepared by adding concentrated HCl solution (5 M) drop-wise to Na_2CO_3 solid in a stoppered flask with only one outlet. The outlet was connected with a glass tube bubble the CO_2 through the reaction mixture at a flow rate 90 mL/L.

Equipment

A 400 W Osram Tungsten Halogen lamp was used as a source for solar simulator light. The lamp spectrum is a

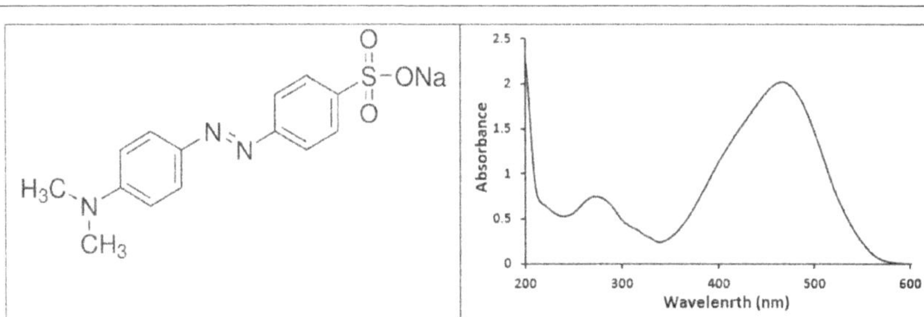

Fig. 1 Molecular structure and UV–vis absorption spectrum of methyl orange

bell curve typical with little (~5 %) in the UV region, just like natural solar light that reaches earth. A light meter (Model lx-102) from Lutron was used to measure the radiation intensity at the reaction mixture surface. A Shimadzu UV-1601 spectrophotometer was used to measure remaining methyl orange concentration using calibration curves, pre-prepared at different pH values, as methyl orange spectra may change with pH value.

The electronic absorption spectra were measured on a Shimadzu UV-1601 spectrophotometer for ZnO powders as suspensions in minimal water amounts. Photoluminescence (PL) Emission Spectra were measured for aqueous suspensions of ZnO powder on a Perkin-Elmer LS50 Luminescence Spectrometer. Excitation wavelength 325 nm was used. XRD patterns were measured on a Philips XRD XPERTPRO diffracto-meter with Cu K_α radiation (λ = 1.5418 Å) located in the labs of Dansuk Industrial Co., LTD., South Korea. Field Emission-Scanning Electron Micrographs (FE-SEM) were measured on a Jeol Model JSM-6700 F microscope, in the labs of Dansuk Industrial Co., LTD. South Korea. Atomic absorption spectra (AAS) were used to measure zinc ions resulting from possible degradation of ZnO. The AAS results were measured on an ICE3000 Thermoscientific Atomic Absorption Spectrophotometer equipped with a zinc lamp.

Catalytic experiment

Photo-catalytic experiments were conducted under direct irradiation from the solar simulator lamp. Water samples pre-contaminated with known concentrations of methyl orange were placed inside a 250 mL beaker. Known nominal amounts of the catalyst ZnO powder were added. The mixture was magnetically stirred with a magnetic bar for 15 min in the dark, to allow adsorption equilibrium and to assess amounts of adsorbed methyl orange on the solid catalyst. The pH of the reaction mixture was controlled by adding drops of dilute HCl or NaOH solutions. The solar simulator lamp, vertically clamped above the solution with an adjustable stand, was then switched on with continuous stirring. The desired irradiation intensity on the mixture surface was achieved by controlling the lamp distance. The reaction time was calculated the time the lamp was switched on. Certain experiments were conducted in duplicate to check the reproducibility of the process.

The reaction progress was followed by measuring the amount of remaining methyl orange with time. This was performed by syringing out small aliquots of reaction mixture at certain times. The aliquots were then centrifuged at high speed (5000 rpm) for 5 min. The liquid phase was then carefully syringed out and analyzed spectrophotometrically at 480 nm.

Results and discussion

Zinc oxide powder characterization

Solid state electronic absorption spectra were measured for the prepared ZnO nano-powder as aqueous suspension. ZnO showed absorption with a maximum at ~368 nm (equivalent to 3.37 eV), Fig. 2. The wide band gap is presumably due to small average particle size, since smaller particles exhibit wider band gap values [41].

The photoluminescence emission spectrum was measured for lab-prepared ZnO powder as dispersion in water, using excitation wavelength 325 nm. The ZnO suspension showed an emission peak at ~385 nm (~3.2 eV), Fig. 3. The other two emission peaks at ~445 nm and ~483 nm are attributed to the presence of oxygen vacancies which cause crystal imperfections, as reported earlier [42]. The value of the band gap is not far different from that measured by electronic absorption spectra discussed above.

Figure 4 shows the XRD patterns for ZnO nano-powder. The ZnO clearly involves a wurtzite form, based on comparison with earlier literature results [43]. Based on Scherrer equation approximations, the average particle size was calculated to be ~19 nm.

SEM was used to study the surface morphology and to further estimate the particle size of prepared ZnO powders, Fig. 5. The micrograph showed elongated nano-rods (with rice-shape) of ZnO agglomerates. The agglomerates involved nano-particles of less than 20 nm size.

Methyl orange photo-degradation

Exposure of aqueous solutions of methyl orange to solar simulator lamp, in the presence of ZnO nano-powder, caused appreciable de-colorization of methyl orange solution in soundly short times. Control experiments conducted in the dark, using catalyst while keeping other conditions the same, showed no detectable de-colorization. This means that no degradation occurred in the dark, and that the ZnO powder adsorbs only little fraction of the contaminant. Control experiments conducted with irradiation in the absence of ZnO did not show any noticeable de-colorization with prolonged exposure. This indicates the necessity of the ZnO particles to activate the methyl orange

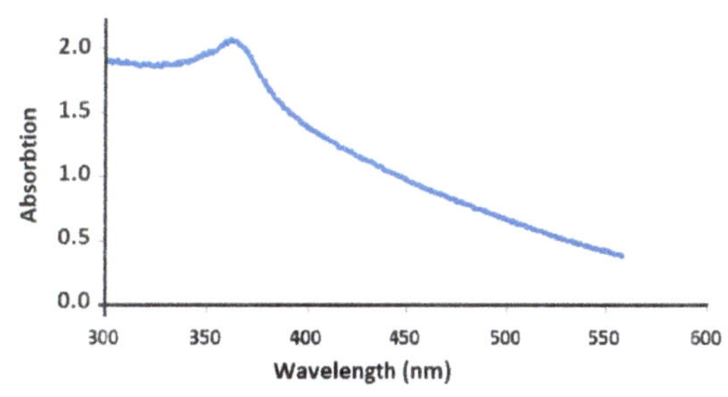

Fig. 2 Electronic absorption spectrum for lab-prepared ZnO powder (aqueous suspension)

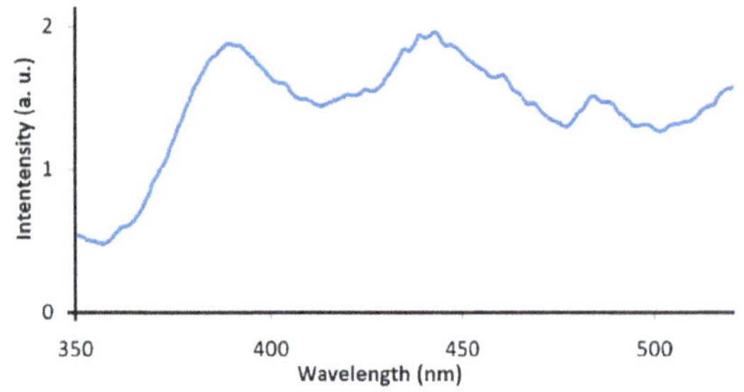

Fig. 3 Photoluminescence emission spectrum measured for ZnO powder (aqueous suspension)

degradation. Using a cut-off filter (that blocks light 400 nm and shorter) caused severe lowering in methyl orange degradation. Collectively, these results indicate that light waves shorter than 400 nm are the driving force for the degradation of methyl orange, and that the ZnO particles are needed to observe the degradation process. Degradation is thus due to the shorter wave length tail available in the lamp light. With a band gap more than 3.2 eV, ZnO powder catalyst employs photons with wavelength shorter than 400 nm in the photo-degradation process.

Therefore, methyl orange de-colorization here, even in case of incomplete process, is due to complete mineralization of the degraded molecules. This was evident from the disappearance of absorbance bands in the range 200–300 nm (characteristic for the phenyl group) and the range 400–500 nm (characteristic for the azo group). When left for enough time, complete removal and complete mineralization were observed, as shown in Fig. 6 below. Therefore, the reacted phenyl group is believed to be completely degraded leaving no organic products. The reacted azo group is also believed to escape as N_2 gas [44, 45]. Complete photo-mineralization of methyl orange molecules lost under the working conditions is well documented [37, 46–54].

In order to assess the ability of ZnO to photo-degrade aqueous methyl orange under simulated natural conditions

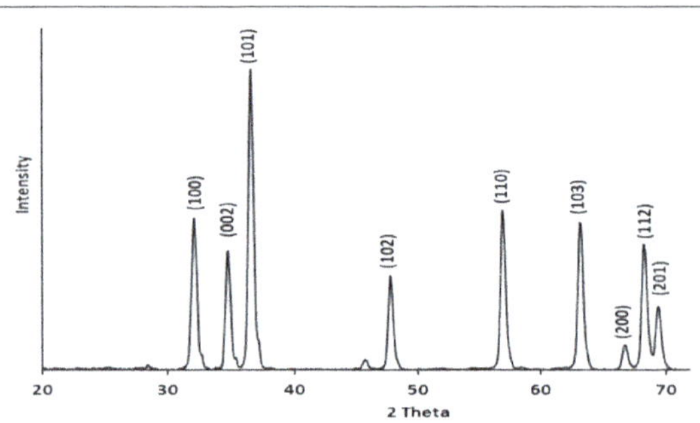

Fig. 4 XRD pattern measured for lab-prepared ZnO powder

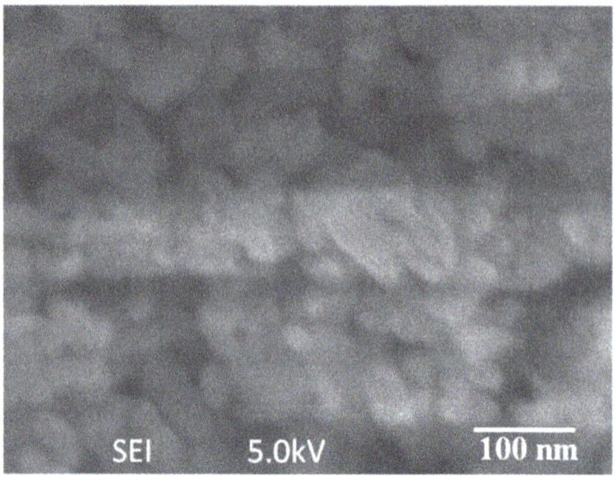

Fig. 5 SEM micrograph of lab-prepared ZnO powder

different parameters were investigated here. Effects of different reaction parameters, such as pH, catalyst concentration and contaminant concentration, on rate of photo-degradation were reported earlier [55]. The parameters (initial nominal pH, methyl orange concentration and ZnO amount) have been revisited here together with other new parameters (aqueous CO_2 concentration, temperature, light intensity and catalyst reuse).

The remaining methyl orange concentrations were plotted with exposure time. The catalytic efficiency is better understood in terms of turnover number, T.N. (degraded molecules/Zn atoms) and quantum yield, Q.Y., (degraded molecules/total incident photons) measured after 30 min exposure to radiation.

Effect of pH on photo-degradation process

Because the amphoteric nature of ZnO, it is necessary to study the effect of the pH value on the methyl orange photo-degradation process. This is also necessary as

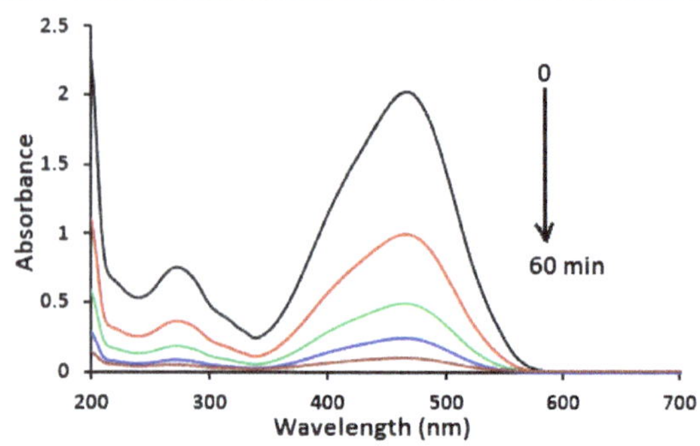

Fig. 6 Electronic absorption spectra showing continued mineralization of methyl orange under photo-degradation conditions. Reaction was conducted using methyl orange solution (100 mL, 10 ppm), at 20 °C, under 19.0 mW/cm^2 total radiation intensity, pH ~7, and ZnO (0.1 g)

natural waters normally have pH values in the range 5–8 [56, 57].

The pH value affects the ZnO surface OH groups [58], the methylene orange and the aqueous solution species. The pH value affects the generation of the oxidizing species (•OH, $O_2\bullet^-$, H_2O_2 and $HO_2\bullet$) that result in the reaction system [59, 60]. The nature of methyl orange molecule varies with pH value, as stated above. ZnO has a point of zero charge at pH 9.0, above which the ZnO surface is predominantly negatively charged [13]. The electrical properties of the ZnO surface may thus vary with the pH.

Experiments were carried out at pH values of (2.5, 5, 7, 9 and 11), Fig. 7. The slightly acidic solution (pH ~5) showed highest T.N. and Q.Y. values, followed by neutral solution. Both solutions with pH 5 and 7 showed complete removal of methyl orange after 60 min of irradiation. As discussed above removal of methyl orange involves complete mineralization, which shows the practicality of using the photo-degradation in natural systems. More acidic or basic solutions (less 2.5 or higher than 9) showed T.N. and Q.Y. values nearly half of those under mild solutions. Table 1 summarizes these results.

In basic media, ZnO becomes $Zn(OH)_2$ form with lower semiconducting properties [61]. Under lower pH conditions the lowering in removal efficiency is possibly due to the dissolution of ZnO into Zn^{2+} ions [62], and in highly basic media the ZnO yields zincate ion ZnO_2^{-2} [63]. The results show that the optimum photo-degradation is close to natural water conditions (neutral to slightly acidic), which adds to the credibility of using ZnO catalyst system. Therefore, unless otherwise stated, all results described here-in-after were obtained under initial nominal pH 7.

Table 1 Effect of pH on photo-degradation of aqueous methyl orange. Reactions were conducted using methyl orange solutions (100 mL, 10 ppm) and ZnO (0.1 g) at 20 °C under total radiation intensity 19.0 mW/cm^2

pH	~7	~5	~2.5	~9	~11
T.N.	1.62×10^{-3}	1.94×10^{-3}	1.17×10^{-3}	8.42×10^{-4}	6.71×10^{-4}
Q.Y.	4.36×10^{-4}	4.28×10^{-4}	2.92×10^{-4}	2.12×10^{-4}	1.74×10^{-4}
% Degradation	100 %	100 %	73 %	60 %	48 %

Effect of temperature

At temperatures in the range 20–40 °C, the ZnO catalyst showed sound activity, reaching up to 85 % methyl orange removal within 60 min. At lower temperatures, ~ 10 °C, the reaction went slower, reaching up to 65 % removal within 60 min. Figure 8 shows effect of working temperature on the methyl orange phtodegradation reaction profiles. If left for longer time, methyl orange is expected to continue even at lower temperatures. Table 2 summarizes values of TN, QY and degradation% measured at different temperatures. The results show the applicability of using the ZnO system in removing methyl orange with simulated solar light. In this work, unless otherwise stated, all study was performed at 20 °C.

If higher temperatures (above 45 °C) are used, the reaction goes slower. This is due to possible escape of the oxygen molecules dissolved inside oxygen. The oxygen molecules are involved with the mechanism of photodegradation reaction. Similar results were observed in earlier reports [53].

Effect of CO_2 and other gas flows

The effect of CO_2 flow on methyl orange photo-degradation was investigated by measuring the reaction profiles for the process while passing a flow of CO_2 gas. The stream of CO_2 (90 mL/min), while keeping all other

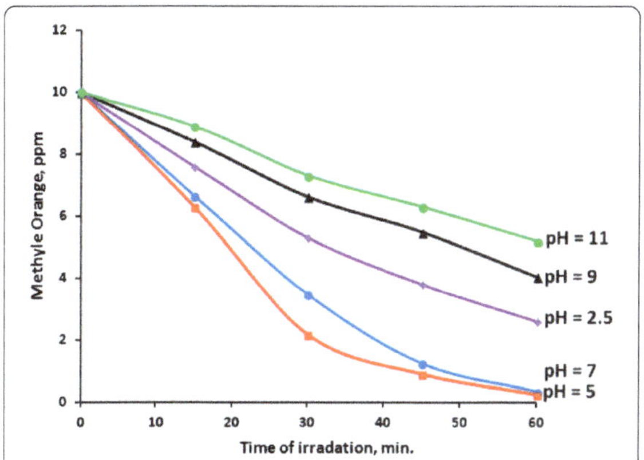

Fig. 7 Effect of pH on photo-degradation of aqueous methyl orange. Reactions were conducted using methyl orange solutions (100 mL, 10 ppm) and ZnO (0.1 g) at 20 °C under total radiation intensity 19.0 mW/cm^2

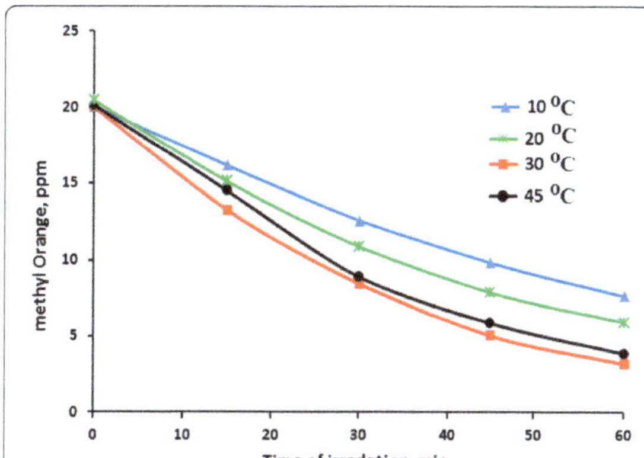

Fig. 8 Effect of temperature on methyl orange photo-degradation. Reactions were conducted using methyl orange solution (100 mL, 20 ppm) at different temperatures, using ZnO catalyst (0.1 g) under total irradiation intensity of 19.0 mW/cm^2 at pH ~7

Table 2 Effect of temperature on methyl orange photo-degradation. Reactions were conducted using methyl orange solution (100 mL, 20 ppm) at different temperatures, using ZnO catalyst (0.1 g) under total irradiation intensity of 19.0 mW/cm^2 at pH ~7

Temp.	10 °C	20 °C	30 °C	45 °C
T.N.	1.86×10^{-3}	2.38×10^{-3}	2.87×10^{-3}	2.80×10^{-3}
Q.Y.	3.52×10^{-4}	4.28×10^{-4}	5.44×10^{-4}	5.29×10^{-4}
% Degradation	62 %	70 %	84 %	81 %

Table 3 Effect of gas streams on methyl orange photo-degradation. Reactions were conducted using methyl orange solution (100 mL, 20 ppm) under 19.0 mW/cm^2 irradiation using ZnO (0.1 g) with continuous stirring at 20 °C

	Exposed to air only	Air flow	N_2 flow open system	CO_2 and air flows together	CO_2 flow
T.N.	2.87×10^{-3}	1.72×10^{-3}	1.44×10^{-3}	0.75×10^{-3}	1.03×10^{-3}
Q.Y.	5.44×10^{-4}	3.25×10^{-4}	2.72×10^{-4}	1.42×10^{-4}	1.95×10^{-4}
% Degradation	84 %	52 %	50 %	25 %	19 %

reaction parameters the same, significantly slowed down the removal of the methyl orange, as shown in Fig. 9. Table 3 summarizes values of TN, QY and degradation% while using CO_2 gas stream. The mode of action of CO_2 on lowering the reaction rate is not due to lowering the solution pH, as the pH was lowered only slightly, from 6.8 (the nominal used pH) to 6.4, after 60 min. As discussed above the pH in the range 5–8 does not inhibit methyl orange removal process. Alternatively, the mode of action of CO_2 is thus due to its ability to react with the radicals formed during the photo-degradation process. As reported earlier, *"CO_2 may interact with some free radical species and may either propagate or inhibit free radical chain reactions"* [64]. In this work the CO_2 clearly inhibits photo-degradation of methyl orange by interacting with the free radicals believed to be formed during the reaction process. The results reflect a warning signal about the negative impact of possible

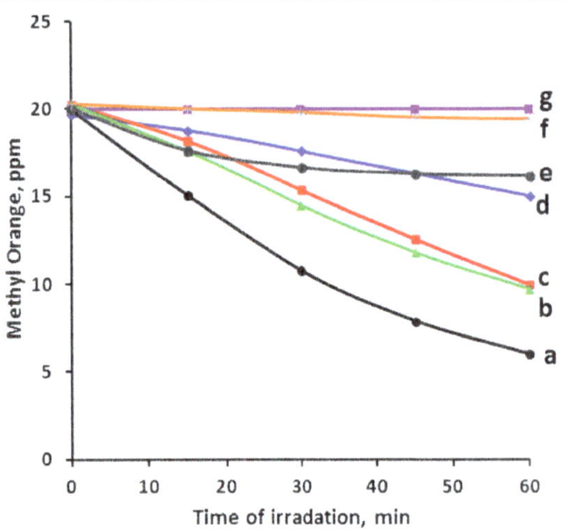

Fig. 9 Effect of gas streams on methyl orange photo-degradation. Reactions were conducted using methyl orange solution (100 mL, 20 ppm) under 19.0 mW/cm^2 irradiation using ZnO (0.1 g) with continuous stirring at 20 °C with different gas flows: (**a**) exposed to air only, (**b**) air flow, (**c**) N_2 flow open system, (**d**) CO_2 and air flows together, (**e**) CO_2 flow, (**f**) closed system with nitrogen flow, (**g**) N_2 and CO_2 flows together

CO_2 higher concentrations in natural waters, which would result from increased atmospheric CO_2 concentration. Having natural waters with higher CO_2 concentrations may negatively affect future water purification processes.

CO_2 gas stream may arguably affect photodegradation rate by removing oxygen dissolved in the reaction mixture. This was investigated using two continuous streams of CO_2 and air together. Figure 9 shows that using the air (1000 mL/min) stream with the CO_2 stream (90 mL/min) did not show significant enhancement in photo-degradation reaction rate. This result further confirms the discussion above, where CO_2 captures the free radicals necessary for the photodegradation to occur.

Adding a stream of air alone did not increase the reaction rate. Figure 9 shows that the air stream lowered the reaction rate by about 25 % compared to experiments conducted under normal air. In a well known mechanism [40], oxygen molecule is assumed to abstract one electron from the excited ZnO particle leading to $O_2{\bullet}^-$ radical anion species as explained in the equation [$e^- + O_2 \rightarrow O_2{\bullet}^-$]. The $O_2{\bullet}^-$ species is believed to react with the other H_2O_2 resulting species to yield the chemically active OH$^\cdot$ radical as in the equation [$H_2O_2 + O_2{\bullet}^- \rightarrow OH^{\bullet} + OH^- + O_2$]. This radical is assumed to react with an organic contaminant molecule and degrade it.

Therefore, the presence of O_2 in water is necessary. However, as the results here show, excess of O_2 in water inhibits the photodegradation reaction. This is due to the adverse effect of excess O_2 which blocks $OH^{\bullet}$ radical as shown in equation [$H_2O_2 + O_2{\bullet}^- \rightarrow OH^{\bullet} + OH^- + O_2$].

Adding nitrogen to the reaction mixture together with CO_2 practically stopped the reaction progress (Fig. 9). The effect is perhaps dual in nature, where the CO_2 behaves as scavenger, as discussed above, while the nitrogen lowers concentration of oxygen that is necessary for the reaction to proceed. Adding a nitrogen flow (240 mL/min) to the reaction mixture, while exposed to atmospheric air, slowed down the process, but did not stop it completely. Nitrogen lowers concentrations of oxygen in the reaction but traces are left therein which are enough for the reaction to occur. All reactions above were conducted under exposure to atmospheric air. This is evident because complete coverage from air while under nitrogen stream caused complete reaction inhibition.

Effect of contaminant concentration

The effect of methyl orange concentration (10, 20, 30 and 40 ppm) on its photodegradation process was studied, Fig. 10. Values of percent methyl orange removal, after 60 min, were 100 % for 10 ppm, 70 % for 20 ppm, 66 % for 30 ppm, 45 % for 40 ppm, as summarized in Table 4. Despite the lowering in removal percentage with higher contaminant concentration, the average reaction rate increased. Values of T.N. and Q.Y. show comparable values for the 20, 30, and 40 ppm concentrations. Lower values were observed for the 10 ppm concentration, which is due to the fact that all added methyl orange molecules were mineralized with no more left. This naturally yields lower TN and QY values at lower contaminant concentrations. The results indicate the suitability of ZnO catalyst to function over a relatively wide range of contaminant concentrations. More importantly, the catalyst completely activates mineralization of low contaminant concentrations, which are more likely to occur in nature [37, 53].

Effect of catalyst nominal amount on photo-degradation process

Catalyst amount may affect photo-degradation processes. The effect of catalyst nominal amount on the photodegradation of methyl orange was investigated using different amounts of ZnO (0.05, 0.10, 0.20 or 0.30 g) in 100 mL solution of 10 ppm methyl orange, under 19.0 mW/cm^2 irradiation intensity. Figure 11 shows that the average reaction rate was unchanged with

Table 4 Effect of contaminant concentration on its photo-degradation. Reactions were conducted using different contaminant concentrations in aqueous solution (100 mL), pH ~7, at 20 °C with ZnO (0.1 g) under 19.0 mW/cm^2 irradiation intensity

	10 ppm	20 ppm	30 ppm	40 ppm
T.N.	1.73×10^{-3}	2.38×10^{-3}	2.37×10^{-3}	2.29×10^{-3}
Q.Y.	4.36×10^{-4}	4.28×10^{-4}	4.48×10^{-4}	4.17×10^{-4}
% Degradation	100 %	70 %	66 %	45 %

catalyst nominal amount. The T.N. value decreased with increasing ZnO amount, as shown in Table 5. This means that the relative efficiency of the catalyst is lowered by increasing catalyst loading. Similar results were observed in other photo-degradation processes [37, 53, 54, 65, 66]. This is attributed to the increased blocking of light with higher catalyst loading. With more catalyst particles, the short wave tail photons are not able to enter the reaction mixture, and the ZnO particles in the reaction mixture do not receive photons. Similar behaviors have been observed in earlier studies [14, 64, 65].

The QY value showed an increase with increasing nominal catalyst amount at the beginning, but then slightly decreased. Again the lowering in QY is due to the blocking of light by the abundant ZnO particles at the mixture surface which prevent photons from reaching other catalyst sites [14, 37, 53, 54, 65–67]. Agglomeration of smaller ZnO particles into larger ones, in case of higher concentrations, may also play a role, as the total number of surface active sites may decrease [67]. The results indicate that using smaller amounts of catalyst enhanced catalyst efficiency without lowering the average reaction rate or the removal percentage. This is

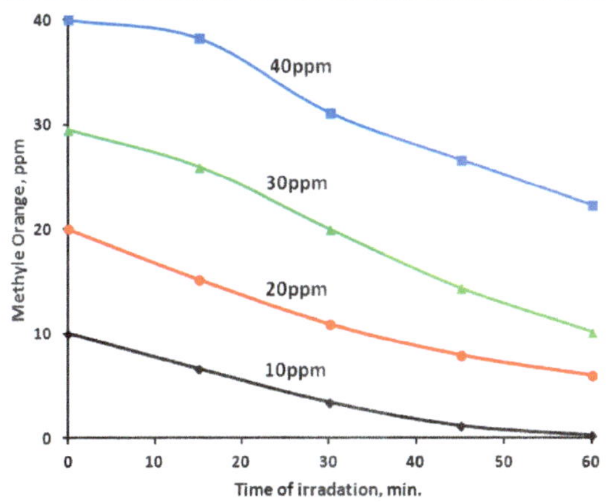

Fig. 10 Effect of contaminant concentration on its photo-degradation. Reactions were conducted using different contaminant concentrations in aqueous solution (100 mL), pH ~7, at 20 °C with ZnO (0.1 g) under 19.0 mW/cm^2 irradiation intensity

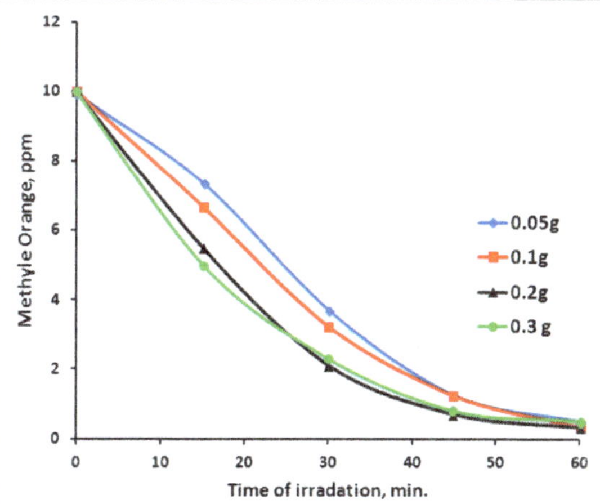

Fig. 11 Effect of catalyst amount on methyl orange photo-degradation. Reactions were conducted using methyl orange solution (100 mL, 10 ppm) at 20 °C pH ~7, under 19.0 mW/cm^2

Table 5 Effect of catalyst amount on methyl orange photodegradation. Reactions were conducted using methyl orange solution (100 mL, 10 ppm) at 20 °C pH ~7, under 19.0 mW/cm^2

	0.05 g	0.10 g	0.20 g	0.3 g
T.N.	3.10×10^{-3}	1.68×10^{-3}	9.82×10^{-4}	9.57×10^{-4}
Q.Y.	2.93×10^{-4}	3.19×10^{-4}	3.72×10^{-4}	3.62×19^{-4}
% Degradation	95 %	100 %	100 %	100 %

a positive feature of the ZnO catalyst described here, as in case of treating natural waters, smaller amounts of catalyst will be highly favored.

Effect of light intensity on the photodegraation process

The effect of incident light intensity on photodegradation rate of methyl orange was investigated, using solutions (100 mL each) with two different concentrations (10 and 20 ppm). Experiments were conducted under different light intensities using 0.10 g of ZnO lab prepared powder. In each contaminant concentration, four different light intensities (1.90, 5.12, 8.78 and 19.0 mW/cm^2) were used. This range includes the average reported daylight intensity of 120 W/m^2 (12 mW/cm^2) [68]. Figure 12 shows how methyl orange removal percentage changed with illumination intensity in a period of 30 min for each contaminant concentration. For the 10 ppm concentration case, up to 100 % removal was observed for the higher radiation intensities (5.12, 8.78, and 19 mW/cm^2), and up to 50 % removal for the lower intensity (1.9 mW/cm^2), in 30 min. For the 20 ppm concentration case, up to 70 % contaminant removal was observed in 30 min (at the higher radiation intensities, and up to 35 % at the lower irradiation intensity). The results indicate the applicability of using ZnO in removing methyl orange from contaminated water even under radiation intensities lower than normal day light.

Table 6 Effect of light intensity on methyl orange photodegradation. Reactions were conducted using two different methyl orange concentrations in 100 mL solution at pH ~7 with ZnO (0.1 g) at 20 °C

10 ppm				
	1.90 mW/cm^2	5.12 mW/cm^2	8.78 mW/cm^2	19.0 mW/cm^2
T.N.	6.96×10^{-4}	1.5×10^{-3}	1.58×10^{-3}	1.73×10^{-3}
Q.Y.	1.42×10^{-3}	1.35×10^{-3}	6.57×10^{-4}	4.36×10^{-4}
% Degradation	54 %	95 %	96 %	100 %
20 ppm				
	1.90 mW/cm^2	5.12 mW/cm^2	8.78 mW/cm^2	19.0 mW/cm^2
T.N.	7.96×10^{-4}	1.86×10^{-3}	1.99×10^{-3}	2.38×10^{-3}
Q.Y.	1.62×10^{-3}	1.41×10^{-3}	8.76×10^{-4}	4.28×10^{-4}
% Degradation	34 %	58 %	65 %	70 %

Values of TN and QY calculated after 30 min for each case are shown in Table 6. In case of 10 ppm, the lower irradiation intensity (1.9 mW/cm^2) showed lower TN value (about 50 %) than its higher intensity counterparts (5.12, 8.78, and 19 mW/cm^2). From the Table and the Figure, it can be seen that under 5.12 mW/cm^2 or higher, the removal percentage reaches approximately constant value. With lower intensity, lower TN value should be expected, as less photons are available for the catalyst sites. However, as radiation intensity is increased above 5.12 mW/cm^2, efficiency of light harvesting becomes less. This is evident from values of QY, which decreased when using higher irradiation intensities.

For the 20 ppm methyl orange concentration, similar behavior occurred, but the irradiation intensity 5.12 mW/cm^2 showed highest QY. Collectively the results suggest

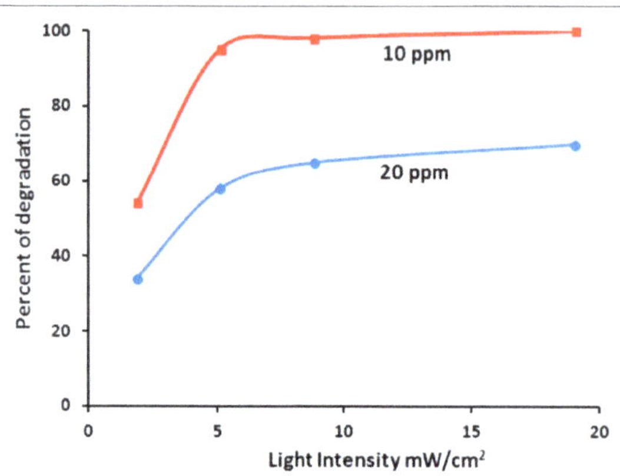

Fig. 12 Effect of light intensity on methyl orange photodegradation. Reactions were conducted using two different methyl orange concentrations in 100 mL solution at pH ~7 with ZnO (0.1 g) at 20 °C

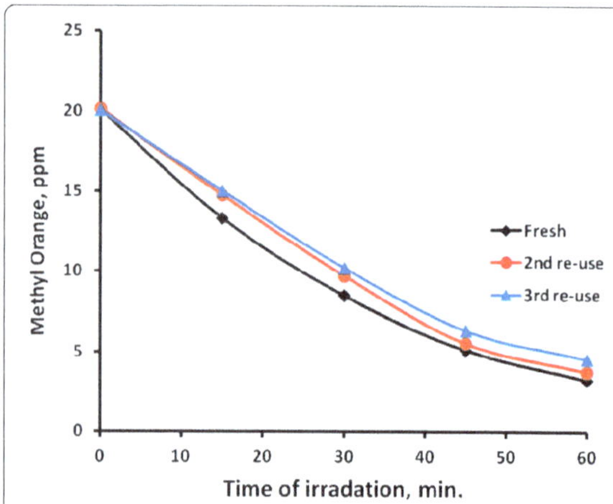

Fig. 13 Effect of catalyst reuse on methyl orange photo-degradation. Reactions were conducted using fresh methyl orange solutions (100 mL, 20 ppm) in multiple use of the ZnO catalyst (0.1 g) at 20 °C, pH 7 under 19.0 mW/cm^2 irradiation intensity

that it is not necessary to use high irradiation intensities to remove methyl orange from water. This adds to the applicability of using ZnO in natural water purification processes in different environments with different light intensities.

Catalyst re-use experiments

Reusability of the ZnO catalyst for methyl orange photodegradation in water was studied, by adding fresh amount of methyl orange to the stirred solution after earlier reaction cessation. Figure 13 shows reaction profiles for three time reuse experiments. The Figure shows that at the beginning of each reuse experiment, the measured amount of the methyl orange was 20 ppm. This is due to complete removal of the earlier methyl orange contaminant in the preceding study, as the reaction was left for enough time. In each experiment, after 60 min time of exposure, more than 80 % removal was achieved, showing only low loss of efficiency with reuse.

The amount of Zn^{2+} ions resulting from dissolution of the used ZnO catalyst (with different amounts 0.05–0.3 g per 100 mL solution) during photo-degradation experiments in neutral media was measured by AAS, and was found to be 6 ppm, when the mixture was left overnight. In case of more acidic media the amount was higher, up to 8 ppm. This indicates that only a small fraction of ZnO dissolved under the working conditions. Based on literature [69] the value for solubility of Zn ions resulting from nano-scale ZnO is about 7 ppm. The WHO recommended upper limit for Zn ions is ~5 ppm [70]. The Zn^{2+} ions dissolved in this work is not far from the recommended WHO threshold limits. The results add to the credibility of using ZnO in purification of natural waters.

Conclusion

Nano-scale ZnO particles can be effectively used as catalysts for complete mineralization of methyl orange in water with solar simulated light. The catalyst can be effectively used under different working conditions (including temperature and pH) that resemble natural waters, and can thus be investigated at larger scale in natural water purification. Adding streams of air, CO_2 gas, and/or N_2 gases may affect the reaction progress and may inhibit the reaction.

Competing interests

The authors declare that they have no competing interests.

Authors' contributions

AZ participated in supervising research, catalytic experimental design, experimental work, data analysis and writing up. AZ performed catalytic experiments. DP and GC conducted advanced characterization. MH participated with writing up, library search and research ideas. The preparations and catalytic study were performed in H. S. H. laboratory. He participated in writing up, provided technical solutions and new ideas. All authors read and approved the final manuscript.

Acknowledgement

The thrust of this work has been done at SSERL, Department of Chemistry, ANU. The authors wish to thank the technical staff at ANU for help. XRD and SEM measurements were performed in the laboratories of Dansuk Industrial Co., LTD., South Korea.

Author details

[1]SSERL, Department of Chemistry, An-Najah National University, Nablus, Palestine. [2]College of Pharmacy and Nutrition, University of Saskatchewan, 116 Thorvaldson Building, Saskatoon S7N 5C9, Canada. [3]Dansuk Industrial Co, LTD. #1239-5, Jeongwang-Dong, Shiheung-Si, Kyonggi-Do 429-913, South Korea. [4]Institut de Chimie de la Matie're Condense'ie de Bordeaux (ICMCB), 87 Avenue du Dr. A Schweitzer, Pessac 33608, France.

References

1. Bianco Prevot A, Baiocchi C, Brussino MC, Pramauro E, Savarino P, Augugliaro V, et al. Photocatalytic degradation of acid blue 80 in aqueous solutions containing TiO_2 suspensions. Environ Sci Technol. 2001;35:971–6.
2. McMullan G, Meehan C, Conneely A, Kirby N, Robinson T, Nigam P, et al. Microbial decolourisation and degradation of textile dyes. Appl Microbiol Biotechnol. 2001;56:81–7.
3. Pearce C, Lloyd J, Guthrie J. The removal of colour from textile wastewater using whole bacterial cells: a review. Dyes and Pigments. 2003;58:179–96.
4. Marcucci M, Nosenzo G, Capannelli G, Ciabatti I, Corrieri D, Ciardelli G. Treatment and reuse of textile effluents based on new ultrafiltration and other membrane technologies. Desalination. 2001;138:75–82.
5. Robinson T, McMullan G, Marchant R, Nigam P. Remediation of dyes in textile effluent: a critical review on current treatment technologies with a proposed alternative. Bioresour Technol. 2001;77:247–55.
6. Tahir S, Rauf N. Removal of a cationic dye from aqueous solutions by adsorption onto bentonite clay. Chemosphere. 2006;63:1842–8.
7. Arslan I, Akmehmet Balcioğlu I, Tuhkanen T. Oxidative treatment of simulated dyehouse effluent by UV and near-UV light assisted Fenton's reagent. Chemosphere. 1999;39:2767–83.
8. Kuo W. Decolorizing dye wastewater with Fenton's reagent. Water Res. 1992;26:881–6.
9. Rice RG. Applications of ozone for industrial wastewater treatment—a review. Ozone Sci Eng. 1996;18:477–515.
10. Dodd MC, Buffle M-O, Von Gunten U. Oxidation of antibacterial molecules by aqueous ozone: moiety-specific reaction kinetics and application to ozone-based wastewater treatment. Environ Sci Technol. 2006;40:1969–77.
11. Glaze WH, Kang J-W, Chapin DH. The chemistry of water treatment processes involving ozone, hydrogen peroxide and ultraviolet radiation. Environ Sci Technol. 1987;39(10):3409–20.
12. Herrmann J-M. Heterogeneous photocatalysis: fundamentals and applications to the removal of various types of aqueous pollutants. Catal Today. 1999;53:115–29.
13. Daneshvar N, Salari D, Khataee A. Photocatalytic degradation of azo dye acid red 14 in water on ZnO as an alternative catalyst to TiO_2. J Photochem Photobiol A Chem. 2004;162:317–22.
14. Mai F, Chen C, Chen J, Liu S. Photodegradation of methyl green using visible irradiation in ZnO suspensions: determination of the reaction pathway and identification of intermediates by a high-performance liquid chromatography–photodiode array-electrospray ionization-mass spectrometry method. J Chromatogr A. 2008;1189:355–65.
15. Turchi CS, Ollis DF. Photocatalytic degradation of organic water contaminants: mechanisms involving hydroxyl radical attack. J Catal. 1990;122:178–92.
16. Umebayashi T, Yamaki T, Tanaka S, Asai K. Visible light-induced degradation of methylene blue on S-doped TiO2. Chem Lett. 2003;32:330–1.
17. Tayade RJ, Surolia PK, Kulkarni RG, Jasra RV. Photocatalytic degradation of dyes and organic contaminants in water using nanocrystalline anatase and rutile TiO_2. Sci Technol Adv Mater. 2007;8:455–62.
18. Ding Z, Zhu H, Lu G, Greenfield P. Photocatalytic properties of Titania pillared clays by different drying methods. J Colloid Interface Sci. 1999;209:193–9.
19. Fox MA, Dulay MT. Heterogeneous photocatalysis. Chem Rev. 1993;93:341–57.

20. Hagfeldt A, Graetzel M. Light-induced redox reactions in nanocrystalline systems. Chem Rev. 1995;95:49–68.
21. Hoffmann MR, Martin ST, Choi W, Bahnemann DW. Environmental applications of semiconductor photocatalysis. Chem Rev. 1995;95:69–96.
22. Panayotov DA, Yates JT. Spectroscopic detection of hydrogen atom spillover from Au nanoparticles supported on TiO_2: use of conduction band electrons. J Phys Chem C. 2007;111:2959–64.
23. Hong W-K, Sohn JI, Hwang D-K, Kwon S-S, Jo G, Song S, et al. Tunable electronic transport characteristics of surface-architecture-controlled ZnO nanowire field effect transistors. Nano Lett. 2008;8:950–6.
24. Dorfman A, Kumar N, Hahm J-i. Nanoscale ZnO-enhanced fluorescence detection of protein interactions. Adv Mater. 2006;18:2685–90.
25. Bao J, Zimmler MA, Capasso F, Wang X, Ren Z. Broadband ZnO single-nanowire light-emitting diode. Nano Lett. 2006;6:1719–22.
26. Law M, Greene LE, Johnson JC, Saykally R, Yang P. Nanowire dye-sensitized solar cells. Nat Mater. 2005;4:455–9.
27. Sakthivel S, Neppolian B, Shankar M, Arabindoo B, Palanichamy M, Murugesan V. Solar photocatalytic degradation of azo dye: comparison of photocatalytic efficiency of ZnO and TiO_2. Sol Energy Mater Sol Cells. 2003;77:65–82.
28. Gouvea CA, Wypych F, Moraes SG, Duran N, Nagata N, Peralta-Zamora P. Semiconductor-assisted photocatalytic degradation of reactive dyes in aqueous solution. Chemosphere. 2000;40:433–40.
29. Lizama C, Freer J, Baeza J, Mansilla HD. Optimized photodegradation of reactive blue 19 on TiO2 and ZnO suspensions. Catal Today. 2002;76:235–46.
30. Lachheb H, Puzenat E, Houas A, Ksibi M, Elaloui E, Guillard C, et al. Photocatalytic degradation of various types of dyes (Alizarin S, Crocein Orange G, Methyl Red, Congo Red, Methylene Blue) in water by UV-irradiated titania. Appl Catal Environ. 2002;39:75–90.
31. Kandavelu V, Kastien H, Thampi KR. Photocatalytic degradation of isothiazolin-3-ones in water and emulsion paints containing nanocrystalline TiO_2 and ZnO catalysts. Appl Catal Environ. 2004;48:101–11.
32. MSDS. Material Safety Data Sheet,Methyl orange MSDS, Fisher Scientific, 1 Reagent Lane, Fair Lawn, NJ 07410. 2000.
33. Sandberg RG, Henderson GH, White RD, Eyring EM. Kinetics of acid dissociation-ion recombination of aqueous methyl orange. J Phys Chem. 1972;76:4023–5.
34. Windholz M, Budavari S. The merck index. Merck and Co. Rahway; 1983.
35. Maynard C. Riegel's Handbook of Industrial Chemistry. In Book Riegel's Handbook of Industrial Chemistry (Editor ed.^eds.). City: JA Kent, ed; 1983.
36. Shih Y-H, Tso C-P, Tung L-Y. Rapid degradation of methyl orange with nanoscale zerovalent iron particles. Nanotechnology. 2010;7:16–7.
37. Hilal HS, Al-Nour GY, Zyoud A, Helal MH, Saadeddin I. Pristine and supported ZnO-based catalysts for phenazopyridine degradation with direct solar light. Solid State Sci. 2010;12:578–86.
38. Hilal SH, Nour G, Zyoud A. Photo-degradation of Methyl Orange with Direct Solar Light Using ZnO and Activated Carbon-supported ZnO. In: Water purification. New York: Nova Science Publishers, Inc; 2009. p. 227–46.
39. Hejjawi S. TiO_2 and ZnO photocatalysts for degradation of widespread pharmaceutical wastes: Effect of particle size and support. MSc Thesis, An-Najah N. University. 2013.
40. Amer H. ZnO nano-particle catalysts in contaminant degradation processes with solar light naked and supported systems. MSc Thesis, An-Najah N. University. 2012.
41. Gupta A, Bhatti H, Kumar D, Verma N, Tandon R. Nano and bulk crystals of ZnO: synthesis and characterization. Digest Int J Nanomat Biostruct. 2006;1:1–9.
42. Lopez-Romero S. Growth and characterization of ZnO cross-like structures by hydrothermal method. Matéria (Rio de Janeiro). 2009;14:977–82.
43. Akhtar MJ, Ahamed M, Kumar S, Khan MM, Ahmad J, Alrokayan SA. Zinc oxide nanoparticles selectively induce apoptosis in human cancer cells through reactive oxygen species. Int J Nanomedicine. 2012;7:845.
44. Dai K, Chen H, Peng T, Ke D, Yi H. Photocatalytic degradation of methyl orange in aqueous suspension of mesoporous Titania nanoparticles. Chemosphere. 2007;69:1361–7.
45. Attia AJ, Kadhim SH, Hussein FH. Photocatalytic degradation of textile dyeing wastewater using titanium dioxide and zinc oxide. J Chem. 2008;5:219–23.
46. Chen C, Wang Z, Ruan S, Zou B, Zhao M, Wu F. Photocatalytic degradation of CI Acid Orange 52 in the presence of Zn-doped TiO_2 prepared by a stearic acid gel method. Dyes Pigments. 2008;77:204–9.
47. Zhou G, Deng J. Preparation and photocatalytic performance of Ag/ZnO nano-composites. Mater Sci Semicond Process. 2007;10:90–6.
48. Wang H, Xie C, Zhang W, Cai S, Yang Z, Gui Y. Comparison of dye degradation efficiency using ZnO powders with various size scales. J Hazard Mater. 2007;141:645–52.
49. Yu D, Cai R, Liu Z. Studies on the photodegradation of rhodamine dyes on nanometer-sized zinc oxide. Spectrochim Acta A Mol Biomol Spectrosc. 2004;60:1617–24.
50. Daneshvar N, Aber S, Dorraji MS, Khataee A, Rasoulifard M. Preparation and investigation of photocatalytic properties of ZnO nanocrystals: effect of operational parameters and kinetic study. Evaluation. 2008;900:6.
51. Shvalagin V, Stroyuk A, Kotenko I, Kuchmii SY. Photocatalytic formation of porous CdS/ZnO nanospheres and CdS nanotubes. Theor Exp Chem. 2007;43:229–34.
52. Byrappa K, Subramani A, Ananda S, Rai KL, Sunitha M, Basavalingu B, et al. Impregnation of ZnO onto activated carbon under hydrothermal conditions and its photocatalytic properties. J Mater Sci. 2006;41:1355–62.
53. Zyoud AH, Zaatar N, Saadeddin I, Ali C, Park D, Campet G, et al. CdS-sensitized TiO_2 in phenazopyridine photo-degradation: Catalyst efficiency, stability and feasibility assessment. J Hazard Mater. 2010;173:318–25.
54. Zyoud A, Zaatar N, Saadeddin I, Helal MH, Campet G, Hakim M, et al. Alternative natural dyes in water purification: anthocyanin as TiO_2-sensitizer in methyl orange photo-degradation. Solid State Sci. 2011;13:1268–75.
55. Hilal SH, Nour G, Zyoud A. Photo-degradation of methyl orange with direct solar light using ZnO and activated carbon-supported ZnO. Chapter Book Water Purif. 2009;Chapter 6:227–46.
56. Neal C, Hill T, Alexander S, Reynolds B, Hill S, Dixon AJ, et al. Stream water quality in acid sensitive UK upland areas; an example of potential water quality remediation based on groundwater manipulation. Hydrol Earth Syst Sci Discuss. 1997;1:185–96.
57. Hem JD. Study and interpretation of the chemical characteristics of natural water. Water Supply Paper 2254, Department of the Interior, US Geological Survey; Alexandria, 1985.
58. Zhang F, Zhao J, Shen T, Hidaka H, Pelizzetti E, Serpone N. TiO_2-assisted photodegradation of dye pollutants II. Adsorption and degradation kinetics of eosin in TiO_2 dispersions under visible light irradiation. Appl Catal Environ. 1998;15:147–56.
59. Chang C, Hsieh Y, Cheng K, Hsieh L, Cheng T, Yao K. Effect of pH on Fenton process using estimation of hydroxyl radical with salicylic acid as trapping reagent. 2008.
60. Zepp RG, Faust BC, Hoigne J. Hydroxyl radical formation in aqueous reactions (pH 3–8) of iron (II) with hydrogen peroxide: the photo-Fenton reaction. Environ Sci Technol. 1992;26:313–9.
61. Velmurugan R, Swaminathan M. An efficient nanostructured ZnO for dye sensitized degradation of reactive red 120 dye under solar light. Sol Energy Mater Sol Cells. 2011;95:942–50.
62. Marci G, Augugliaro V, Lopez-Munoz MJ, Martin C, Palmisano L, Rives V, et al. Preparation characterization and photocatalytic activity of polycrystalline ZnO/TiO2 systems. 2. Surface, bulk characterization, and 4-nitrophenol photodegradation in liquid–solid regime. J Phys Chem B. 2001;105:1033–40.
63. Laudise ER, Kolb E, Laboralories BT, Hiti IM, Jeriey N. The solubility of zincite in basic hydrothermal solvents. Amer Mineral. 1963;48:642.
64. Vesela A, Wilhelm J. The role of carbon dioxide in free radical reactions in organism. Physiol Res. 2002;51:335–40.
65. Zyoud AH, Hilal HS. Silica-supported CdS-sensitized TiO_2 particles in photo-driven water purification: Assessment of efficiency, stability and recovery future perspectives. Chapter in a book, Water Purification, Novascience Pub, NY (in Press, 2008) 2009.
66. Hilal HS, Nour GY, Zyoud A. Photodegradation of Methyl orange and phenazopyridine HCl with direct solar light using ZnO and activated carbonsupported ZnO, Water Purification Novascience Publ, NY. 2009. p. 227e246.
67. Chen C-C. Degradation pathways of ethyl violet by photocatalytic reaction with ZnO dispersions. J Mol Catal A Chem. 2007;264:82–92.
68. Guide W. Guide to Meteorological Instruments and Methods of Observation. In: Book Guide to Meteorological Instruments and Methods of Observation. Genf, Schweiz: Secretariat of the WMO; 2006.
69. Reed RB, Ladner DA, Higgins CP, Westerhoff P, Ranville JF. Solubility of nano-zinc oxide in environmentally and biologically important matrices. Environ Toxicol Chem. 2012;31:93–9.
70. Krenkel P. Water quality management. Elsevier; Burlington, e-Book 2012.

The impacts of land cover types on urban outdoor thermal environment: the case of Beijing, China

Hai Yan[1,2] and Li Dong[1*]

Abstract

Background: This study investigated the microclimatic behavior of different land cover types in urban parks and, the correlation between air temperature and land cover composition to understand how land cover affects outdoor thermal environment during hot summer.

Methods: To address this issue, air temperatures were measured on four different land cover types at four observation sites inside an urban park in Beijing, China, meanwhile, the land cover composition of each site was quantified with CAD, by drawing corresponding areas on the aerial photographs.

Results: The results showed that the average air temperature difference among four land cover types was large during the day and small during the night. At noon, the average air temperature differed significantly among four land cover types, whereas on night, there was no significant difference among different land cover types. Results of the linear regression indicated that during daytime, there was a strong negative correlation between air temperature and percent tree cover; while at nighttime, a significant negative correlation was observed between air temperature and percent lawn cover. It was shown that as the percent tree cover increased by 10 %, the air temperature decreased by 0.26 °C during daytime, while as the percent lawn cover increased by 10 %, the air temperature decreased by 0.56 °C during nighttime.

Conclusions: Results of this study help to clarify the effects of land cover on urban outdoor thermal environment, and can provide assistance to urban planner and designer for improving green space planning and design in the future.

Keywords: Urban heat island, Urban park, Vegetation, Air temperature, Land cover

Introduction

In the last decades, a great concentration of people around urban areas took place worldwide. The urbanization process, with its fast population increase, creates changes in the urban climate [1]. A distinct feature of urban climate is the urban heat island (UHI) effect, in which the urban air temperature is higher than the air temperature of the surrounding rural or suburban areas [2]. UHI has significant negative effects on the buildings energy consumption, outdoor air quality, living environment, and habitability of cities [3, 4]. With increasing urbanization, the urban heat island will affect a larger number of urban residents. Therefore, there is a pressing need for urban researchers to evaluate strategies that may mitigate against further increases in temperatures in urban areas.

Among all cooling measures, planting of vegetation in urban areas is one of the simplest and most effective strategies to mitigate the UHI effect [5, 6]. Urban green areas can ameliorate UHI effect by the combined impact of shading and evapotranspiration. A series of field measurement studies show that vegetated areas are likely to be cooler than their surrounding urban built environment [7–10]. This vegetated cool patch within the warmer built-up environment is referred to as a "park cool island" (PCI). In a study, by Jansson et al. [11], temperatures of an urban vegetated park and its surroundings in central Stockholm were measured during three summer days, the results indicated that the PCI intensity was in the range of 0.5–0.8 °C during the day and reached a maximum of 2 °C at sunset. In Mexico City, Jauregui [12] found that the air temperature of a large irrigated park was 3–4 °C cooler than its built-up surroundings. Similar results were also obtained from a study of two urban parks in Singapore

* Correspondence: dongli@bjfu.edu.cn
[1]College of Landscape Architecture, Beijing Forestry University, Beijing 100083, China
Full list of author information is available at the end of the article

[13]. The cooling effect of urban parks in cities has been confirmed by the above studies. However, the physical constitution of the parks, such as the type of pavements, the amount of tree and grass cover and the floristic structure of vegetation can be expected to affect the cooling effect [14]. Cao et al. [15], based on remote sensing data, studied the effects of park characteristics on the formation of PCI in Nagoya, and found that PCI intensity is clearly related to the area of tree and shrub inside the park, and that grass has negative impact on PCI formation. Comparing the temperatures of 61 parks during the summer at noon in Taipei City, Chang et al. [16] found that parks with more than 50 % paved coverage and little tree and shrub cover were on average warmer than their surroundings. The land cover composition of a park has been shown to positively correlate with the magnitude of differences in air temperature.

From these findings, it can be inferred that park characteristics, especially in regard to the type of land cover and the proportion of different land cover types may have a significant effect on outdoor air temperature [17, 18]. Therefore, knowledge of the relationship between air temperature and land cover is critical in improving landscape design strategies to ameliorate urban thermal environment. However, the quantifiable effect and statistical relationship between air temperature and land cover in a park have not been established and thus limit the design of optimal parks with remarkable PCI effect. In the present study, we investigated the thermal performance of different land cover types, and how the feature of land cover composition influences local air temperature in the city of Beijing, China. The work focused on humidity and hot summer days, when the green areas are more frequently used by the citizens in the study area.

The objectives of this study were:

(1) to examine diurnal variations in air temperature of different land cover types;
(2) to compare the air temperature difference among various land cover types;
(3) to quantify the relationship between air temperature and land cover composition during daytime and nighttime in summer.

Methods

Study area and site description

Beijing is located in the northern part of the North China Plain. It is the second largest city in China with a total population of 19.6 million by the end of 2010. It has a monsoon influenced humid continental climate characterized by hot and humid summers and generally cold, windy and dry winters. According to the climatological normals (1971–2000), January is the coldest month with an average temperature of −3.7 °C, while July is the hottest month with an average temperature of 26.2 °C. The main wind direction is from southeast to northeast in summer and in reverse during winter. Since 1978, Beijing's urban population and yearly construction area have been gradually increasing, leading to significant modifications in the underlying surface properties and notable increase in the intensity of the UHI effect.

This study was conducted in the Beijing Olympic Forestry Park, which is in the northern part of the city and surrounded by residential and commercial buildings. The park covers 680 ha; about 70 % of the total area is vegetated area and 10 % is water area. Observations were conducted simultaneously on four fixed sites. The locations of the four observation sites are indicated in Fig. 1, and site A, one of the measurement sites, is outside the park and the other three sites (B, C and D) are inside the park. At each observation site we selected four types of land cover, i.e. trees area, lawn area, paved area and water area as sample points to conduct air temperature measurements. The method similar to Krüger et al. [19] was utilized to obtain land cover pattern of each observation site, which were made with CAD, by drawing corresponding areas on the aerial photographs. Each observation site represents an area of 49,000 m^2 (approximately a 125 m radius around the center of each observation site). Table 1 shows the percentages of the four categories of land cover for each observation site.

Air temperature measurements

Measurements were carried out simultaneously at four observation sites on 18th, 27th, 28th, July of 2010. Atmospheric conditions on the measuring days were fairly clear and windless. During the observations, air temperature was measured once every two hours from 8:00 to 20:00 h. The major instruments used in the measurement were Testo humidity temperature meters. The measurements were taken at 1.5 m above the ground, which is approximately the level where a person of mean height breathes in. At each measurement point, we waited until the wind speed slowed below 2 m/s and wait for an additional few minutes for the temperature measurement to stabilize before taking the air temperature data.

Data analysis

In the data analysis, 14:00 h and 20:00 h were selected to represent the daytime and nighttime, respectively. Statistical analyses were performed to test the influence of land cover on air temperature using one-way ANOVA, and multiple comparisons were made using the Turkey HSD method. Simple correlation analysis was also performed to study the relations between local air temperature and land cover patterns of each observation site during daytime and nighttime. Statistical analysis was performed by

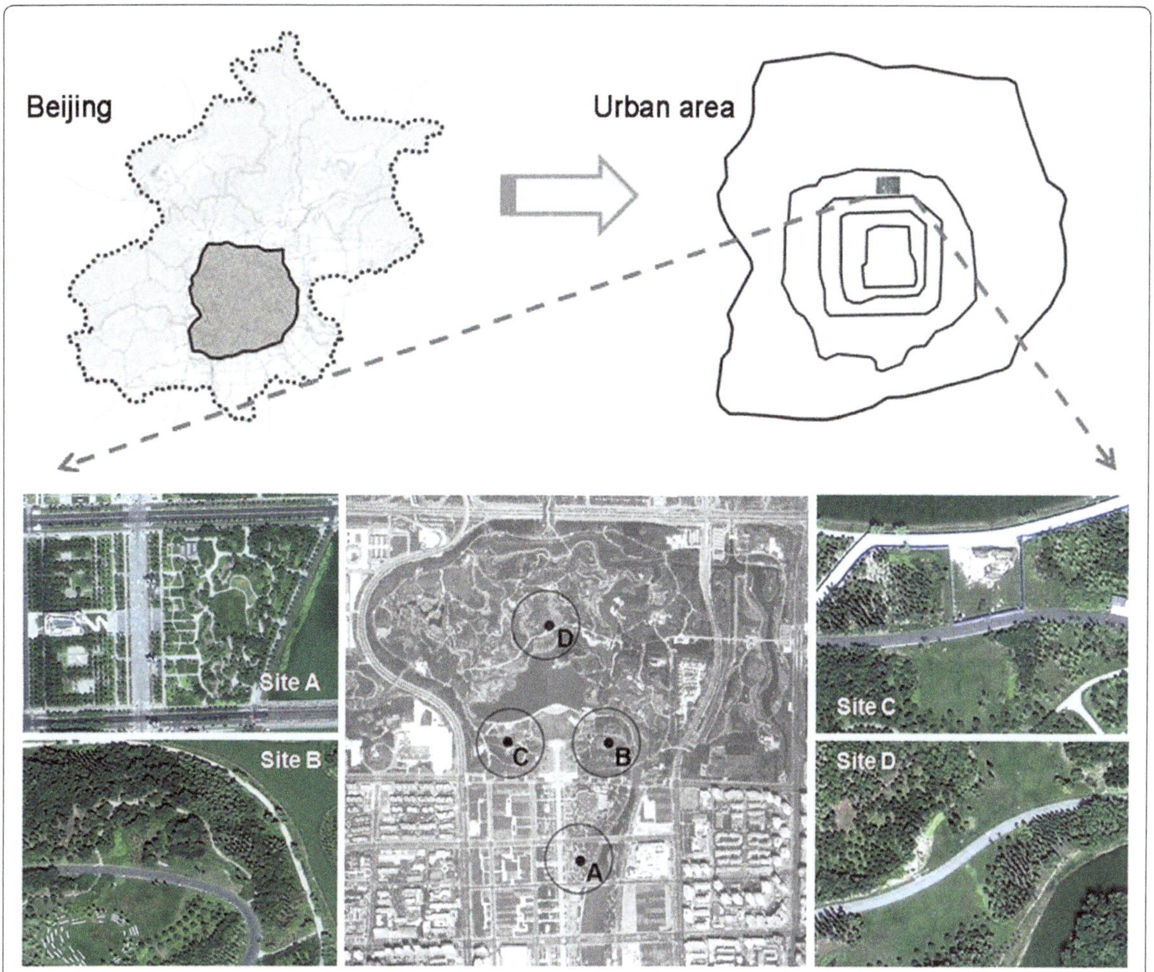

Fig. 1 Location and aerial view of the observation sites

running the SPSS/PC + software package (SPSS, Inc.) on a personal computer. P values of less than 0.05 were regarded as statistically significant.

Results and discussion

Temperature difference among land cover types

Figure 2 shows the air temperature variation of different land cover types during hot summer. Temperature difference among land cover types was minimal in the morning, increased during the hot hours of the day and then decreased toward the evening. In general, three main temperature patterns could be observed: the paved area had the highest temperature values, the lawn area was slightly cooler than the paved area and, air temperatures were lowest in the water area and trees area. It is evident that the air temperature of all four land cover types reached the highest value at 14:00 h, and the highest temperature value is in the order of paved area > lawn area > water area > trees area. They were 37.5 °C in the paved area, 36.5 °Cin the lawn area, 34.7 °Cin the water area and 34.5 °Cin the trees area. In the late afternoon, air temperature of lawn area dropped fastest among the four land cover types, which was likely to became the same with that of trees area at about 19:00 h, and reached the minimum (36.1 °C) at 20:00 h.

Table 1 Land cover percentages for each observation site (%)

Location	Wood area	Lawn area	Paved area	Water area
Site A	20.1	24.9	44.7	10.3
Site B	47.0	33.5	10.4	9.1
Site C	52.6	26.9	8.1	12.4
Site D	59.4	24.1	5.6	10.9

Considering the air temperature difference of each land cover type during different time periods, daytime and nighttime data were analyzed separately. In this study,

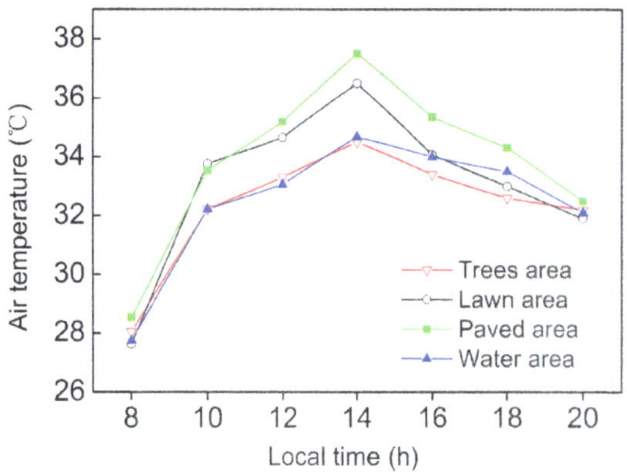

Fig. 2 The diurnal variation of air temperature at four types of land cover during hot summer

temperature at 14:00 h and 20:00 were selected to represent the data of daytime and nighttime, respectively. Figure 3 illustrates the average air temperatures of each land cover type during the two time periods. At 14:00 h, difference in average air temperatures was significant among different land cover types. The average air temperature of paved area (37.1 °C) was significantly higher than that of water area (35.3 °C) and trees area (34.3 °C), meanwhile, temperature of lawn area (36.1 °C) and water area were markedly higher than that of trees area. Previous studies carried out in Nanjing by Huang et al. [20] also found similar temperature differences among different land cover types. During daytime, the effect of solar radiation was the main reason for this temperature behavior. The lower air temperature in trees area was the result of good shading provided by dense canopy, which was able to intercept much more incoming solar radiation when compared to open paved area and lawn area [21]. Both paved area and lawn area were constantly exposed to direct solar radiation, resulting in increased temperature. At 20:00 h, the paved area was still

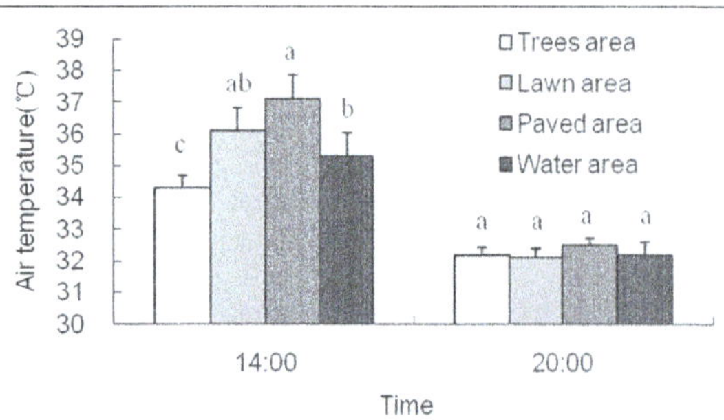

Fig. 3 Average air temperature of four land cover types at two time periods. Lowercase letters indicate significantly different means based on a Tukey HSD multiple comparisons test at 0.05 level. Values in each column with the same letter are not significantly different among land covers

found to be the warmest one, while the lawn became the coolest site. However, there was no significant difference in average air temperatures among four land cover types at this time. It was also found that the maximum nighttime temperature difference (0.4 °C) among various land cover types is lower than that of the daytime period (2.8 °C). During daytime, the large temperature difference was mainly contributed by the high air temperature which was located at open paved area and the low temperature which was located at shaded areas with vegetation; whereas, during nighttime, the former site cool down at a faster rate as compared with the latter, since there was no obstruction to block the nighttime net long-wave loss without vegetation.

Relationship between local air temperature and land cover pattern

To compare the difference of air temperature in four observation sites, we used the average air temperature of four land cover types to represent that of the observation sites namely local temperature effect. Figure 4 shows the result of comparisons among the average air temperatures of four observation sites. At 14:00 h, the average temperature ranged from 35.0 to 36.3 °C at four sites. The hottest place was site A which is located outside the southern entrance of the park, with an average air temperature reaching 36.3 °C. This area has the largest proportion of paved area (44.7 %) and the lowest proportion of trees area (20.1 %). Furthermore, this location is surrounded by some offices and commercial buildings. The continuous heating of the pavement surface by solar radiation and the release of anthropogenic heat contribute to the high air temperature here. The lowest average temperature, 35.0 °C, was obtained at site D, which is located at the center of the park and has the highest proportion of vegetation area (59.4 %). At 20:00 h, the air temperature of site D became the hottest while that of site B became the coldest. These results could be explained by the vegetation character of the corresponding sites. The vegetation in site D is denser and thicker than the vegetation in site B, resulting in a lower sky view factor, which creates better shading efficiency during the day but prevents radiation cooling during the night. In Tel Aviv, a similar result was observed by Potchter et al. [22], indicating that the grass park with few trees tended to be warmer during the day, compared to its surrounding, than 2 other parks with greater tree cover. However, during nighttime the park that contains dense, medium sized trees can create uncomfortable climatic conditions owing to the reduction of wind velocity and increase in relative humidity. This implies that variation in the composition of land cover within a park, such as the amount of tree cover and lawn cover can be expected to affect air temperature. Therefore, we further examined the correlation between air temperature and land cover pattern of each observation site to clarify

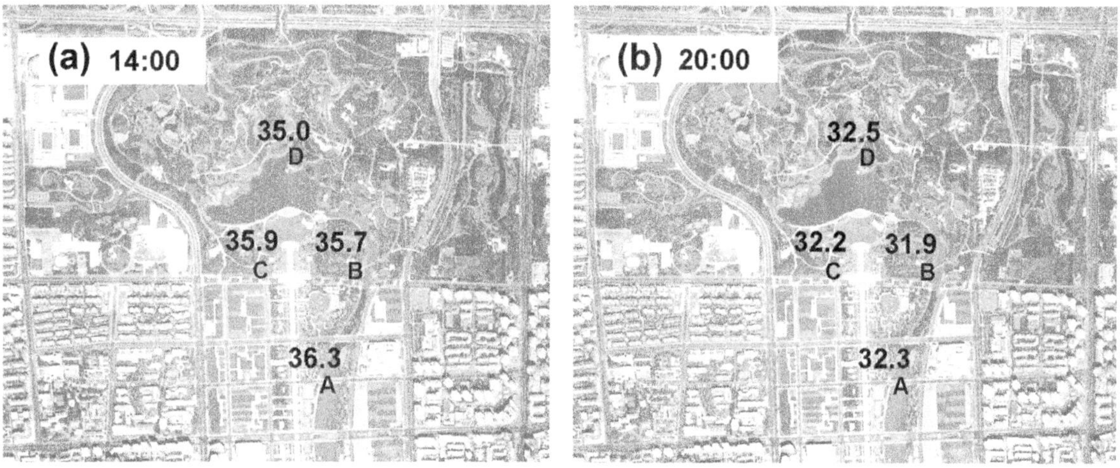

Fig. 4 Mean air temperature of different observation sites considering all the field work days (**a**) at 14:00h, (**b**) at 20:00h

how land cover influenced local air temperatures in the city of Beijing.

Figure 5 shows the correlation between air temperature and the coverage of trees area, lawn area, paved area, and water area within a 125 m in radius of each observation site, represented by the time at 14:00 h and 20:00 h. In spite of the limited size of our field sample, the results pointed out a negative correlation between the air temperature and the percent of tree cover at 14:00 h, as shown in Fig. 5a. About 69.9 % of the variation in air temperature could be explained by the percent tree cover. The air temperature decreased by 0.26 °C as the tree cover ratio increased by 10 %. The result indicated that during daytime, when there was solar radiation, the more the tree coverage, the lower the air temperature is. The vegetation can provide shade and the cooling effect by evapotranspiration; therefore, increasing the tree cover ratio in urban area can mitigate the heat island effect and drop the ambient air temperature. During nighttime, the correlation between air temperature and tree cover was found to be

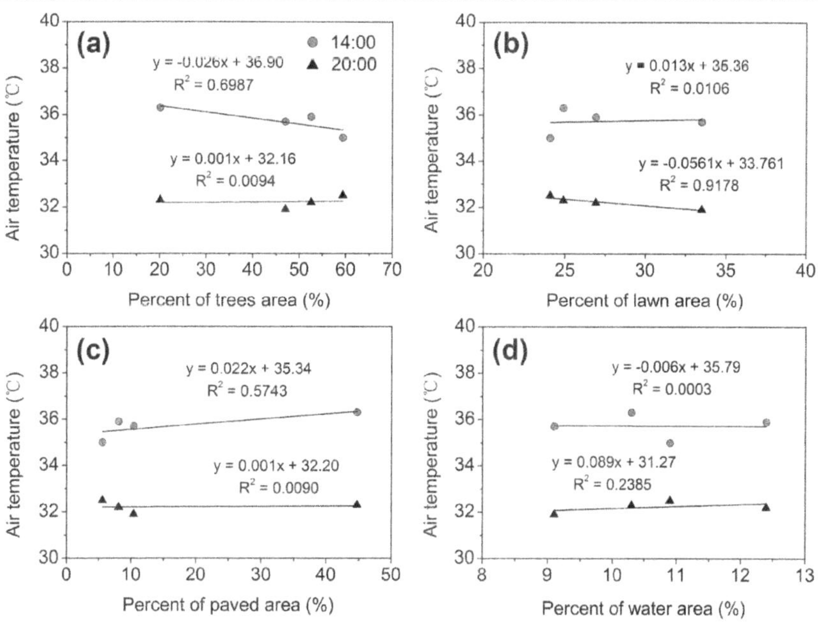

Fig. 5 Relationship between air temperature and land cover ratio with regression line (**a**) trees area (%), (**b**) lawn area (%), (**c**) paved area (%), (**d**) water area (%)

weaker when solar radiation as the main heat source no longer exists. In addition, it shows clearly the change of correlation from negative correlation in the afternoon measurement time to positive correlation in the night measurement time. It means that the tree has an effect on reducing air temperature by shading during hot daytime, however, the tree also reduces the net long-wave loss during nighttime, which in turn, retain and even elevate the air temperature. There was a weak positive correlation between air temperature and lawn cover at 14:00 h, while the lawn cover had the most significant influence on the air temperature at 20:00 h, with a coefficient much higher than others (Fig. 5b). The considerable cooling effect of lawn at night result presumably from its high humidity and exposure to the open sky, which enhances upwelling radiation loss at night. According to the result of this study shown in Fig. 5c, the air temperature always has a positive correlation with paved cover ratio. The air temperature increased by 0.22 °C and 0.01 °C at 14:00 and 20:00 h, respectively, as the paved cover ratio increased by 10 %. At noon in summer, large proportion of paved surfaces absorbs and reflects much incoming radiance, resulting in increased temperature. It also shows that the correlation between air temperature and water cover ratio was pretty poor (Fig. 5d). This result is similar to the one found by Cao et al. [15], which showed that the water body played an unimportant role on PCI formation. This may be due to the fact that the water area was only a very small percentage of the total land cover of each observation site. In general, tree cover and lawn cover are the most main factors which can influence local air temperature during daytime and nighttime, respectively.

Conclusions

In this paper, we investigated the diurnal variations in air temperature among four types of land cover. The correlations between air temperature and land cover pattern were also discussed. The following conclusions could be drawn:

1) The air temperature difference among four land cover types was more significant during the day than during the night. At noon, the average air temperature differed significantly among four land cover types, which is lower on trees area than on paved area, lawn area, or water area; whereas on night, there was no significant difference among four land cover types.
2) It was also found that the average temperature of each observation site was closely related to the land cover composition. The site with large proportions of paved cover and little vegetation had a very high daytime air temperature, while the site with large proportions of tree cover had a low daytime air temperature. At night, however, an opposite trend was observed.
3) The effect of land cover composition on air temperature demonstrated a diurnal variation and was also dependent on land cover type. We found that site difference in average air temperature at 14:00 h was better predicted by percent tree cover, while average air temperature at 20:00 h was better predicted by percent lawn cover. It was shown that with a 10 % increase in the percent tree cover, the air temperature decreased by 0.26 °C during daytime in summer, by contrast, as the percent lawn cover increased by 10 %, the air temperature decreased by 0.56 °C during nighttime in summer.

This study extended our scientific understanding of the effects of land cover, especial the land cover composition on air temperature in summer. In addition, the findings have important implications for urban green space planning and design. In order to ameliorate the outdoor thermal environment, planners and designers must consider the composition and configuration of the land cover. However, it should be noted that this study was conducted only for one urban green space during a single summer season. Therefore, future work should expand this research to consider more land cover in different metropolitan areas, and expanding the analyses to also include different seasons.

Competing interests
The authors declare that they have no competing interests.

Authors' contributions
HY carried out the design of the study, the numerical analysis, and drafted the manuscript. LD participated in its design and coordination and helped to draft the manuscript. All authors read and approved the final manuscript.

Acknowledgments
We sincerely thank two anonymous reviewers for their constructive comments and suggestions. This research was supported by the Research Foundation of Talented Scholars of Zhejiang A & F University (NO. 2014FR063).

Author details
[1]College of Landscape Architecture, Beijing Forestry University, Beijing 100083, China. [2]School of Landscape Architecture, Zhejiang Agriculture and Forestry University, Lin'an, Zhejiang 311300, China.

References
1. Kalnay E, Cai M. Impact of urbanization and land-use change on climate. Nature. 2003;423:528–31.
2. Oke TR. The energetic basis of the urban heat island. Q J Roy Meteorol Soc. 1982;108:1–24.
3. Roshan G, Ghanghermeh A, Orosa JA. Thermal comfort and forecast of energy consumption in Northwest Iran. Arab J Geosci. 2014;7(9):3657–74.
4. Orosa JA, Costa ÁM, Rodríguez-Fernández Á, Roshan G. Effect of climate change on outdoor thermal comfort in humid climates. J Environ Healt Sci Eng. 2014;12:46.
5. Ca VT, Asaeda T, Abu EM. Reductions in air conditioning energy caused by a nearby park. Energ Buildings. 1998;29(1):83–92.
6. Gill SE, Handley JF, Ennos AR, Pauleit S. Adapting cities for climate change: the role of the green infrastructure. Built Environ. 2007;33(1):115–33.
7. Spronken-Smith RA, Oke TR. The thermal regime of urban parks in two cities with different summer climates. Int J Remote Sens. 1998;19(1):2085–104.

8. Makhelouf A. The effect of green spaces on urban climate and pollution. Iran J Environ Healt Sci Eng. 2009;6(1):35–40.
9. Hamada S, Ohta T. Seasonal variations in the cooling effect of urban green areas on surrounding urban areas. Urban For Urban Gree. 2010;9(1):15–24.
10. Oliveira S, Andrade H, Vaz T. The cooling effect of green spaces as a contribution to the mitigation of urban heat: a case study in Lisbon. J Build Environ. 2011;46(11):2186–94.
11. Jansson C, Jansson PE, Gustafsson D. Near surface climate in an urban vegetated park and its surroundings. Theor Appl Climatol. 2007;89(3–4):185–93.
12. Jauregui E. Influence of a large urban park on temperature and convective precipitation in a tropical city. Energ Buildings. 1991;15(3–4):457–63.
13. Chen Y, Wong NH. Thermal benefits of city parks. Energ Buildings. 2006;38(2):105–20.
14. Barradas VL. Air temperature and humidity and human comfort index of some city parks of Mexico City. Int J Biometeorol. 1991;35(1):24–8.
15. Cao X, Onishi A, Chen J. Quantifying the cool island intensity of urban parks using ASTER and IKONOS data. Landscape Urban Plan. 2010;96(4):224–31.
16. Chang C, Li M, Chang S. A preliminary study on the local cool island intensity of Taipei city parks. Landscape Urban Plan. 2007;80(4):386–95.
17. Yan H, Fan S, Guo C, Wu F, Zhang N, Dong L. Assessing the effects of landscape design parameters on intra-urban air temperature variability: the case of Beijing, China. Build Environ. 2014;76:44–53.
18. Yan H, Fan S, Guo C, Hu J, Dong L. Quantifying the impact of land cover composition on intra-Urban air temperature variations at a mid-latitude city. Plos one. 2014;9(7):e102124.
19. Krüger E, Givoni B. Outdoor measurements and temperature comparisons of seven monitoring stations: preliminary studies in Curitiba, Brazil. Build Environ. 2007;42(4):1685–98.
20. Huang L, Li J, Zhao D, Zhu J. A fieldwork study on the diurnal changes of urban microclimate in four types of ground cover and urban heat island of Nanjing, China. Build Environ. 2008;43(1):7–17.
21. Shashua-Bar L, Hoffman ME. Vegetation as a climatic component in the design of an urban street: an empirical model for predicting the cooling effect of urban green areas with trees. Energ Buildings. 2000;31(3):221–35.
22. Potchter O, Cohen P, Bitan A. Climatic behavior of various urban parks during hot and humid summer in the Mediterranean city of Tel Aviv, Israel. Int J Climatol. 2006;26(12):1695–711.

Ultrafiltration of natural organic matter from water by vertically aligned carbon nanotube membrane

Ali Jafari[1], Amir Hossein Mahvi[2,1,3*], Simin Nasseri[2,1], Alimorad Rashidi[4], Ramin Nabizadeh[1] and Reza Rezaee[5]

Abstract

In this study vertically aligned carbon nanotubes (VA-CNT) was grown on anodized aluminum oxide (AAO) substrate. The synthesized AAO-CNT membrane was characterized using Raman spectroscopy, field emission scanning electron microscopy (FESEM), contact angle and BET. The pure water flux, humic acid (HA) (as representative of natural organic matters) rejection and fouling mechanism were also evaluated. The fabricated membrane has pore density of 1.3×10^{10} pores per cm^2, average pore size of 20 ± 3 nm and contact angle of 85 ± 8°. A significant pure water flux of 3600 ± 100 $L/m^2.h$ was obtained at 1 bar of pressure by this membrane due to the frictionless structure of CNTs. High contact angle exhibited the hydrophobic property of the membrane. It was revealed that HA is primarily rejected by adsorption in the membrane pores due to hydrophobic interactions with HA. Flux decline occurred rapidly through both cross flow and dead end filtration of the HA. Based on the blocking laws, internal pore constriction is dominant fouling mechanism in which HA adsorbs in membrane pores results in pores blockage and flux decline.

Keywords: Membrane, Carbon nanotube, Fouling, Natural organic matter, Ultrafiltration

Introduction

Natural organic matters (NOMs) are known as problematic substances in environment and health. Nowadays their various direct and indirect effects are well understood. They own different characteristics in terms of reactivity, structure and they enter to water bodies through various natural and man-made sources [1]. NOMs are present to different extents in waters [2, 3]. Typical ranges of 0.1–0.2 mg/L and 1–20 mg/L of NOM based on total organic carbon (TOC) have been reported for ground and surface waters, respectively. However, the TOC concentrations can be very higher (100–200 mg/L) in colored waters of swamps and marshes [4, 5].

These substances form hazardous disinfection byproducts (DBPs) such as trihalomethanes (THMs) in reaction with chlorine. NOM is often made of two fractions, namely hydrophobic and hydrophilic. Hydrophobic and hydrophilic fractions have the potential of THMs and haloacetic acids (HAAs) formation, respectively. Hydrophobic components are humic acid and fulvic acid and the hydrophilic components are proteins, amino acids and carbohydrates [4, 5].

Hydrophobic compounds have the greatest effect on DBPs formation. Furthermore, some hydrophobic substances may intrinsically be much more toxic than the chlorinated components [6].

The presence of NOMs have other problems such as negative effect on the water quality and treatment process, increasing the coagulants and disinfectants demand, biological growth in distribution network, decomposition of organic matter within the network and creating a slimy layer on the pipes [5, 7]. In addition, NOM adversely affects the membrane performance in water purification [8].

Different methods with varying efficiencies such as chemical coagulation and precipitation, ion exchange, adsorption, electrocoagulation, advanced oxidation and membrane process have been applied for NOM mitigation [5, 9–14]. Although in some cases enhanced coagulation has been proposed for NOMs removal, but large application of coagulants, pH modification problems and large amount of produced sludge are the main related obstacles of this method.

* Correspondence: ahmahvi@yahoo.com
[2]Center for Water Quality Research (CWQR), Institute for Environmental Research (IER), Tehran University of Medical Sciences, Tehran, Iran
[1]Department of Environmental Health Engineering, School of Public Health, Tehran University of Medical Sciences, Tehran, Iran
Full list of author information is available at the end of the article

Furthermore, adsorption as a known process in water treatment, have been studied and applied for NOM removal using various materials. In addition to activated carbon materials, new nano adsorbents such as CNTs and zero valent iron nanoparticles have also been studied as promising adsorbents [15, 16], but the questions related to release of nanomaterials and regeneration costs are the main drawback of adsorption application.

Membranes are used for NOMs fractions removal from aqueous solution as one of the important processes in water treatment. Membrane process is of interest due to no changes in the structure of pollutants, no intermediates addition to water, no adverse environmental effects, no need of chemicals and easy navigation [17].

The major obstacles associated with the membrane are energy consuming and fouling problem. Researchers are attempting to change the structure of conventional polymeric membranes or developed new membranes with higher permeability and higher pollutant rejection.

In this regard, carbon nanotubes (CNTs) have been considered for membrane synthesis due to their exceptional properties and high adsorption capabilities [18, 19]. Due to porous structure of the tubes and high surface area, a wide range of contaminants have been effectively removed by CNTs [20].

Promising results show that CNTs in membranes structure have higher flux, higher performance, less fouling, less required cleaning, higher thermal stability, higher consistency and lower energy requirement than conventional polymeric membranes [21–23].

Carbon nanotube membranes can be synthesized by various methods. One of these techniques is template carbonization to synthesize CNTs with desired diameter and high purity. In this method, the situation is prepared in such a way that the CNTs grow inside the channels of anodic aluminum oxide (AAO) template [23]. Thus, the membrane is created through growing CNT arrays and known as vertically aligned carbon nanotubes (VA-CNT) membrane.

One of the most important advantages of the VA-CNT membrane is high flux of water through the CNTs due to low length to the high density of nanotubes [21]. The first plan of VA-CNT membranes was developed by Hinds research team that CNTs were grown on iron as a catalyst using chemical vapor deposition (CVD) method [21]. It has been reported that hydrophobic channel of CNT is smooth and frictionless that facilitate the rapid movement of water [21]. Accordingly, in recent years, CNTs have been mixed with polymers in order to improve the performance of polymeric membranes with higher flux and less fouling [24–29].

To our knowledge, relatively few studies have been conducted in the development of vertically aligned CNT membranes for water purification. With regard to promising results related to CNTs application for membrane synthesis, present work is going to synthesize and characterize the VA-CNT membrane through AAO technique and investigate for NOMs rejection from water.

Materials and methods

Membrane experimental set up

The schematic diagram of the experimental setup is shown in Fig. 1. It consists of a 2-L feed tank, membrane module with the effective area of 1.4 cm^2, feeding pump, cooling system, valves, gauges and flow meters.

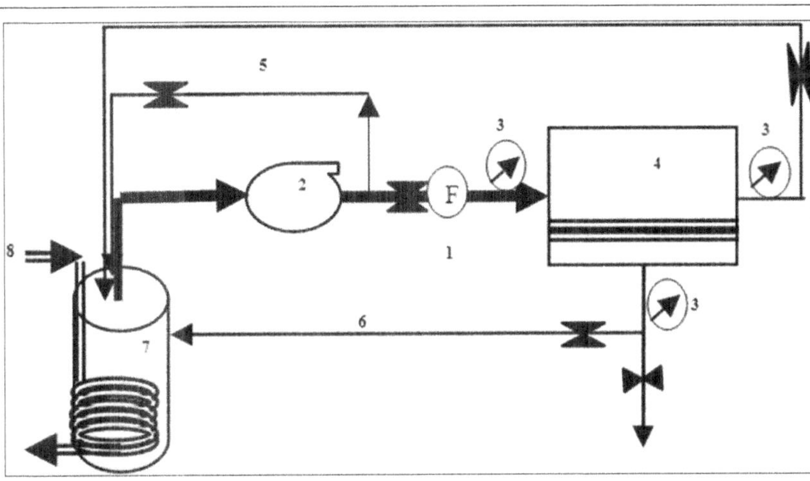

Fig. 1 Simplified schematic of experimental set-up unit. 1. Flow meter 2. Low pressure pump 3. Gauges 4. Membrane module 5. Recirculation (bypass) line 6. Concentrate line 7. Feed tank 8. Cooling circuit

Synthesis, preparation and characterization of membrane
All the chemicals reagents were of reagent grade and no further purification was done. The fabricated membrane was synthesized via anodic aluminum oxide (AAO) method through a two-step process (anodizing and growth of CNTs in the porous AAO).

In this study, a similar procedure as Gilani et al. was used for membrane synthesis and preparation [22, 30].

High purity (99.99) aluminum (Al) foil of 300 μm thickness was cut in small rectangular pieces. The foils were sonicated in acetone solution and then rinsed with double distilled water in order to degrease and subsequently dried in room temperature. Then, Al plates were electropolished in ethanol and perchloric acid (60 %) mixture solution (4/1 v/v) under constant cell voltage of 20 V for 2 min. The back surface of the plates was protected by an insulting tape.

The anodizing process started using oxalate acid (0.3 M) as electrolyte solution and under voltage of 40 volts for 2 h. Separation of the oxide layer was conducted using a mixture of phosphoric acid (6 % wt) and chromic acid (1.8 wt %) for 2 h at 65 °C.

Aluminum foil was re-anodized for 58 h under identical manner used for first anodization step. Then the unoxidized part was removed by putting in saturated mercuric chloride. The barrier layer was removed by soaking the template in phosphoric acid (5 wt %) at temperatures of 50 °C for 3 h [22, 30]. Deposition of CNTs onto the interior walls of the template was conducted by placing the AAO in CVD furnace. The temperature of the furnace was gradually increased to 650 °C at a rate of 5 °C/min. Meanwhile, a controlled argon flow (200 ml/min) was induced to the furnace. A mixture of acetylene and argon was inserted into the furnace as the carbon precursor and carrier gas, respectively with a ratio of 0.01 for 12 h. After the carbon deposition, the acetylene flow was turned off, under the condition of argon flow the reactor was allowed to cool to room temperature for 12 h. Finally, the synthesized membrane was washed in ethanol and dried in vacuum oven at 60 °C [22, 30].

Membrane characteristics were performed using Raman spectroscopy, FESEM, contact angle, and BET. Field emission scanning electron microscopy (FESEM) (Hitachi-S4160) was used to characterize the uniformity and morphology of the AAO–CNT membrane. The specific surface area of the AAO–CNTs was determined using the Brunauer–Emmett–Teller (BET) method by ASAP 2010 (Micromertics Inc., Norcross, GA).

Raman spectrum was used to observe the uniformity of graphite structure of the growing CNTs in the membrane using a Raman spectrometer (Almega Thermo Nicolet Dispersive). Contact angle as an important factor in membrane characterization was measured by a contact angle analyzer (OCA 15 plus, dataphysics Instruments, Germany) using the sessile drop technique.

Solutions and analytical measurements
A laboratory grade humic acid (Acros Organics Company, NJ – USA) was used in this study as NOM model to evaluate the performance and removal mechanism by synthesized VA-CNT-AAO membrane. A known amount of HA powder was dissolved in distilled water and pH was adjusted around 7 for all experiments. The concentration of HA was reported as the term of TOC, as a surrogate measure using a TOC analyzer (TOC-VCPH, Shimadzu, Japan). For this purpose different samples (feed, permeate and concentrate) were taken at defined interval times and analyzed for TOC concentration.

Generally, in membrane process, materials may be removed from water by adsorption and/or repulsion mechanisms. The portion of desorbed or adsorbed solutes on the membrane surface is important in fouling and flux analysis.

From a practical standpoint, to investigate the removal mechanism, a certain volume of synthetic solution was placed in the feed tank (Fig. 1). Then, the system was operated in closed loop condition where permeate and concentrate were recycled back to the feed tank at constant transmembrane pressure (TMP) of 1 bar. A cooling circuit was applied to feed tank to maintain the temperature of the feed solution at a constant value of 25 ± 0.5 °C. Sampling was performed at specified intervals from feed tank, permeate and retentate flows for further analysis. All experiments were conducted in duplicate. The observed percentage of HA rejection (%) was calculated as Eq. 1.

$$\%R = \left(\frac{Cf-Cp}{Cf}\right) \times 100 \qquad (1)$$

Where C_f and C_p are TOC concentrations in feed solution and permeate, respectively.

The adsorbed mass of TOC is equal to initial TOC mass in the feed tank minus the sum of TOC mass in the feed tank and cumulative samples of permeate at the end of experiment period, as determined by following mass balance equation (Eq. 2).

$$A.\ Mads = CfiVfi\text{–}\left[CffVff + \sum CpVp\right] \qquad (2)$$

Where A is the effective membrane area. M_{ads} is the adsorbed mass of TOC per surface area of membrane. C_{fi}, C_{ff} and Cp are the initial concentration of TOC, final concentration of TOC in the feed tank and concentration of TOC in permeate respectively. V_{fi}, V_{ff} and V_p are the initial volume of feed solution in the tank, final volume of solution in the tank and volume of permeate, respectively.

Results and discussion

Membrane characteristics

Figures 2a and b illustrate the cross section and surface FESEM image of the membrane respectively. A through hole membrane is clearly shown in Fig. 2a. This image also depicts the direction of cavities and grown CNTs in the holes. The anodizing process and operation conditions (namely voltage, electrolyte concentration and time) effectively influence the properties of the channels [31].

The straight form of the channels indicates the well ordering of CNTs in this fabricated membrane. Fig. 2b shows the pores of the synthesized membrane (dark points). From analysis of FESEM image using the ImageJ analyzer [32] a highly uniform distribution of pores arrangement and nearly uniform pore size (≈20 nm) was created which is in the range of a UF membrane. As seen in Fig. 2b, the surface of the membrane looks uneven. Appling low voltages for AAO synthesis usually results in lower pore sizes and higher pore densities. This property has been shown in other similar works [22, 30]. Therefore, in low voltages due to higher spaces between the pores, the surface is rougher. Cleaning and polishing the surface of aluminum foil can relatively decrease the total surface roughness, but during the anodizing process and growing the CNTs near the top surface, the roughness increases. Although such a roughness may be defined as an advantage for some applications [31] due to higher surface area as an important factor in adsorption process, this can not be of interest for water purification. In particular, high roughness affects the membrane performance in water purification that results in fouling problem.

As depicted in Fig. 3, two strong peaks appeared in the Raman spectrum. The first peak is at around 1351 cm^{-1} (disordered D line band) and the next peak is about 1602 cm^{-1} (ordered G band). From the shift of the Raman spectrum peaks (D and G) the ratio of their intensities (IG/ID) is about one which shows the good structure of CNTs formed in the porous AAO and free from amorphous carbon which is consistent with other researchers [22, 33]. Compare to CNTs grown by other methods, commonly growing on metal cores as catalyst, growing of CNTs in AAO template produce higher purity CNTs with less amporph carbons. Accordingly the need of further purification is not necessary for AAO-CNTs. Nevertheless, this technique produces nearly uniform CNTs in the membrane structure.

Contact angles of several droplets on the surface of the membrane were measured and the average was reported (Table 1). Results showed that AAO-CNT membrane has a hydrophobic behavior as the result of high contact angle. Fig. 4 shows the droplet of pure water on the surface of the membrane and the contact to the surface. Generally, grown VA-CNTs on different substrates may somewhat change the hydrophilicity behavior and contact angle of the VA-CNT membrane due to surface chemical structure and method of synthesis [34]. Since CNTs intrinsically have hydrophobic properties, it has been revealed that membranes fabricated by unmodified or non-functionalized VA-CNTs have close contact angles and are primarily hydrophobe (Table 1). Functionalization of VA-CNT membrane can change the membrane properties and introduce function groups on the CNTs [30].

Permeation analysis

Pure water flux, (J_0) was calculated using the following equation (Eq. 3):

$$J_0 = V/At \tag{3}$$

where V is the total volume of permeated pure water, A is the effective membrane area, and t is the operation time.

The pure water permeability for the VA-CNT membrane was 3600 ± 100 $L/m^2.h$ at TMP of 1 bar. This value is several times than conventional UF membranes for water process. A high practical flux of a commercial UF membrane was reported to be 800 $L/m^2.h$-bar flux [35]. Furthermore, due to frictionless structure of VA- CNT channels, it has been reported that fluid flow

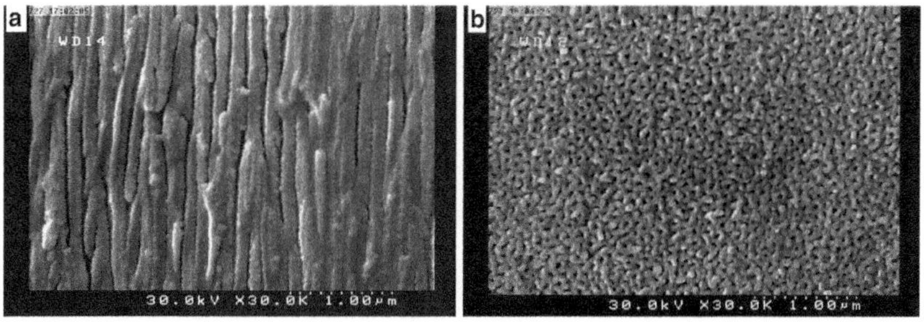

Fig. 2 FESEM image of AAO-CNT membrane. **a** cross section of the membrane and **b** surface area image of the membrane

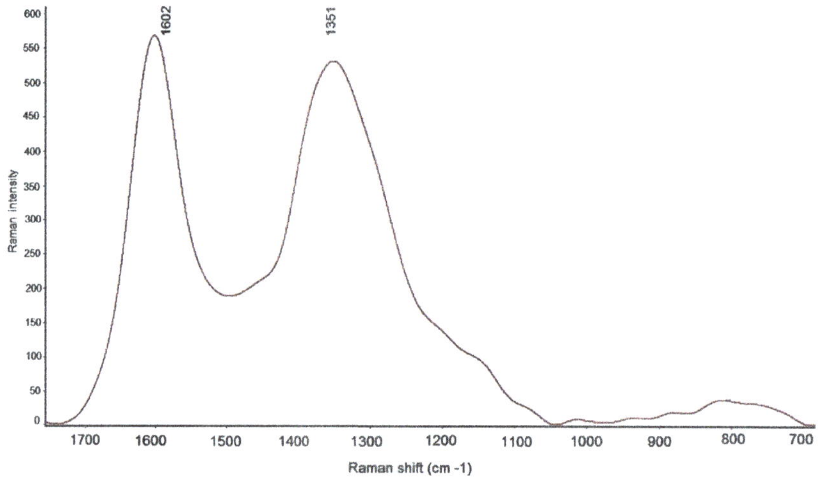

Fig. 3 Raman spectrum for AAO-CNT membrane

can be 4–5 times faster than conventional flows [36]. This dramatic velocity can facilitate the application of CNTs channel for other fields.

However, the flux of VA-CNT is significantly higher than that of similar polymeric membranes. In spite of lower pore density, lower pore diameter and higher thickness of aligned CNT membranes, a higher flux (3–4 orders of magnitude) than polymeric UF membrane have been reported [37, 38]. Besides pore size different parameters such as membrane thickness, method of preparation, size distribution can influence the flux of VA-CNT membranes that should be considered for comparing membrane permeabilities. Higher pore diameter (~20 nm) and lower thickness of the membrane result in higher flux in this study. In spite of low pore number of the synthesized membrane a high flux was observed due to lower thickness and also a guarantee of vertically aligned CNTs standing. As shown in Fig. 2a, aligned structure of CNTs in AAO template can facilitate transport of water through the membrane. The number of pores per unit of membrane surface can also affect the membrane flux significantly in combined with other parameters (e.g. membrane structure, thickness and pore number) [21].

Table 1 VA-CNT membrane characteristics compared to other related works

	This work	Youngbin Baek. et al [37]	Seung-Min Park. et al [38]
Materials	CNT-AAO	CNT-epoxy	CNT-epoxy
Pore density (pore/ cm^2) $*10^{10}$	1.3	6.8	6.8
Average pore size (nm)	20 ± 3	4.8 ± 0.9	4.87 ± 0.87
Pore volume (cm^3/g)	0.425	Nd[a]	Nd
BET surface area (m^2/g)	220.4	Nd	Nd
Contact angle (degree)	85 ± 8	74.6 ± 2.8	92.1
Porosity	0.18 ± 0.4	Nd	Nd
Thickness (μ)	~120 ± 20	~200	200 ± 50
Flux(L/m^2.h) at 1 bar	3600 ± 100	1100 ± 130	1000 ± 100

[a]Not defined

TOC Removal mechanism

In cross flow filtration of HA, flux declined after a short period of filtration (Fig. 5). The flux declined to near 0.6 of initial flux (J_0) after 5 min of filtration (40 % of flux decline). The flux decrease continues to more than 90 % of J_0 after 60 min of filtration. Interaction of hydrophobic surface of membrane with HA results in plugging of the pores and consequently rapid flux decrease [38].

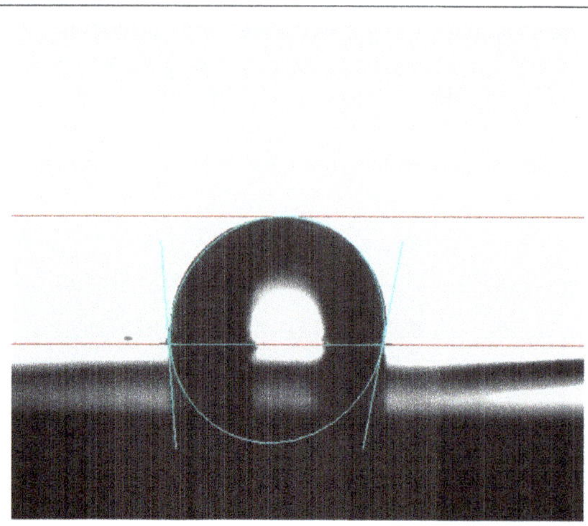
Fig. 4 Contact angle image for AAO-CNT membrane surface

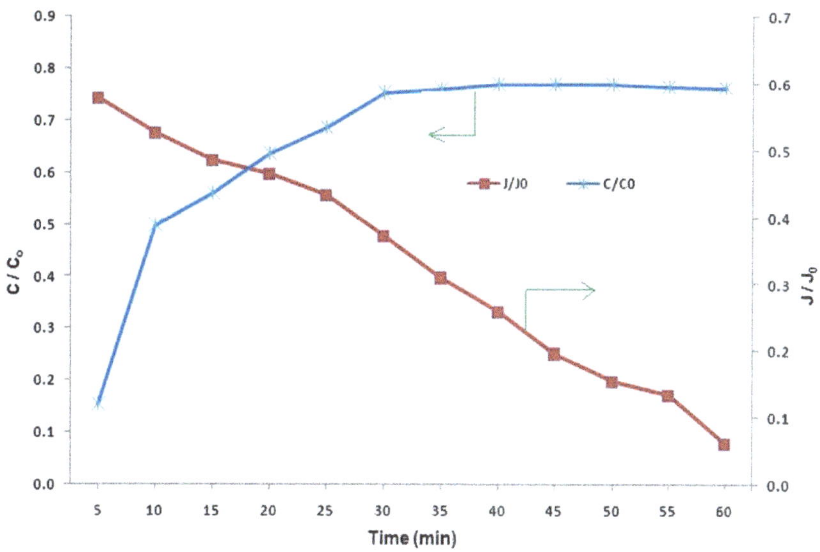

Fig. 5 Trend of TOC concentrations in permeate and flux in cross flow operation for initial TOC of 5 ± 0.3 mg/L, pH of 7.0 ± 0.2 at TMP of 1 bar

Principally, adsorption of NOM by CNT is a rapid process and the adsorption capacity is quickly exhausted. From this study, using mass balance equation (Eq. 1), 61 % of the loaded TOC was adsorbed on the VA-AAO-CNT membrane and only 11 % was repulsed. It was also calculated that 30 ± 0.5 g TOC was adsorbed per square meter of the membrane at a constant TMP of 1 bar for 60 min of filtration. Although adsorption may be an effective rejection mechanism during the initial steps of AAO-CNT membrane operation, but due to quick flux decline during the process, it is not an efficient mechanism in long-term filtration. However it may be preferred for some biochemical and biomedical applications for retention of toxin from plasma, some trace contaminants such as endocrine disrupting compounds (EDC) bisphenol A or heavy metals [39–41].

Anyway, determination of removal mechanism is very important. Therefore, making a decision about the best mechanism for removing a specific contaminant or whether depends on several factors. In some cases, the superior removal mechanism may be adsorption or repulsion of pollutants by the membrane, so the adsorption or repulsion capacities can be increased by inducing certain functional groups or by imposing certain conditions. It was revealed that functionalized CNTs with carboxylic groups can somewhat decrease the adsorption on the membrane [42]. From this study materials similar with HA substances can effectively be adsorbed on the CNT membrane types.

Fouling mechanism analysis

Blocking laws as one of the most popular models were applied to characterize the fouling mechanisms in this study. These empirical models were presented by Hermia [43]:

$$\frac{d^2t}{dv^2} = \mathrm{k}\left(\frac{\mathrm{dt}}{\mathrm{dv}}\right)^{\mathrm{n}} \tag{4}$$

Where t is time (s), V is volume (L) k is blocking law filtration coefficient (units depends on n) and n is blocking law filtration exponent (dimensionless) that expressing the fouling regime. Based on the n values different modes of fouling namely pore sealing ($n = 2$), internal pore constriction ($n = 1.5$), pore sealing with super position ($n = 1$) and cake filtration ($n = 0$) can be expressed. To determine the mechanism responsible for fouling, the experiment was conducted under dead end condition at constant pressure of 1 bar. At certain intervals, permeate volumes were recorded. Data was tabulated in a spreadsheet for analysis.

Using the Eq. 4 by plotting log $\mathrm{d^2t/dv^2}$) versus (dt/dv) the slope of the line is constant value (n) that represent the fouling mechanism [44].

In dead end filtration of HA, about 50 % of rejection occurs at first 10 min of operation (Fig. 6). As previously noted, high affinity of CNTs to HA results in rapid adsorption and fast depletion of adsorption capacity. In other word, due to increase in accumulation of HA in the solution, HA penetrate into the membrane, attach to adsorption sites and pass through the membrane. This trend is nearly similar to whatever occurs in the tangential operation, although in cross flow mode the rejection is higher as the operation time elapsing due to the cross

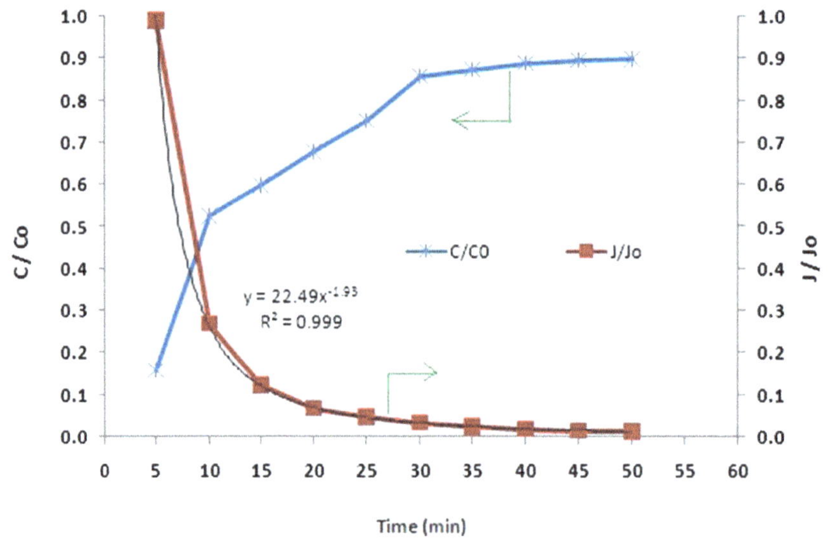

Fig. 6 Flux decline and TOC rejection trend in dead end filtration of HA at TMP of 1 bar and initial TOC = 5 ± 0.3 5 mg/L and pH of 7 ± 0.2

flow velocity, in which, some of deposited HA is swept away from the membrane surface.

In this operation mode, the flux declines rapidly (Fig. 6). About 80 % of decline occurs at first 10 min of filtration and after 20 min, it reduce to 90 % that differs from what ever seen in cross flow mode. Increasing of HA in bulk solution due to its accumulation in dead end filtration, result in rapid blocking of the pores and rapid flux decline. Generally, a 90 % of the flux decline occurred at 57 min of filtration in cross flow operation, while this percentage of flux reduction happened after about 15 min of filtration for dead end mode.

From Fig. 7 based on the equation obtained by plotting the log (d^2t/dv^2) versus log (dt/dv) the line slope (n) is 1.55. Accordingly, fouling mechanism of the membrane can be expressed by pore constriction or standard blocking filtration law that is defined as the reduction of the cross- sectional area of the membrane pores due to adsorption of HA.

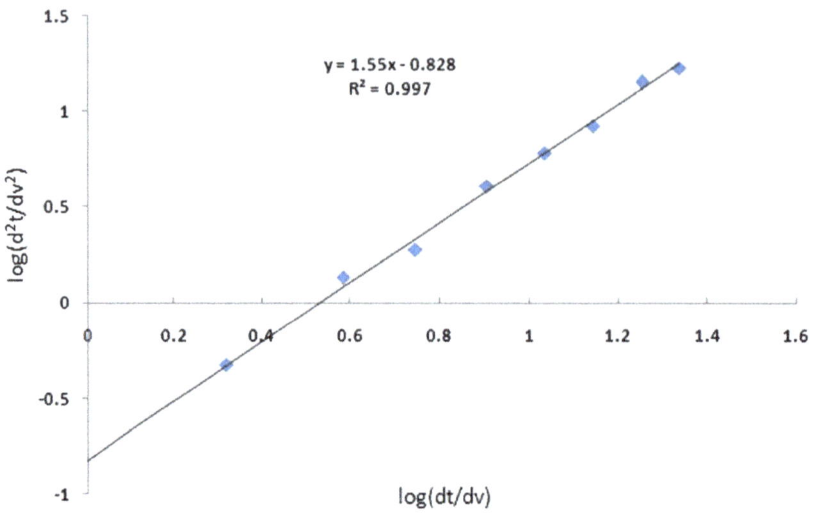

Fig. 7 Fouling analysis for HA filtration. Operating conditions: TMP = 1 bar, TOC =5 ± 0.3 mg/ L, pH = 7 ± 0.2

Sufficient small size of the pollutant that penetrate into the membrane and the adsorption affinity of the pollutant to membrane material have been considered as the main factors for pore constriction phenomenon [44]. Primarily rapid adsorption of HA into the membrane pores decrease the pore size and subsequently results in rapid flux decline. Such an adsorption through the membrane pores and channels (Fig. 2a) makes the cleaning difficult and lowers the membrane reversibility to some extent, otherwise, an effective cleaning technique should be developed.

The conditions, mainly membrane characteristics, can reveal different fouling mechanisms [45]. In fouling analysis, a combination of mechanisms may also occur in a filtration process. In some researches, intermediate blocking followed by cake filtration reported under experimental conditions [46]. In general, attempts to reduce the existing fouling by different methods and changing the removal mechanism from adsorption to electrostatic repulsion are of favor to overcome the problem. For existing membrane inducing the negative charges, can be a solution for reduction of fouling.

Conclusion

Despite of high contact angle and high hydrophobic property of the fabricated CNT-AAO membrane, pure water flux is considerably higher than that of common types of polymeric membranes. Due to high affinity, the membrane rapidly absorbs HA and consequently rapid flux decline occurs because of internal pore constriction as dominant fouling mechanism. It is important to be noted that a challenge related to present fabricated membrane is its frangibility. It is a critical obstacle for larger surface area application and high driven pressures for municipal and industrial applications. However, its application for some laboratory purposes may be beneficial to absorb some materials with the same characteristics as HA. Further studies can focus on methods of the AAO-CNT membranes fabrication with higher tolerability and flexibility for other pollutants removal from water.

Competing interests

The authors declare that they have no competing interests.

Authors' contributions

AJ has participated in all stages of the study (design of the study, conducting the experiments, analyzing the data and preparation of the manuscript). AHM participated in the design of the study, revision of the manuscript and intellectual helping in different stages of the study. SN participated in design of the study, final deeply revision of the manuscript and intellectual helping thorough the study. AMR participated in synthesis process and preparation of the membrane and interpretation of membrane characteristics. RN carried out statistical and technical analysis of data, participated in design of the study. RR participated in data collection and carried out technical analysis and manuscript preparation. All authors read and approved the final manuscript.

Acknowledgments

This research was part of a PhD dissertation of the first author and has been financially supported by a grant (NO, 22715-46-02-92) from Center for Water Quality Research (CWQR), Institute for Environmental Research, Tehran University of Medical Sciences, Tehran, Iran. Therefore, the authors greatly acknowledge the CWQR for the support of this research. The authors also thank the Laboratory staff of department of Environmental Health Engineering.

Author details

[1]Department of Environmental Health Engineering, School of Public Health, Tehran University of Medical Sciences, Tehran, Iran. [2]Center for Water Quality Research (CWQR), Institute for Environmental Research (IER), Tehran University of Medical Sciences, Tehran, Iran. [3]Center for Solid Waste Research (CSWR), Institute for Environmental Research (IER), Tehran University of Medical Sciences, Tehran, Iran. [4]Nanotechnology Research Institute of Petroleum Industry (RIPI), West Blvd. Azadi Sport Complex, Tehran, Iran. [5]Kurdistan Environmental Health Research Center, Kurdistan University of Medical Sciences, Sanandaj, Iran.

References

1. Matilainen A, Vepsäläinen M, Sillanpää M. Natural organic matter removal by coagulation during drinking water treatment: A review. Adv Colloid Interface Sci. 2010;159:189–97.
2. Karnik BS, Davies SH, Baumann MJ, Masten SJ. The effects of combined ozonation and filtration on disinfection by-product formation. Water Res. 2005;39:2839–50.
3. Zazouli M, Nasseri S, Mahvi A, Mesdaghinia A, Younecian M, Gholami M. Determination of hydrophobic and hydrophilic fractions of natural organic matter in raw water of Jalalieh and Tehranspars water treatment plants (Tehran). J Appl Sci. 2007;7:2651–5.
4. Kim H-C, Yu M-J. Characerization of natural organic matter in conventional water treatment process for selection of treatment processes focused on DBPs control. Water Res. 2005;39:4779–89.
5. Crittenden JC, Trussel RR, W HD, J HK, GT: Warer treatment: Principles and design. 2nd edition: John Wiley & sons Inc., New Jersey; 2005
6. Chen C, Zhang X, Zhu L, Liu J, He W, Han H. Disinfection by-products and their precursors in a water treatment plant in North China: seasonal changes and fraction analysis. Sci Total Environ. 2008;397:140–7.
7. Anu Matilainen ETG, Tanja L, Leif H, Amit B, Mika S. An overview of the methods used in the characterisation of natural organic matter (NOM) in relation to drinking water treatment. Chemosphere. 2011;83:1431–42.
8. Zazouli M, Ulbricht M, Nasseri S, Susanto H. Effect of hydrophilic and hydrophobic organic matter on amoxicillin and cephalexin residuals rejection from water by nanofiltration. Iranian J Environ Health Sci Eng. 2010;7:15–24.
9. Moussavi S, Ehrampoush M, Mahvi A, Ahmadian M, Rahimi S. Adsorption of Humic Acid from Aqueous Solution on Single-Walled Carbon Nanotubes. Asian J Chem. 2013;25.
10. Moussavi S, Ehrampoush M, Mahvi A, Rahimi S, Ahmadian M. Efficiency of Multi-Walled Carbon Nanotubes in Adsorbing Humic Acid from Aqueous Solutions. Asian J Chem. 2014;26:821–6.
11. Bazrafshan E, Biglari H, Mahvi AH. Humic acid removal from aqueous environments by electrocoagulation process using iron electrodes. J Chem. 2012;9:2453–61.
12. Mahvi A, Maleki A, Rezaee R, Safari M. Reduction of humic substances in water by application of ultrasound waves and ultraviolet irradiation. Iranian J Environ Health Sci Eng. 2009;6:233–40.
13. Zazouli M, Nasseri S, Mahvi A, Gholami M, Mesdaghinia A, Younesian M. Retention of humic acid from water by nanofiltration membrane and influence of solution chemistry on membrane performance. Iranian J Environ Health Sci Eng. 2008;5:11–8.
14. Rezaee R, Maleki A, Jafari A, Mazloomi S, Zandsalimi Y, Mahvi AH. Application of response surface methodology for optimization of natural organic matter degradation by UV/H2O2 advanced oxidation process. J Environ Health Sci Eng. 2014;12:67.
15. Alipour V, Nasseri S, Nodehi RN, Mahvi AH, Rashidi A. Preparation and application of oyster shell supported zero valent nano scale iron for

removal of natural organic matter from aqueous solutions. J Environ Health Sci Eng. 2014;12:146.
16. Naghizadeh A, Nasseri S, Mahvi AH, Nabizadeh R, Kalantary RR, Rashidi A. Continuous adsorption of natural organic matters in a column packed with carbon nanotubes. J Environ Health Sci Eng. 2013;11:14.
17. Peter-Varbanets M, Zurbrügg C, Swartz C, Pronk W. Decentralized systems for potable water and the potential of membrane technology. Water Res. 2009;43:245–65.
18. Chin CJM, Shih LC, Tsai HJ, Liu TK. Adsorption of oxylene and p-xylene from water by SWCNTs. Carbon. 2007;45:1254–60.
19. Xuemei Rena CC, Masaaki N, Xiangke W. Carbon nanotubes as adsorbents in environmental pollution management: A review. Chem Eng J. 2011;170:395–410.
20. Upadhyayula VKK, Deng S, Mitchell MC, Smith GB. Application of carbon nanotube technology for removal of contaminants in drinking water: A review. Sci Total Environ. 2009;408:1–13.
21. Ahn CH, Baek Y, Lee C, Kim SO, Kim S, Lee S,Kim S-H, Bae SS, Park J, Yoon J: Carbon nanotube-based membranes: Fabrication and application to desalination. J ind Eng Chem. 2012;18:1551–9.
22. Gilani N, Daryan JT, Rashidi A, Omidkhah MR. Separation of methane–nitrogen mixtures using synthesis vertically aligned carbon nanotube membranes. Appl Surf Sci. 2012;258:4819–25.
23. Hou PX, Liu C, Shi C, Cheng HM. Carbon nanotubes prepared by anodic aluminum oxide template method. Chin Sci Bull. 2012;1–18.
24. Celik E, Park H, Choi H. Carbon nanotube blended polyethersulfone membranes for fouling control in water treatment. Water Res. 2011;45:274–82.
25. Kim E-S, Hwang G, Gamal El-Din M, Liu Y. Development of nanosilver and multi-walled carbon nanotubes thin film nanocomposite membrane for enhanced water treatment. J Membra Sci. 2012;394–395:37–48.
26. Majeed S, Fierro D, Buhr K, Wind J, Du B, Boschetti-de-Fierro A, Abetz V: Multi-walled carbon nanotubes (MWCNTs) mixed polyacrylonitrile (PAN) ultrafiltration membranes. J Membra Sci. 2012;403–404:101–9.
27. Qiu S, Wu L, Pan X, Zhang L, Chen H, Gao C. Preparation and properties of functionalized carbon nanotube/PSF blend ultrafiltration membranes. J Membra Sci. 2009;342:165–72.
28. Rahimpour A, Jahanshahi M, Khalili S, Mollahosseini A, Zirepour A, Rajaeian B. Novel functionalized carbon nanotubes for improving the surface properties and performance of polyethersulfone (PES) membrane. Desalination. 2012;286:99–107.
29. Vatanpour V, Madaeni SS, Moradian R, Zinadini S, Astinchap B. Fabrication and characterization of novel antifouling nanofiltration membrane prepared from oxidized multiwalled carbon nanotube/polyethersulfone nanocomposite. J Membra Sci. 2011;375:284–94.
30. Gilani N, Towfighi J, Rashidi A, Mohammadi T, Omidkhah MR, Sadeghian A. Investigation of H2S separation from H2S/CH4 mixtures using functionalized and non-functionalized vertically aligned carbon nanotube membranes. Appl Surf Sci. 2013;270:115–23.
31. Poinern GEJ, Ali N, Fawcett D. Progress in nano-engineered anodic aluminum oxide membrane development. Materials. 2011;4:487–526.
32. Abràmoff MD, Magalhães PJ, Ram SJ. Image processing with ImageJ. Biophotonics Int. 2004;11:36–43.
33. Chen X, Cendrowski K, Srenscek-Nazzal J, Rümmeli M, Kalenczuk RJ, Chen H, Chu PK, Borowiak-Palen E: Fabrication method of parallel mesoporous carbon nanotubes. Colloids Surf A Physicochem Eng Asp. 2011;377:150–5.
34. Rana K, Kucukayan-Dogu G, Bengu E. Growth of vertically aligned carbon nanotubes over self-ordered nano-porous alumina films and their surface properties. Appl Surf Sci. 2012;258:7112–7.
35. Salahi A, Abbasi M, Mohammadi T. Permeate flux decline during UF of oily wastewater: Experimental and modeling. Desalination. 2010;251:153–60.
36. Majumder M, Chopra N, Andrews R, Hinds BJ. Nanoscale hydrodynamics: enhanced flow in carbon nanotubes. Nature. 2005;438:44–4.
37. Baek Y, Kim C, Seo DK, Kim T, Lee JS, Kim YH, Ahn KH, Bae SS, Lee SC, Lim J, Lee K, Yoon J: High performance and antifouling vertically aligned carbon nanotube membrane for water purification. J Membra Sci. 2014;460:171–7.
38. Park S-M, Jung J, Lee S, Baek Y, Yoon J, Seo DK,Kim YH: Fouling and rejection behavior of carbon nanotube membranes. Desalination. 2014;343:180–6.
39. Avramescu M-E, Sager W, Borneman Z, Wessling M. Adsorptive membranes for bilirubin removal. J Chromatogr B. 2004;803:215–23.
40. Jamshidi Gohari R, Lau W, Matsuura T, Halakoo E, Ismail A. Adsorptive removal of Pb (II) from aqueous solution by novel PES/HMO ultrafiltration mixed matrix membrane. Sep Purif Technol. 2013;120:59–68.
41. Liu L, Zheng G, Yang F. Adsorptive removal and oxidation of organic pollutants from water using a novel membrane. Chem Eng J. 2010;156:553–6.
42. Naghizadeh A, Nasseri S, Rashidi A, Kalantary RR, Nabizadeh R, Mahvi A. Adsorption kinetics and thermodynamics of hydrophobic natural organic matter (NOM) removal from aqueous solution by multi-wall carbon nanotubes. Water Sci Technol: Water Supply. 2013;13:273–85.
43. Hermia J. Constant pressure blocking filtration law application to powder-law non-Newtonian fluid. Trans Inst Chem Eng. 1982;60:183–7.
44. Crittenden JC, Trussell RR, Hand DW, Howe KJ, Tchobanoglous G: MWH's Water Treatment: Principles and Design. 3rd edition, John Wiley & sons Inc, New Jersey; 2012.
45. Susanto H, Ulbricht M. High-performance thin-layer hydrogel composite membranes for ultrafiltration of natural organic matter. Water Res. 2008;42:2827–35.
46. Heo J, Kim H, Her N, Lee S, Park Y-G, Yoon Y. Natural organic matter removal in single-walled carbon nanotubes–ultrafiltration membrane systems. Desalination. 2012;298:75–84.

Wastewater treatment using integrated anaerobic baffled reactor and Bio-rack wetland planted with *Phragmites* sp. and *Typha* sp.

Shervin Jamshidi[1], Abbas Akbarzadeh[2], Kwang-Sung Woo[3] and Alireza Valipour[3*]

Abstract

The purpose of this study is to examine the potential use of anaerobic baffled reactor (ABR) followed by Bio-rack wetland planted with *Phragmites* sp. and *Typha* sp. for treating domestic wastewater generated by small communities (751 mg COD/L, 500 SCOD mg/L, 348 mg BOD_5/L). Two parallel laboratory-scale models showed that the process planted with *Phragmites* sp. and *Typha* sp. are capable of removing COD by 87% & 86%, SCOD by 90% & 88%, BOD_5 by 93% & 92%, TSS by 88% & 86%, TN by 79% & 77%, PO_4-P by 21% & 14% at an overall HRT of 21 (843 g COD/m^3/day & 392 g BOD_5/m^3/day) and 27 (622 g COD/m^3/day & 302 g BOD_5/m^3/day) hours, respectively. Microbial analysis indicated a high reduction in the MPN of total coliform and TVC as high as 99% at the outlet end of the processes. The vegetated system using *Phragmites* sp. showed significantly greater ($p < 0.05$) pollutant removal efficiencies due to its extensive root and mass growth rate ($p < 0.05$) of the plant compared to *Typha* sp. The *Phragmites* sp. indicated a higher relative growth rate (3.92%) than *Typha* sp. (0.90%). Microorganisms immobilized on the surface of the Bio-rack media (mean TVC: 2.33×10^7 cfu/cm^2) were isolated, identified and observed using scanning electron microscopy (SEM). This study illustrated that the present integrated processes could be an ideal approach for promoting a sustainable decentralization, however, *Phragmites* sp. would be more efficient rather than *Typha* sp.

Keywords: Anaerobic baffled reactor, Bio-rack wetland system, *Phragmites* sp, *Typha* sp, Domestic wastewater treatment

Background

Decentralized wastewater treatment systems (DEWATS) are appropriate for low-density communities and varying site conditions, and are more cost-effective than centralized practices. However, the efficiency of these systems depends on the attributes, and design criteria of the selected process [1]. Therefore, it is imperative to conduct research in order to develop a feasible and sustainable treatment technique for decentralization.

Anaerobic baffled reactor (ABR) reported to be a promising solution in domestic wastewater treatment [2-4]. The system recognized by incorporating the advantages of upflow anaerobic sludge blanket (UASB) and phase separation. It consists of alternating hanging and standing baffles, which compartmentalizes the reactor [5]. This practice leads the flow into intimate contact with the biomass [6,7], resulting in partial separation of acidogenesis and methanogenesis longitudinally down the reactor, and more stable operation [8-10]. It has been shown to provide higher resilience to hydraulic and organic shock loads, higher treatment rate, longer biomass retention times, and lower sludge yields than other anaerobic treatment systems [5]. Previous hydrodynamic studies revealed that the low dead space (7% to 30%) occurred in ABR [7]. Nasr et al. [2] reported removal efficiencies of 76% for total chemical oxygen demand (COD), and 55% for biochemical oxygen demand (BOD_5) in ABR treating domestic wastewater at a hydraulic retention time (HRT) of 12 hours. Bodkhe [11] used a modified ABR in order to achieve 84% COD, and 87% BOD_5 in treating municipal wastewater at a HRT of 6 hours. Feng et al. [12] used a bamboo carrier ABR to treat sewage achieving 69% COD reduction at a HRT of 18 hours. Despite the significant advantages and efforts made worldwide, typically the effluent of ABR technique is totally nutrients rich, oxygen deficit, and containing high concentration of unacceptable pathogen [2]. This would surely deteriorate the quality

* Correspondence: alirezavalipour.envi@gmail.com
[3]Department of Civil Engineering, Yeungnam University, Gyungsan, South Korea
Full list of author information is available at the end of the article

of surface waters in rural areas. In fact, it requires post treatment for removing the remaining organic matters, nutrients and pathogens.

In the recent years, the application of constructed wetlands for wastewater treatment has received greater attention since they offer a cost effective and an environmentally sound approach [13]. In that order, the possible applications of integrated anaerobic pretreated-constructed wetlands have been introduced as a promising model for DEWATS [14-16]. The major mechanism associated in constructed wetland for pollutant removal is the interaction between the bacterial metabolism and plant uptake, respectively, termed as rhizoremediation and phytoextraction [17]. Plants transfer oxygen to their root system and release a fraction of this oxygen into the rhizosphere for aerobic bacterial activity [18]. The type of aquatic plant species can also act as an important biotic factor in the treatment efficiency of constructed wetlands [19]. In that order, among various aquatic weeds, *Phragmites* sp. and *Typha* sp. are two well-known macrophytes demonstrated as potentially valuable vegetation in the natural purification process [20]. Nevertheless, the use of constructed wetlands, either as a standalone or combined solution, could be restricted by choking, clogging, slow mass transfer, poor root penetration into the multilayer soil column, high area requirement and capital investment. It is implied that conventional decentralized treatment processes are required to be optimized and upgraded to prevail over the limitations.

In our earlier recent work, the application of ABR has been studied comprehensively to optimize its design and operation in pollutant removal from domestic wastewater (~350-750 mg COD/L), and it was simulated by artificial neural network [9,10]. On the other hand, the Bio-rack system (BRS) is one of the latest evolutions of wetland technologies that developed to overcome the drawbacks of conventional wetland processes [21]. This is a robust biological practice that can be applied to the efficient and reliable elimination of pollutants, even under unfavorable influent conditions stressed by high total dissolved solids and heavy metal [21,22]. Analytical data which collected during the treatment of domestic wastewater (COD ≤440 mg/L, $BOD_5 \leq 238$ mg/L) showed that this process able to reduce up to 80% COD, and 90% BOD_5 at a HRT of 10 hours [21]. The process is designed by incorporating the advantages of engineered attached growth (using a support matrix of the Bio-racks) and phytoremediation systems. The Bio-rack technique provides a desirable condition for plant root growth, efficient oxygen diffusion, and a distinguished surface area for a superior microbial population responsible for organic degradation at much low area requirement and capital cost [23]. The interrelationships between the plants and microorganisms associated with biofilms attached to the racks, stems, roots, and water column form a high rate wetland system. A further study also revealed the efficiency of this method planted with *Thalia dealbata*, *Acorus calamus*, *Zizania latifolia* and *Iris sibirica* for river water treatment [24,25]. Marchand *et al.* [26] successfully applied a Bio-racks filled with a homogeneous mix of gravels and perlite for the removal of copper ion from synthetic Cu-contaminated wastewaters using *Phragmites australis*, *Juncus articulatus* and *Phalaris arundinacea*.

Hence, it is recommended that using Bio-rack wetland upgraded with ABR should be considered as a novel scientific advancement and integrated approach. This innovation has not been documented before; its performance would be controversial and requires to be optimized thoroughly. This study is aimed to develop and examine the performance of an integrated process of ABR and BRS for effective treatment of domestic wastewater which could be implemented in decentralization practices. The potential ability of two aquatic plants, included *Phragmites sp.* and *Typha sp.*, in wetland phytoremediation were also compared to find the most efficient and well matched vegetation in the combined ABR and BRS. This is important to have a comparative assessment on the use of aquatic weeds in the phytoremediation systems, where the most suitable macrophytes are available.

Materials and methods

The characteristic of wastewater

The overall characteristic of domestic wastewater during the study period was as follows: pH 7.44 ± 0.12, total chemical oxygen demand (COD) 751 ± 43 mg/L, soluble chemical oxygen demand (SCOD) 500 ± 45 mg/L, biochemical oxygen demand (BOD_5) 348 ± 26 mg/L, dissolved oxygen (DO) 0.19 ± 0.07 mg/L, total suspended solids (TSS) 528 ± 41 mg/L, total nitrogen (TN) 64.65 ± 5.14 mg/L, phosphate (PO_4-P) 13.7 ± 1 mg/L, total coliform $5.27 \times 10^7 \pm 1.8 \times 10^7$ MPN/100ml, and total viable count (TVC) $3.30 \times 10^7 \pm 6.53 \times 10^6$cfu/ml.

Chemicals and instrumentation

The chemicals used in this study were of analytical grade (from Merck, Germany) as follows: Borax, Bromocresol green (5%), Citric acid, Ferroin indicator, Formaldehyde solution, Methyl red (1%), Starch, Ag_2SO_4, $CaCl_2$, $C_{20}H_{14}O_4$, C_2H_5OH, $CuSO_4.5H_2O$, $FeCl_3.6H_2O$, $Fe(NH_4)_2(SO_4)_2.6H_2O$, H_3BO_3, HCl, $HgSO_4$, H_2SO_4, $K_2Cr_2O_7$, KI, KH_2PO_4, K_2HPO_4, K_2SO_4, $MnSO_4.4H_2O$, NaCl, $NaHCO_3$, NaN_3, NaOH, Na_2SO_4, $Na_2S_2O_3.5H_2O$, $Na_2HPO_4.7H_2O$, $Na_2S_2O_3.5H_2O$, $(NH_4)_6Mo_7O_{24}.4H_2O$, $(NH_4)_2S_2O_8$, NH_4Cl, $MgSO_4.7H_2O$, Nutrient agar, and MacConkey broth.

The sample pH was measured by a pH-meter model 75P (Istek, Korea). COD tests were performed by using the open-reflux digestor model EME6/CEB (Electrothermal, UK). TN was examined via the semimicro Kjeldahl setup. UV-visible spectrophotometer model P/N BUV40X00

(PerkinElmer, USA) was used to measure PO_4-P. Steroscan 440 scanning electron microscope (SEM, Leica, Cambridge, UK) was used during observation of active biomass on the support matrix (Bio-rack).

Pilot plant setup

Two bench scale anaerobic baffled reactors (ABR) in parallel followed by horizontal flow Bio-rack system (BRS) vegetated with *Phragmites* sp. and *Typha* sp. were set-up on the premises of Water and Wastewater Research Centre (WWRC), Water Research Institute (WRI), Tehran, Iran. The pilot plants were comprised of three major sections including storage tanks (70 L), constant head tanks (20 L), and wetland units (Figure 1).

Each Plexiglas anaerobic baffled reactor (Length: 0.94 m, Width: 0.16 m, Height: 0.5 m) with 60 L net volume, consists of equally six compartments. The compartments were arranged by further vertical baffles dividing upflow-to-downflow parts by a ratio of 3:1 to affect the fluid dynamics in the sludge bed [7]. In this process, the wastewater force to flow under and over the baffles from one compartment to the next as it passes from the inlet to the outlet. The biogas formed during the anaerobic fermentation was released by the exhaust valves located on the top of the reactor.

The wetland systems (Bio-rack units) included a rectangular tank measuring 0.32 m × 0.3 m × 0.6 m (L × W × H), an effective depth of 0.54 m, and a 50 L void volume in the presence of vegetation and other internals. Unique feature of this system is the presence of 15 vertical PVC pipes (a 500 mm effective height × 60 mm outer diameter), free of soil strata, assembled as a rack and called Bio-rack. The pipes contained numerous surface perforations (20 mm diameter) for liquid transportation. These Bio-racks are involved in the treatment process by holding vegetation and providing an abundant attachment site for microbial growth. In this practice, the wastewater is distributed uniformly and then flows horizontally through the support matrix (Bio-racks), stems and roots of the plants to treat by physical and biological processes. The occupied area and specific surface of the matrix Bio-rack were 0.06 m^2 and 55 m^2/m^3 effective volume (57 m^2/m^3 filled volume), respectively. Sixty *Phragmites* sp. and thirty *Typha* sp. plants were held in the support matrix of the Bio-rack at the initial stage of the plantation. The lower number of *Typha* sp. was used because these plans are larger in size compared to *Phragmites* sp. The inlet and outlet arrangements were made as per standard practices.

Start-up and acclimatization

The experiments were initiated with the batch mode of merely anaerobic baffled reactors by seeding the mixture of cow dung and sewage sludge at the ratio of 1:2 (50% v/V) on effluent wastewater in each compartment for 2 weeks. The content of the reactors was recycled for homogeneity in the same period. Subsequently, the two comparable anaerobic baffled reactors in combination with Bio-rack systems were operated through serial exposure of sewage starting from 25% loading rate, which was increased gradually to 100% at an overall HRT of 44 hours over a 25 day period. In this stage, the systems continued to perform for more 45 days until the reduction in the percentage of COD reached a constant level, which was considered as the acclimatization period. Initially, the plant density was low and gradually the plant growth and reached their maximum possible number as bacterial growth was enhanced. In that order, the ratio of the volatile fatty acids to total alkalinity concentration was observed to be maintained below 0.3 at the outlet end of the ABR during studies.

It is noteworthy to say that the *Phragmites* sp. and *Typha* sp. were obtained from marshy lands of Tehran Province and Malayer County, respectively. Sampling was accomplished with simple hand tools. The underground parts (roots and bulbs) of the plants were carefully dug up, and the soil removed with care. A plastic collection container containing water marsh was used for transferring the sampled plants and minimizing their damage through several mechanisms. In the lab, the

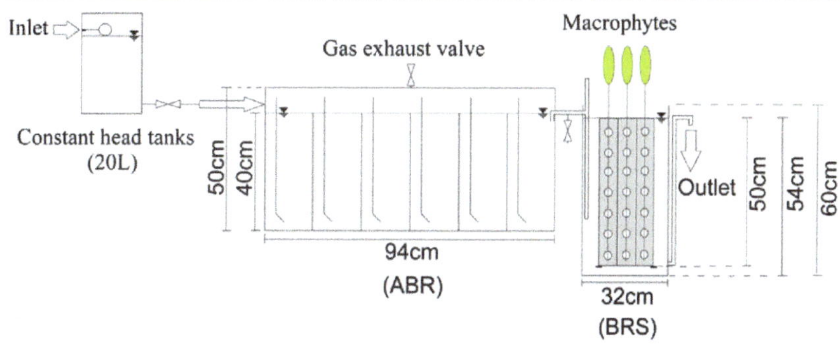

Figure 1 Schematic diagram of the integrated treatment systems (ABR: anaerobic baffled reactor (ABR), BRS: bio-rack system).

roots of sampled plants were washed with tap water to remove any remaining adsorbed soil particles before preliminary plantation. The type of the plants determined with the help of the National Botanical Garden, Teharan, Iran.

Operational procedure

The integrated systems of ABR and Bio-rack wetland vegetated with *Phragmites* sp. and *Typha* sp. were operated in an ambient air temperature (25-29°C), where sunlight could effectively penetrate. Temperatures were not controlled except to prevent the effect of cold weather. After the acclimatization period, the experiments were initiated during February 2012 to 2013 to determine the state of present processes denoted by hydraulic retention time (HRT), treatment performance and plant growth with the intention of organic pollutant elimination considering the effluent discharge norms specified by the national pollution control board of Iran (COD <100 mg/L, and $BOD_5 < 30$ mg/L), that is required for discharge into natural water resources. Under steady state condition, the systems were operated in six phases (Table 1). The daily flow was calculated by taking into account the theoretical HRT of ABR, and subsequently examined the HRT of wetland unit through each phase. The theoretical HRT, t (hours), of each treatment unit was established from the following equation:

$$t = \frac{V}{Q} \tag{1}$$

where V (L) is the void volume of the reactor, and Q (L/hour) is the design flow rate. Wastewater flow (L/day) expresses the design wastewater flow over a 24 hour period. Overall HRT indicates the sum of retention time both ABR and wetland system.

The inflow rates were fixed accordingly to 65, 80, 96, 114, 126 and 144 L/day for overall HRTs of 41, 33, 27, 23, 21 and 18 hours, respectively. The systems are operated at each retention time for 60 days, during which the effluent characteristics with an almost constant percentage reduction were achieved.

Additionally, the old plants were removed periodically and new plants were retained or allowed to grow during experimentations. In general, the roots of young plants can display greater ability to absorb impurities and release oxygen than old plants due to the age of the plants and tissues. Therefore, it is important to use healthy young plants for the more efficient contaminant removal [27]. Sodium bicarbonate is a buffer used to stabilize pH as per requirement in ABR.

Wastewater sampling and analysis

Raw wastewater samples were collected from a residential source of WWRC, WRI, Iran, on a daily basis for performance evaluation. The samples from the inlet and outlet of the reactors was analyzed every 24 h at 10 am for pH, COD, SCOD, BOD_5, TSS, TN, PO_4-P and MPN of coliform bacteria according to the standard method [28]. In that order, the samples were merely filtered through Whatmann 42 before testing of SCOD and BOD_5. The microbial population presented in the inlet and outlet, plant root surface, and Bio-rack surface were examined to determine the total viable count (TVC) using the pour plate technique [28]. The active attached biomass on the surface of Bio-racks was observed by using scanning electron microscope (SEM) as per the standard procedure [29]. Bacteria presented on the support matrix (Bio-racks) were merely isolated on nutrient agar medium and the Gram-negative bacterial identification was done using Mini API (BioMérieux, France).

Botanical aspects

The morphological characteristics of *Phragmatis* sp. and *Typha* sp. in terms of the number of leaves, size of the

Table 1 Experimental conditions implied in wastewater treatment

Phase Item	I	II	III	IV	V	VI
Operation period (day)	60	60	60	60	60	60
Overall HRT (hours)	41	33	27	24	21	18
HRT_{ABR} (hours)	22	18	15	13	11	10
HRT_{BRS} (hours)	19	15	12	11	9	8
Q (L/day)	65	80	96	114	126	144
OLR						
(g COD/day)	50 ± 2.63	61 ± 3.02	68 ± 2.02	85 ± 6.02	93 ± 6.46	113 ± 2.56
(g BOD_5/day)	23 ± 1.96	29 ± 2.60	33 ± 2.09	40 ± 3.51	43 ± 3.07	50 ± 4.11
(g COD/m^3/day)*	455 ± 24	553 ± 27	622 ± 18	769 ± 55	843 ± 59	1024 ± 23
(g BOD_5/m^3/day)*	205 ± 18	260 ± 24	302 ± 19	361 ± 32	392 ± 28	452 ± 37

HRT: hydraulic retention time; Q: flow rate; OLR: organic loading rate *based on the sum of effective volume both ABR and BRS.

leaves, number of roots, longest root, dry weight, and ash weight were analyzed every 15 days over a 3 month period throughout the six phases of the HRT evaluation to monitor morphological changes in the plants as per standard practice [30].

Statistical analysis

The data of 365 consecutive days were analyzed to examine the performance of two integrated systems. Treatment efficiency was calculated as the percentage of removal for each parameter as follows:

$$\text{Removal efficiency } (\%) = \frac{\text{Ci}-\text{Ce}}{\text{Ci}} \times 100 \quad (2)$$

where C_i and C_e are the influent and effluent concentrations. Organic loading rates, OLR (g/day), were calculated by multiplying the discharge flow (L/day) and the organic concentrations (g/L). Relative growth rate of the plants is calculated using the following equation:

$$\text{Relative growth rate } (\%) = \frac{\ln \text{W2} - \ln \text{W1}}{\text{t2}-\text{t1}} \times 100 \quad (3)$$

where W_1 and W_2 are the dry weight of plants at times t_1 and t_2. Statistical analysis of the data to compare integrated systems on the organic load removal and morphological characteristics of plants growth were done through the variance (ANOVA) and Duncan test using SPSS software [31]. Performance differences were deemed to be significant if $p < 0.05$.

Results and discussions

This investigation discusses the possibility application of the Bio-rack wetland system as a post-treatment of anaerobic baffled reactor through single specimens of *Phragmites sp.* or *Typha sp.* for DEWATS. In the previous study, the performance of ABR throughout eight-compartment treating domestic wastewater was assessed, simulated, and optimum configuration was determined [9,10]. The ABR toward the treatment of domestic wastewater (750 mg COD/L) clearly showed a stable performance under different hydraulic retention times by having a high compartments number (more than 5). Therefore, the six-compartment ABR was selected in the present study to ensure an effective pre-treatment condition in treating domestic wastewater.

Organic pollutant removal

Since, the constancy of any biological process thoroughly depends on the hydraulic and organic loading rates; the experiments were performed to estimate the satisfactory hydraulic retention time (HRT) of the whole integrated process of ABR followed by Bio-rack system using *Phragmites* sp. (ABR-BRSUP) and *Typha* sp. (ABR-BRSUT).

The SCOD and BOD_5 concentration of the treated effluent was below 60 and 30 mg/L at overall HRTs above 21 and 27 hours, in the treatment systems planted by *Phragmites* sp. and *Typha* sp., respectively (Figure 2). Likewise, the COD concentration was exceeded Irans's permissible limit at below 21 (95 mg COD/L) and 27 (97 mg COD/L) hours HRTs. An ANOVA and Duncan test done on the performance data in terms of BOD_5 removal indicate that the differences exist between the performances of these two processes; p-value was less than 0.05 merely at overall HRT of 21 and 18 hours (Table 2). The supremacy of the Bio-rack wetland vegetated with *Phragmites* sp. would be significant in lower retention times. Therefore, overall HRTs of 21 and 27 hours are considered to achieve a satisfactory organic removal performance in ABR-BRSUP and ABR-BRSUT, respectively.

Many studies comparing planted systems over unplanted units have been conflicting results regarding the importance of plants in any phytoremediation process [32,33]. In the absence of the rhizomes of the plants, the micro-sites occupied by the wetland unit become anaerobic; lead to a lower rate of impurities elimination. The major advantage associated with the current integrated treatment systems is the presence of the Bio-rack wetland. The Bio-rack process planted with *Phragmites* sp and *Typha* sp. examined to offer, respectively, a lower HRT of 9.5 (COD: 77%, SCOD: 79%, BOD_5: 84% reduction) and 12.5 (COD: 66%, SCOD: 69%, BOD_5: 76% reduction) hours in polishing anaerobic effluent as compared to other relevant literatures [2,14,15]. Kaseva [14] reported average COD removal efficiencies of 56 & 61% at HRT of 1.96 and 1.99 days in the conventional constructed wetlands using *Phragmites* sp. and *Typha* sp., respectively. Mbuligwe [15] was determined the efficiency of conventional constructed wetlands using *Typha* sp. and *Colocasia* sp., respectively, by 79 & 75% COD reduction at 1.2 days HRT. The Bio-rack wetland used in this study also showed a higher removal of organic pollutant compared to the duckweed system, in which 54 & 58% COD, 63 & 64% SCOD and 21 & 63% BOD_5 reduction could be accomplished at 10 and 15 days HRT, respectively [2]. It can be verified that wetland type, efficient oxygen diffusion, and the high accumulation of the attached bacterial populations on the surface of support matrix are the major factors for high level of removal efficiency in the Bio-rack process.

The Bio-rack wetland with *Phragmites* sp. exhibits a higher rate of pollutant reduction owing to the extensive root system of the plant which is responsible for desirable rate of the oxygen transfer efficiency, and greater microbial mass contribution in the treatment unit. However, there was a little difference in the removal of organic pollutant at longer retention times during the operation of

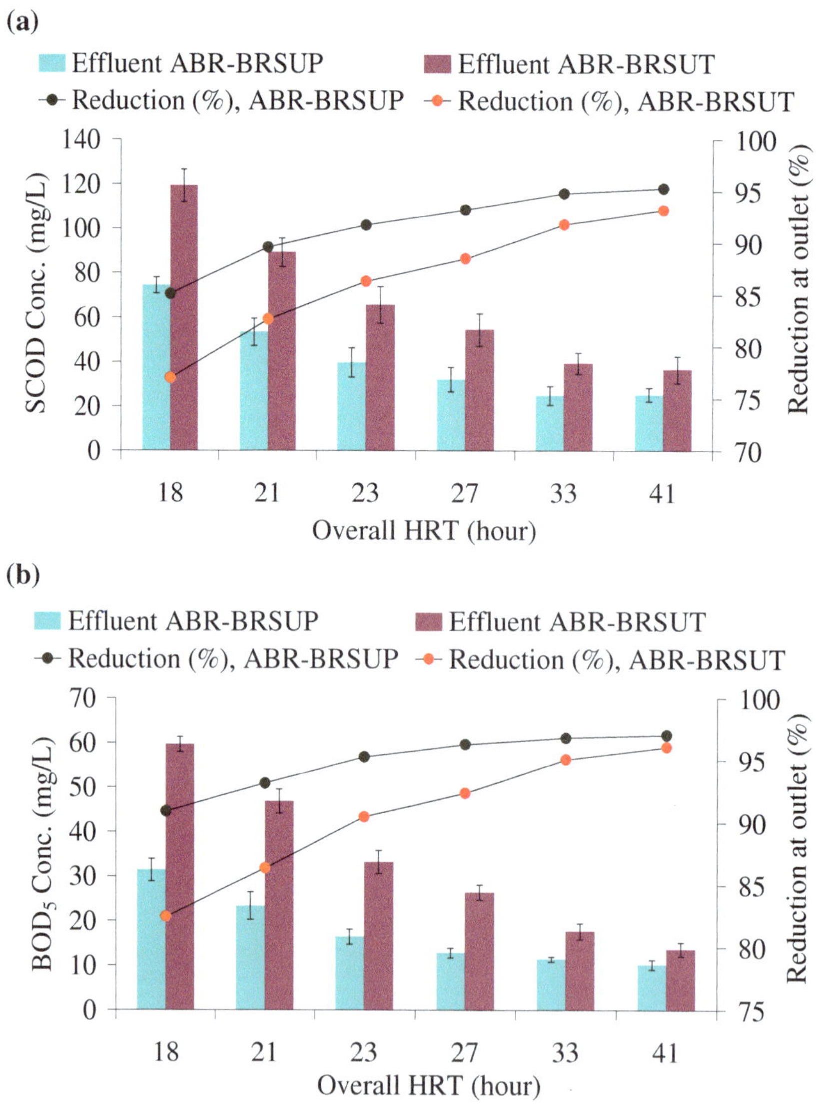

Figure 2 Effluent (a) SCOD and (b) BOD_5 concentrations with five days repetition through the integrated systems.

both treatment processes. The visual observation showed that the *Phragmites* sp. tends to develop a wonderfully root system which occupies thoroughly over the depth of the treatment unit. *Typha* sp. appears to have a shallower root system.

Dissolve oxygen silhouette in the reactor

Adequate dissolved oxygen required for bacterial oxidation is relatively inefficient by a transfer process of atmospheric diffusion, and in the Bio-rack wetland the transfer is likely to be smaller since the dense plant cover reduces surface gas-exchange. Vegetation plays a significant role in transferring oxygen via aerenchyma

Table 2 Organic pollutant removal with five days repetition through the integrated systems

Overall HRT (hour)	BOD_5 removed-g/day (ABR-BRSUP)	BOD_5 removed-g/day (ABR-BRSUT)	P-Value
41	21.85 ± 1.96	21.63 ± 1.90	0.486
33	27.71 ± 2.60	27.21 ± 2.50	0.398
27	31.95 ± 2.2	30.64 ± 2.23	0.102
23	37.85 ± 3.60	35.93 ± 3.56	0.062
21	40.14 ± 2.93	37.19 ± 2.80	0.016
18	45.21 ± 4.20	41.15 ± 4.25	0.007

HRT: hydraulic retention time;
ABR-BRSUP: anaerobic baffled reactor - bio-rack system using *Phragmites* sp.;
ABR-BRSUT: anaerobic baffled reactor - bio-rack system using *Typha* sp.

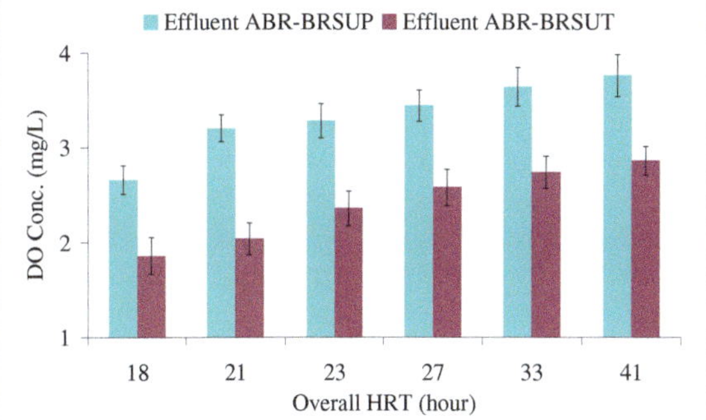

Figure 3 Mean DO values of the processes effluent with five days repetition.

tissue [32]. The dissolved oxygen inside the Bio-rack cells was estimated to be an average of 3.2 and 2.6 mg/L O_2 at overall HRTs of 21 and 27 h in ABR-BRSUP and ABR-BRSUT, respectively (Figure 3). The results suggest that the mechanism of aerobic respiration is a key microbial population in the Bio-rack process due to high rate of oxygen transfer efficiency through the roots. The aerobic bacteria are fast growing microflora causing a greater rate of organic elimination compared to anaerobic microorganism. The higher level of dissolved oxygen in the Bio-rack unit planted with *Phragmites* sp. probably can be explained by type of plant having an extensive root system; allows oxygenation to occur from the roots through the entire depth of the treatment unit.

Treatment performance

A comprehensive evaluation of other parameters was conducted at reasonable overall HRTs of 21 and 27 h (Table 3). Regarding to the results, it can be concluded that high organic loads of BOD_5 and TSS of influent can be efficiently alleviated in ABR as a pretreatment of the Bio-rack wetlands. The data evaluated in the previously reported literature, likewise, specified a possible need of a longer retention period in the Bio-rack wetlands if they use as a standalone method in treating domestic wastewater with high organic pollutant concentrations (COD > 440 mg/L, BOD_5 > 238 mg/L), whenever plants respond positively [21]. Therefore, the appropriateness of the ABR process for primary sanitation can be remarkable to improve the performance of the phytoremediation systems; meanwhile it can also decrease choking and clogging problems associated with quality variations of the influent in the conventional wetland processes. This can be implied by standard deviations shown in Table 3.

Both integrated systems can also be a viable option to reduce nutrient levels by more than 75% TN and 14% PO_4-P. Dissolved oxygen concentration would seem to be more than 2.5 mg/L in the wetland units. *Phragmites* sp. has a great potential distribution of roots enhanced nutrient uptake by the root segments in their favorable environment. Literature based evaluation confirms that the present processes potentially have a higher nutrient reduction of 40-58% TN compared to the anaerobic baffled reactor as a standalone solution [2]. It would emphasize that the application of the Bio-rack wetlands, as a post treatment of ABR can effectively improve the quality of treated domestic wastewater to be discharged to surface waters in rural areas.

The suspended solids are removed throughout the integrated systems via sedimentation and filtration phenomena. The efficiency of nutrient (N,P) removal can be explained adequately by the nitrification/denitrification of rhizoremediation process and plant uptake route. Nitrogen removal is rather high for both integrated systems. Phosphorus removal is notoriously poor in any constructed wetland practices [32]. The anaerobic systems typically increase the soluble amount of phosphate while can hardly be removed efficiently through the phytoremediation techniques. The greater percentage reduction of phosphorus can be attained by incorporating the advantages of using chemical divalent cations as a result

Table 3 Summary of effluents characteristic with five days repetition from two integrated treatment systems

Parameters*	ABR-BRSUP (overall HRT of 21 hours)				ABR-BRSUT (overall HRT of 27 hours)			
	Inlet	Outlet at ABR	Outlet at BRSUP	Overall reduction (%)	Inlet	Outlet at ABR	Outlet at BRSUT	Overall reduction (%)
pH	7.45 ± 0.09	7.10 ± 0.05	7.19 ± 0.04	-	7.50 ± 0.10	7.15 ± 0.06	7.29 ± 0.05	-
DO	0.16 ± 0.05	-	3.2 ± 0.14	-	0.18 ± 0.06	-	2.6 ± 0.20	-
COD	736 ± 51.28	420.4 ± 30.96	95.2 ± 2.28	87.1	713 ± 21.40	290 ± 17.04	97.4 ± 1.52	86.3
SCOD	515 ± 42.51	256 ± 25.26	53.4 ± 6.12	89.6	473 ± 24	173.8 ± 26.25	54.4 ± 7.85	88.5
BOD_5	342 ± 24.36	150 ± 12.32	23.4 ± 3.13	93.2	345.6 ± 22	110 ± 8.12	26.4 ± 1.67	92.4
TSS	523.4 ± 48.22	245 ± 42.66	61 ± 11.71	88.3	521 ± 47	237.2 ± 28.62	71.2 ± 7.33	86.3
TN	67.97 ± 3.88	56.31 ± 5.17	14.02 ± 0.64	79.4	63.45 ± 5.72	51.25 ± 4.61	14.41 ± 0.32	77.3
PO_4-P	13.65 ± 0.65	20.26 ± 1.82	10.73 ± 1.16	21.4	15.30 ± 0.43	22.69 ± 2.25	13.13 ± 1.04	14.2

*All analytical values except pH are based on mg/L.

of superior exchange reaction mechanism. Furthermore, the nutrient elimination would be succeeded by frequent harvesting of plants based on climate condition.

Microbial investigation

The MPN of total coliform and TVC concentrations at the outlet of two integrated processes at overall HRTs of 21 and 27 h are shown in Figure 4. The average reduction of these parameters was observed approximately 99% at the outlet end of the processes. In wetland units, there is a reduction of the TVC level at the outlet, and biological mass is getting attached to the surface of the Bio-racks. This could be phenomena in the initial stage of operation. At steady state condition, there will be uniform growth on the Bio-rack surfaces, and biomass will slough and come out with the flowing water.

The microorganisms create a sort of natural polymer responsible for their adhesion to develop the biofilm and bio-oxidation mechanism [34]. The support matrix (Bio-rack) provides the evidence of enormous TVC concentrations (Figure 4b). TVC concentrations were also found to be high both on the root surface of *Phragmites* sp. and *Typha* sp. It should be realized that *Phragmites* sp. with its extensive root system enhanced bacterial population throughout

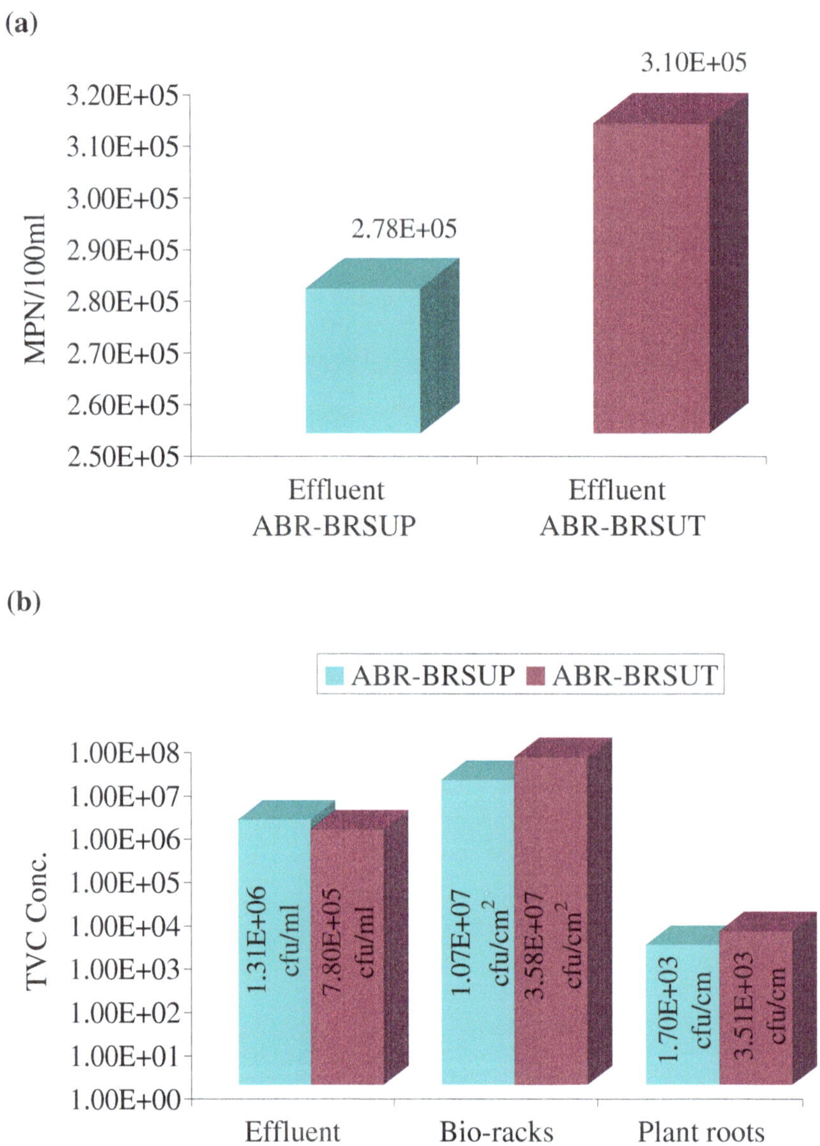

Figure 4 Mean (a) total coliform and (b) total viable count values through the integrated systems.

the Bio-rack unit. In the Bio-rack wetland, the vicinity of the support matrix, stems and roots of the plants are a preferred environment for many micro-organisms to attach and to degrade pollutants in the phytoremediation process.

The biofilm adhesion in the context of bacterial formation was visualized by scanning electron microscope (SEM). The microscopic examinations revealed the bulk of the biomass concentration on the Bio-rack surface media in both ABR-BRSUP and ABR-BRSUT (Figure 5). The biofilm, which were grown on the surface of the Bio-racks, promote somewhat a denser morphology in ABR-BRSUP (overall HRT of 21 hours) compared to ABR-BRSUT (overall HRT of 27 hours). This can be demonstrated by a high flow condition at a low retention

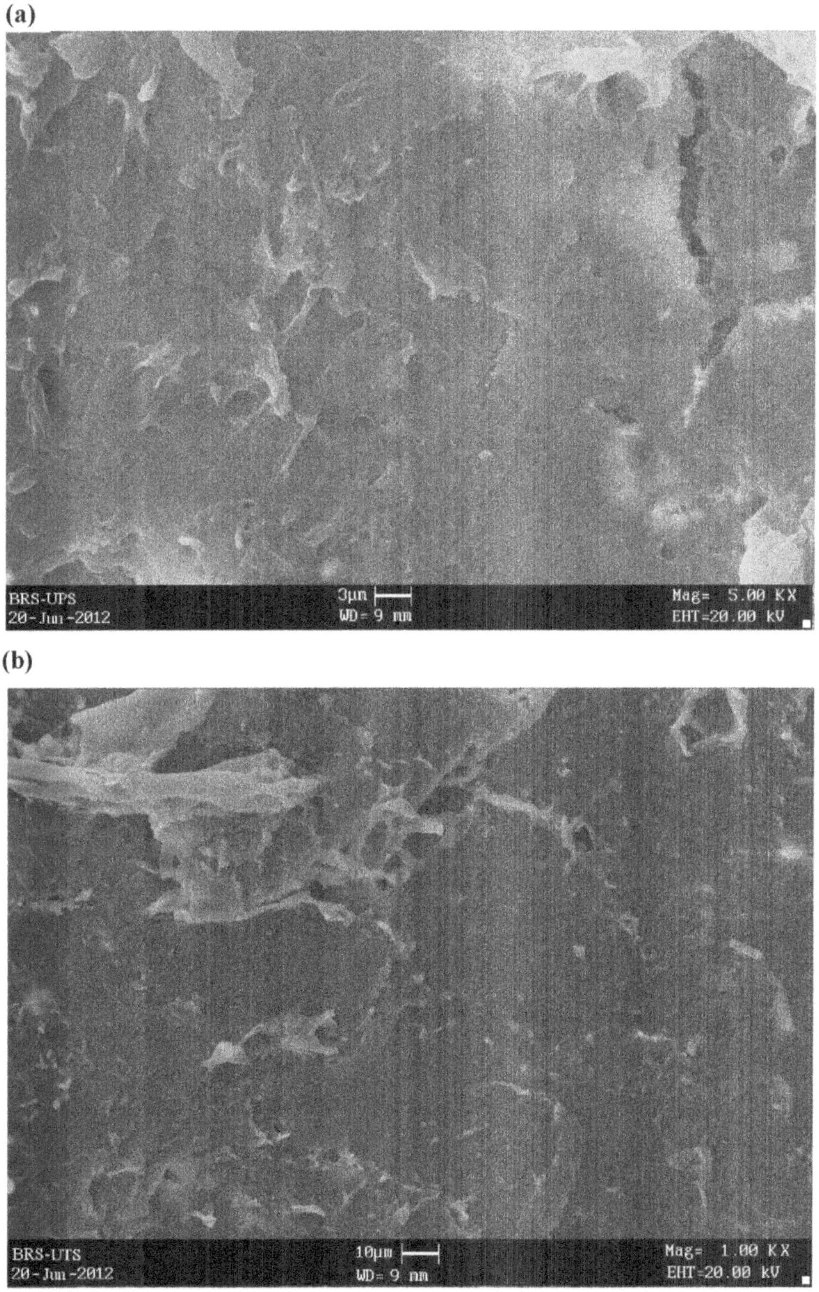

Figure 5 SEM photographs of the biofilm-forming bacteria on the surface of Bio-racks in (a) ABR-BRSUP and (b) ABR-BRSUT.

time where the viscoelastic nature of extracellular biopolymers holding the microcolonies together. In ABR-BRSUT, the morphology of biofilm grown at a low flow discharge exhibit a nearly lower dense and microcolonies are tapered. The high flow condition can also result in the detachment of biofilm, reduce the biofilm bacteria quantity, and increase of effluent bacteria population as a result of a sloughing process. This can be evident from the results on TVC (Figure 4b). Similar phenomena were also reported in the relevant literature [35]. The amount of biofilm formed on the surface of the Bio-rack was estimated to be 7 to 8 and 8 to 9 g/L in BRSUP and BRSUT, respectively.

Correspondingly, the profiling of microflora population on the surface of Bio-racks can show the presence of approximately 12 bacterial strains grown on nutrient agar medium i.e. *Acinetobacter lwoffii, Aeromonas sobria, Escherichia coli, Pseudomonas stutzeri, Aeromonas hydrophila, Citrobacter koseri, Acienetobacter johnsonni, Entrobacter intermedius, Alcaligenes faecalis, Pantoea sp., Pseudomonas putida, Acinetobacter baumanni*; this could verify the results of previous work [21]. It should be noted that there is a possibility of other microbial population, which could not be detected in a nutrient agar medium.

Plant morphological study

A study of the morphological aspects of the vegetation clearly indicated that anaerobically treated domestic sewage had no detrimental effect on the plant morphology, and the yield of the plants was increased (Table 4). In this study, anaerobically treated effluents were enriched with nutrients, particularly nitrogen (Table 3). The absorption and assimilation of nutrients by plants and the natural pH of the treated effluents may be the reasons for positive influence on the plant growth. Relative growth rate of plants also showed that *Phragmites* sp. would be more resilient to grow (3.92%) in the pretreated anaerobic effluent than *Typha* sp. (0.90%). The statistical analysis also indicated that there is a significant difference between plants in their growth ($p < 0.05$), except the longest root which found not significantly different ($p > 0.05$). These findings suggest that the *Phragmites* sp. which has a higher mass growth rate can contribute most to phytoremediation process for pollutant removal within a wetland unit (Table 3). The wetland macrophytes can adapt morphologically to grow in a water-saturated substrate through aerenchyma [36].

Pre-estimation of capital cost

A pre-estimation of economic analysis has been done for 1 m^3/day of sewage inflow based on the results generated by bench scale trials (Table 5). The result of this analysis suggested that the application of the ABR-BRSUP process could lead to 24% less land space than the ABR-BRSUT; making the phytoremediation process more sustainable for DEWATS. The total capital investment of ABR-BRSUP and ABR-BRSUT for an estimated capacity of 1 m^3/day sewage is $US 90, and $US 120, respectively. The purpose of this pre-estimation was merely to verify the advantages within the present integrated treatment systems. However, both processes can provide added benefits of an overall low HRT and high pollutant removal efficiency compared to other reported literatures [2,14,15]. The low HRT in the present integrated systems reduces the land space requirement; makes the treatment method more valuable. A detailed cost analysis of these processes needs to be performed in subsequent pilot and field experiments.

It can be summarized that the anaerobic baffled reactor followed by Bio-rack wetland can accomplish high rate organic degradation; however, the application of *Phragmites* sp. can make the treatment process partially more concise and reliable. Yet, the effluent of this process requires disinfection before discharging into the river. In addition, the effluent can also be soil infiltrated in soak pit, leach fields and mounds or else discharged underground at soil depths.

Conclusions

The studies highlight the performance of an anaerobic baffled reactor followed by Bio-rack wetland planted with *Phragmites* sp. and *Typha* sp. for decentralized treatment of domestic wastewater. These processes are characterized by other integrated treatment practices,

Table 4 Morphology characteristics of the plants at initial step and after 15 days operation (n = 5)

Parameter	BRSUP		BRSUT		P-Value
	Initial	After 15 days	Initial	After 15 days	
Number of leaves	6.2 ± 1.8	10.4 ± 1.14	8.8 ± 1.3	12 ± 1.6	0.0393
Size of leaves (mm^2)	24.3 ± 2.75	26.65 ± 2.17	96.02 ± 22	140.05 ± 20	0.0001
Number of roots	9.8 ± 1.5	28.2 ± 5.8	45.4 ± 17.52	94.6 ± 18.25	0.0005
Longest root (mm)	12.7 ± 1.43	16.42 ± 1.05	19.34 ± 4.2	22.64 ± 5	0.0670
Dry weight (g/plant)	0.65 ± 0.5	1.17 ± 0.6	28.39 ± 1.7	32.49 ± 1.3	0.0014
Ash weight (g/plant)	0.035 ± 0.006	0.114 ± 0.05	3.018 ± 0.42	3.91 ± 0.2	0.0002

Table 5 Pre-estimated capital cost of integrated treatment systems (Q =1m^3/d, COD <100 mg/L, and BOD_5 < 30 mg/L)

Item	ABR-BRSUP		ABR-BRSUT	
	ABR	BRSUP	ABR	BRSUT
Volume (m^3/m^3_{inflow})	0.48	0.41	0.63	0.54
Cost				
US$/$m^3_{inflow}$	30	60	40	80
US$/kg BOD_5 removed	155	480	167	950
Total cost				
US$/$m^3_{inflow}$	90		120	
US$/kg BOD_5 removed	635		1117	

ABR: anaerobic baffled reactor; BRSUP: bio-rack system using *Phragmites* sp.; BRSUT: bio-rack system using *Typha* sp.

where conventional wetland systems have provided in case further polishing of anaerobic effluent and in lieu, a support matrix (Bio-rack) is provided to enrich the aerobic bacteria in the form of biofilm within wetland unit. They eliminate possible limitations of ABR and Bio-rack wetland as standalone solutions, respectively, relating to low nutrient elimination and high organic load restriction. The integrated system planted with *Phragmites* sp. has low space requirement, low capital investment, and most importantly, high degradation of organic pollutants, which was capable of achieving COD, SCOD, and BOD_5 removal as high as 87%, 90% and 93%, respectively, at an overall HRT of 21 h. The integrated process using *Typha* sp. also showed stable and consistent performance in degradation of organic pollutants, where it was possible to remove 86% COD, 89% SCOD, and 92% BOD_5 at an overall HRT of 27 h. Both of these integrated processes are effective for nitrogen removal (77-79%) whereas they are less efficient in removing phosphorus (14 - 21%); divalent cation materials can be incorporated. The relative growth rate could make *Phragmites* (3.92%) a good species for phytoremediation activities than *Typha* sp. (0.90%). *Phragmites* sp. has adapted its root system to extend over the depth of the wetland unit, resulting in higher oxygen transfer efficiency through the roots, better nutrient uptake, and larger surface area for aerobic microbial biofilm to adhere and growth compared to *Typha* sp. This is a principal function of *Phragmites* sp. that can potentially increase pollutant reduction in the treatment unit ($p < 0.05$). It can be concluded that present integrated processes (especially by using *Phragmites* sp.) can be an ideal technology for DEWATS; however, this calls for detail pilot scale and field studies.

Competing interests
We certify that there is no conflict of interest with any financial organization regarding the material discussed in this manuscript.

Authors' contributions
The overall implementation of this study including experimental design, data analysis and manuscript preparation were done by SJ, AA, KW and AV. AV critically reviewed and revised the article. All authors read and approved the final manuscript.

Acknowledgements
The authors wish to thank to the Water Research Institute (WRI)-Water and Wastewater Research Center (WWRC), Tehran, Iran as well as Yeungnam University of KOREA for their valuable assistance in accomplishing this study.

Author details
[1]Department of Environmental Engineering, Faculty of Environment, University of Tehran, Tehran, Iran. [2]Water Research Institute (WRI), Tehran, Iran. [3]Department of Civil Engineering, Yeungnam University, Gyungsan, South Korea.

References
1. Massoud MA, Tarhini A, Nasr JA: **Decentralized approaches to wastewater treatment and management: applicability in developing countries.** *Environ Manage* 2009, **90**:652–659.
2. Nasr FA, Doma HS, Nassar HF: **Treatment of domestic wastewater using an anaerobic baffled reactor followed by a duckweed pond for agricultural purposes.** *Environmentalist* 2009, **29**:270–279.
3. Badalians Gholikandi G, Jamshidi S, Valipour A: **Application of electrolysis upgrading the operation of anaerobic reactors.** *Environ Stud* 2013, **38**:9–16.
4. Yu Y, Lu X, Wu Y: **Performance of an anaerobic baffled filter reactor in the treatment of algae-laden water and the contribution of granular sludge.** *Water* 2014, **6**:122–138.
5. Foxon KM, Pillay S, Lalbahadur T, Rodda N, Holder F, Buckley CA: **The anaerobic baffled reactor (ABR): an appropriate technology for on-site sanitation.** *Water SA* 2004, **30**:44–50.
6. Wang J, Huang Y, Zhao X: **Performance and characteristics of an anaerobic baffled reactor.** *Bioresour Technol* 2004, **93**:205–208.
7. Sarathai Y, Koottatep T, Morel A: **Hydraulic characteristics of an anaerobic baffled reactor as onsite wastewater treatment system.** *J Environ Sci* 2010, **22**:1319–1326.
8. Liu R, Tian Q, Chen J: **The developments of anaerobic baffled reactor for wastewater treatment: a review.** *Afr J Biotechnol* 2010, **9**:1535–1542.
9. Badalians Gholikandi G, Jamshidi S, Ebrahimzade V: **The response of anaerobic baffled reactor in various operational conditions.** *Int J Wastewater Treat Green Chem* 2011, **2**:1–10.
10. Badalians Gholikandi G, Jamshidi S, Hazrati H: **Optimization of anaerobic baffled reactor (ABR) wastewater treatment system using artificial neural network.** *Environ Eng Manage*. in press.
11. Bodkhe SY: **A modified anaerobic baffled reactor for municipal wastewater treatment.** *Environ Manage* 2009, **90**:2488–2493.
12. Feng HJ, Hu LF, Mahmood Q, Qiu CD, Fang CG, Shen DS: **Anaerobic domestic wastewater treatment with bamboo carrier anaerobic baffled reactor.** *Int Biodeterior Biodegrad* 2008, **62**:232–238.
13. Chang JJ, Wu SQ, Dai YR, Liang W, Wu ZB: **Treatment performance of integrated vertical-flow constructed wetland plots for domestic wastewater.** *Ecol Eng* 2012, **44**:152–159.
14. Kaseva ME: **Performance of a sub-surface flow constructed wetland in polishing pre-treated wastewater - a tropical case study.** *Water Res* 2004, **38**:681–687.
15. Mbuligwe SE: **Comparative effectiveness of engineered wetland systems in the treatment of anaerobically pre-treated domestic wastewater.** *Ecol Eng* 2004, **23**:269–284.
16. Singh S, Haberl R, Moog O, Shrestha RR, Shrestha P, Shrestha R: **Performance of an anaerobic baffled reactor and hybrid constructed wetland treating high-strength wastewater in Nepal - a model for DEWATS.** *Ecol Eng* 2009, **35**:654–660.
17. Landmeyer JE: *Introduction to Phytoremediation of Contaminated Groundwater*. New York: Springer; 2012.
18. Stottmeister U, Wiebner A, Kuschk P, Kappelmeyer U, Kastner M, Bederski O, Muller RA, Moormann H: **Effects of plants and microorganisms in**

constructed wetlands for wastewater treatment. *Biotechnol Adv* 2003, **22**:93–117.
19. Valipour A, Azizi S, Raman VK, Jamshidi S, Hamnabard N: The comparative evaluation on the performance of two phytoremediation systems for domestic wastewater treatment. *Environ Sci Eng.* in press.
20. Arivoli A, Mohanraj R: Efficacy of *Typha angustifolia* based vertical flow constructed wetland system in pollutant reduction of domestic wastewater. *Int J Environ Sci* 2013, **3**:1497–1508.
21. Valipour A, Raman VK, Ghole VS: A new approach in wetland systems for domestic wastewater treatment using *Phragmites* sp. *Ecol Eng* 2009, **35**:1797–1803.
22. Valipour A, Raman VK, Ghole VS: Application of patent bio-rack wetland system using *Phragmites* sp. for domestic wastewater treatment in the presence of high total dissolved solids (TDS) and heavy metal salts. *Environ Sci Eng* 2011, **53**:281–288.
23. Valipour A, Raman VK, Badalians Gholikandi G: Comparative evaluation on the performance of bio-rack and shallow pond systems for domestic wastewater treatment. *Environ Sci Eng* 2012, **54**:453–462.
24. Wang J, Zhang L, Lu S, Jin X, Gan S: Contaminant removal from low-concentration polluted river water by the Bio-rack wetlands. *Environ Sci* 2012, **24**:1006–1013.
25. Wang J, Zhang LY, Lu SY, Gan S, Jin XC: Removal of N and P from river water treated by the bio-rack wetland planted with *Thalia dealbata* and *Acorus calamus Linn*. *J Jilin Univ (Earth Sci Ed)* 2012, **42**:408–414.
26. Marchand L, Nsanganwimana F, Oustrière N, Grebenshchykova Z, Lizama-Allende K, Mench M: Copper removal from water using a bio-rack system either unplanted or planted with *Phragmites australis*, *Juncus articulatus* and *Phalaris arundinacea*. *Ecol Eng* 2014, **64**:291–300.
27. Tangahu BV, Abdullah SRS, Basri H, Idris M, Anuar N, Mukhlisin M: A review on heavy metals (As, Pb, and Hg) uptake by plants through phytoremediation. *Int J Chem Eng* 2011, **2011**:1–31.
28. APHA: *Standard Methods for the Examination of Water and Wastewater.* Washington DC: American Public Health Association; 2005.
29. Costley SC, Wallis FM: Bioremediation of heavy metals in a synthetic wastewater using a rotating biological contactor. *Water Res* 2001, **35**:3715–3723.
30. Kalra YP: *Handbook of Reference Methods for Plant Analysis.* Florida: CRC Press; 1998.
31. Ge Z, Zhang H, Zhang Y, Yan C, Zhao Y: Purifying synthetic high-strength wastewater by microalgae *chlorella vulgaris* under various light emitting diode wavelengths and intensities. *J Environ Health Sci Eng* 2013, **11**:1–10.
32. Vymazal J, Kropfelova L: *Wastewater Treatment in Constructed Wetlands with Horizontal Sub-surface Flow.* Dordrecht: Springer; 2008.
33. Karathanasis AD, Potter CL, Coyne MS: Vegetation effects on fecal bacteria, BOD, and suspended solid removal in constructed wetlands treating domestic wastewater. *Ecol Eng* 2003, **20**:157–169.
34. Marques JJ, Souza RR, Souza CS, Rocha ICC: Attached biomass growth and substrate utilization rate in a moving bed biofilm reactor. *Braz J Chem Eng* 2008, **25**:665–670.
35. Lewandowski Z, Beyenal H: Mass transport in heterogeneous biofilms. In *Biofilms in Wastewater Treatment: an Interdisciplinary Approach.* Edited by Wuertz S, Bishop P, Wilderer P. London: IWA Publishing; 2003:147–177.
36. Hondulas JL: *Treatment of Polluted Water Using Wetland Plants in a Floating Habitat.* Gatlinburg, Tennessee: United States Patent: US5337516; 1994.

Influence of urban activity in modifying water parameters, concentration and uptake of heavy metals in *Typha latifolia* L. into a river that crosses an industrial city

Stefan-Adrian Strungaru[1], Mircea Nicoara[1*], Oana Jitar[2†] and Gabriel Plavan[1†]

Abstract

Background: Heavy metals like Cu, Cd, Pb, Ni, Co and Cr can naturally be found almost all over this planet in various amounts. Urban activities such as heavy metal industry, traffic and waste can rapidly increase the metal concentrations in a fresh water ecosystem.

Methods: This study was done in natural conditions to capture as many aspects in heavy metals pollution and bioremediation of Nicolina River, Romania considered a stream model which is under anthropogenic pressure. Water, sediment and leaves samples of *Typha latifolia* L. were collected during October 2013 and analyzed in order to assess certain heavy metals (Cu, Cd, Pb, Ni, Co and Cr) from each sampling site using GF-HR-CS-AAS with platform. Heavy metals in significant concentrations in cattail samples were correlated with the water parameters to show the possibility to use the cattail leaves as indicators in heavy metals pollution with potential in bioremediation because they can be easily harvested in autumn and this species is spread worldwide.

Results: The levels of metals concentrations in leaves were: Cu > Ni > Cr > Pb > Co knowing that copper is an essential element for plants. The sampling time was important to draw the river diagnosis for heavy metal pollution. The samples were collected, from river, after more than 60 days without rain same as a "human patient" prepared for blood test. Cobalt was considered the metal marker because it was an element with the lowest level of usage in the city. Compared with it only lead, cadmium and copper were used intensively in the industrial activities.

Conclusions: *T. latifolia* L. can be use as an indicator for the health of the studied stream and it was noticed that the heavy metals were not accumulated, although the metal uptake was influenced by sediments and water parameters. The alkalinity of the studied river acts as an inhibitor in the bioremediation process of cattail for cadmium and copper. Lead was uptake by leaves and the water parameters influenced it but it wasn't concentrated enough in leaves to propose this species in lead bioremediation process for Nicolina River.

Keywords: Bioremediation, Heavy metals, Environmental interactions, Metal uptake, *Typha latifolia*, Urban activities

* Correspondence: mirmag@uaic.ro
†Equal contributors
[1]Department of Biology, "Alexandru Ioan Cuza" University of Iasi, Faculty of Biology, 700505 Iasi, Romania
Full list of author information is available at the end of the article

Background

Human activities have a high pressure against the environment with damages of all ecosystems. Each living being deserves a healthy and a clean environment to be borne, rise, to reproduce and die. The organisms react different when the concentration of chemical compounds is increasing in the environment, some of them tolerating very fast the changes but the others suffering so much because of this [1]. Food can be easy contaminated with toxic compounds and this problem can produce damage to human health if it is not well monitored [2]. A stream that crosses a city or a small urban area may negatively interact with the anthropogenic activities, with a significant amount of pollutants. Some of these pollutants are represented by heavy metals from the industrial activities [3], the illegal landfills, traffic and industrial wastewaters released into the environment, without a prior treatment.

Heavy metals can persist for a long time in plant and animal tissues, even if they are in small amounts in the environment [4]. The water chemistry has an important role in heavy metal absorption by organisms within aquatic environments and it can be easily influenced by urban activities [5]. The heavy metals pollution in a river can be analyzed for water, sediments and biota. The seston in a river is in a direct relationship with the rainwater that transports these compounds from atmosphere and terrestrial environment very fast [6]. Sediments can directly influence the heavy metal pollution if they are mixed by the water streams [7]. In the aquatic environments, some parameters like pH, redox potential, salinity, other metals and ionic bounds affect the metal absorption in organisms [8]. Biological absorption of heavy metals is a friendly environment technology with large applications in the future. The plants have the capacity in removing toxic metals from water; also some fungus species have high potential in this process [9].

Typha latifolia L. is a wide spread macrophyte that grows very fast in biomass [10], with a high capacity of absorption and accumulation of heavy metals from the environment [11-15]; thus can be used as a bioindicator of heavy metal pollution [16] and in bioremediation processes. *Typha* sp. has the capacity to degraded fast the organic pollutants [17], which is very important in the treatment of the domestic water.

The study was conducted on the analysis and interpretation of the connection between the change of water parameters (pH, salinity, conductivity, ORP, TDS) and heavy metals concentrations (Cu, Cd, Pb, Ni, Co, Cr) in water, sediments and upper parts of *Typha latifolia* L. from Nicolina River, along its course through Iasi City in different areas affected by urban activities like heavy industry. It was studied the capacity of this species in bioremediation of heavy metals and the role as bioindicator for health of studied environment.

Materials and methods

Sampling area description

Nicolina River crosses the Iasi City situated in the eastern side of Romania, along its way to Bahlui River, from the direction South to North. For this study five sampling sites (Figure 1) were selected and they were used as a model in this study. Site_1 is considered the reference sampling site and it is situated outside the city in Dumbrava village, an area without any industrial activities but with the traffic as the main pollution source. Site_2 is situated to the entrance in the city, close to the industrial area called in the past Heavy Equipment Works (CUG), at present days Fortus. Its activity was intensive between 1976 and 2003 period focused on construction of iron and steel heavy parts for nuclear reactors, cargo boats and others. Today only a small part is still active. Site_3 is situated 1 km downstream the industrial complex in a residential area with an intensive traffic. Site_4, located in a residential area and it is surrounded by vegetation and neighborhoods. Site_5 is situated 400 m upstream of the confluence with the Bahlui River. The sampling was conducted in October 2013 after more than 60 days with no rainfall.

The pH, salinity, conductivity, total dissolved solids (TDS) and redox potential (ORP) were measured at each sampling site in situ using a HI 9828 produced by Hanna Instruments, calibrated in the laboratory, 24 h

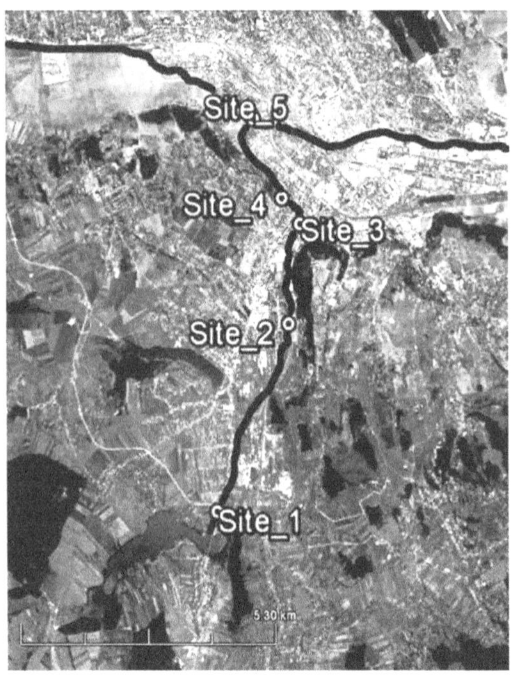

Figure 1 Map of the sampling sites (Google Maps).

before sampling. The period between the measurements at each sampling site was 20–30 minutes.

Water samples preparation

The samples were collected from each sampling site in replicates (n = 3) in 250 ml polyethylene (PE) sterile bottles, prewashed with sampling water and acidified to a pH < 2 with HNO_3 65% Suprapur, Merck for preservation [18,19]. In the laboratory the samples were prepared for microwave mineralization in TFM pressure vessels, carefully mixing 25 ml of water sample with 1.5 ml HNO_3 65% Suprapur. The mixture needed 15 minutes to react before mineralization in 3 steps program of the MWS-2, Berghof following the protocol recommended by producer. After mineralization, the samples were kept in sterile 30 ml PE bottles for metal analysis.

Sediment samples preparation

The sediments were collected in replicates (n = 3) from each sampling site, in a 20 cm column using a polycarbonate (PC) corer, 7 cm diameter. Each sample was stored in PE bags in a cooling box until the preparation for the next step. In laboratory they were slowly dried at 75°C, grinded in fine powder and sorted the small stones. The fine powder was stored in PE bags and shacked for 5 minutes. 0.5 g from each sample were weighted and mixed in TFM pressure vessels with 2 ml HCl 37%, 2 ml HNO_3 65% Suprapur and 1 ml H_2O_2 30% Merck. The mixture needed 25 minutes to react before mineralization in 3 steps program for sediments. After mineralization, the samples were filtered using filter paper for quantitative analysis (ashless) IDL GMBH &CO in 100 ml flasks and washed with ultrapure water until it reached the 100 ml volume for each sample. After filtration and dilution, the samples were kept in the flasks for heavy metal analysis.

***Typha latifolia* L. tissues samples preparation**

The most important for study were the cattail leaves because they can be harvested every year in the same sampling period (October-November, 2013) and they may clean the environment by concentrating the heavy metals. This macrophyte was present in the highest biomass and abundance in the end of vegetation season. It was absent at Site_5. This species was identified in the field as *Typha latifolia* (L.) and they were sampled leaves in replicates (n = 3) from biomass above the water surface from each sampling site. The samples were stored in PE bags in a cooling box. In the laboratory, the samples were washed with ultrapure water, chopped with plastic tools, dried at 85°C and grinded. 0.15 g of each sample were weighted and mixed in TFM pressure vessels with 1 ml HCl 37%, 2 ml HNO_3 65% Suprapur and 0.5 ml H_2O_2 30% Merck. The mixture needed 25 minutes to react before mineralization in 3 steps program for dried plants. After mineralization, the samples were filtered using filter paper for quantitative analysis (ashless) in 50 ml flasks and washed with ultrapure water until was reached a 50 ml volume. After filtration and dilution, the samples were kept in the flasks for metal analysis.

Apparatus optimization for metal analysis and method validation

Metals measurement was performed using a GF-HR-CS-AAS with platform contrAA600, AnalytikJena. For each metal, the AAS was optimized and calibrated using stock solutions for Cu, Cd, Pb, Ni, Co and Cr diluted from standard certificated solutions 1000 mg L^{-1} (Merck) in ultrapure water with 0.05% HNO_3. The samples needed Palladium matrix modifier. It was studied the signal and the spectrum of each sample to avoid the interferences

Table 1 The calibration and quality control results for lead measurements

Pb (217.005 nm)					
Evaluation					
Line	**Int. mode**	**BGC mode**	**Spectr. range**	**Eval. pixels**	**BGC fit**
Pb217	Area	with reference	200	5	dynam.
Compute calibration		**Quality control**			
R^2(adj.): 0.997703286	**Sample**	**Nominal val.**	**Recovery**		
Method SD: 0.38421 µg/L	1	6 µg/l	105.7% OK		
Char.conc.: 0.39746 µg/L	2	6 µg/l	104.3% OK		
	3	6 µg/l	105.9% OK		

Table 2 The calibration and quality control results for copper measurements

Cu (324.754 nm)					
Evaluation					
Line	**Int. mode**	**BGC mode**	**Spectr. range**	**Eval. pixels**	**BGC fit**
Cu324	Area	with reference	200	5	dynam.
Compute calibration linear		**Quality control**			
R^2(adj.): 0.989369193	**Sample**	**Nominal val.**	**Recovery**		
Method SD: 1.83130 µg/L	1	20 µg/l	91.7% OK		
Char.conc.: 0.20960 µg/L	2	20 µg/l	95.8% OK		
	3	20 µg/l	103.2% OK		

Table 3 The calibration and quality control results for cadmium measurements

Cd (228.801 nm)					
Evaluation					
Line	**Int. mode**	**BGC mode**	**Spectr. range**	**Eval. pixels**	**BGC fit**
Cd228	Area	with reference	200	5	dynam.
Compute calibration linear		**Quality control**			
R^2(adj.): 0.989476072	**Sample**	**Nominal val.**	**Recovery**		
Method SD: 0.19918 µg/L	1	3 µg/l	101.2% OK		
Char.conc.: 0.03882 µg/L	2	3 µg/l	97.4% OK		
	3	3 µg/l	97.2% OK		

Table 4 The calibration and quality control results for nickel measurements

Ni (232.003 nm)					
Evaluation					
Line	**Int. mode**	**BGC mode**	**Spectr. range**	**Eval. pixels**	**BGC fit**
Ni232	Area	with reference	200	5	dynam.
Compute calibration linear		**Quality control**			
R^2(adj.): 0.989669840	**Sample**	**Nominal val.**	**Recovery**		
Method SD: 0.71148 µg/L	1	8 µg/l	105.3% OK		
Char.conc.: 1.93116 µg/L	2	8 µg/l	99.1% OK		
	3	8 µg/l	108.1% OK		

Table 5 The calibration and quality control results for chromium measurements

Cr (359.348 nm)					
Evaluation					
Line	**Int. mode**	**BGC mode**	**Spectr. range**	**Eval. pixels**	**BGC fit**
Cr359	Area	with reference	200	5	dynam.
Compute calibration linear		**Quality control**			
R^2(adj.): 0.996788129	**Sample**	**Nominal val.**	**Recovery**		
Method SD: 0.33459 µg/L	1	5 µg/l	93.6% OK		
Char.conc.: 0.43403 µg/L	2	5 µg/l	93.8% OK		
	3	5 µg/l	103.7% OK		

Table 6 The calibration and quality control results for cobalt measurements

Co (240.725 nm)					
Evaluation					
Line	**Int. mode**	**BGC mode**	**Spectr. range**	**Eval. pixels**	**BGC fit**
Co240	Area	with reference	200	5	dynam.
Compute calibration linear		**Quality control**			
R^2(adj.): 0.999345714	**Sample**	**Nominal val.**	**Recovery**		
Method SD: 0.15798 µg/L	1	4 µg/l	106.8% OK		
Char.conc.: 0.26280 µg/L	2	4 µg/l	104.3% OK		
	3	4 µg/l	104.7% OK		

and possible contaminations. During the measurements there were conducted QC (Quality Control) analyzes for each metal using certificated solutions. The linear calibration and the method validation results are presented in Tables 1, 2, 3, 4, 5 and 6 for each studied metal.

Metal concentration factor

The heavy metal concentration factor was calculated according to formula: $CF = [M]_{plant}/[M]_{environment}$ [20], where M is the metal concentration. This factor had been calculated as the report between leaf and sediment concentrations at each sampling site. Its value expressed metal's bioconcentration and level of the pollution.

Statistical analysis

For Normality Test it was performed the Shapiro-Wilk test. Statistical analyses for sediment, biota and *Typha latifolia* L. were performed using the One-Way ANOVA, followed by Tukey HSD test, in order to explain the influence of urban activities on river course. Pearson correlation followed by 2-tailed test of significance was performed between heavy metal from environment and cattail, water parameters and the significant metal concentrated in the cattail samples from all sampling sites. All the statistical analyses were carried out using OriginPro 8 software.

Results

Water analysis

Water parameters analysed provided the first image about the influence of the city. The values of pH (Figure 2) were between 8.17-8.6 different for each sampling site which is characteristic for this area rich in limestone. The lowest value was recorded outside the city, at Site_1 while in the city the pH easily increased with the highest value at Site_4 - area with fine sediments and stones. There

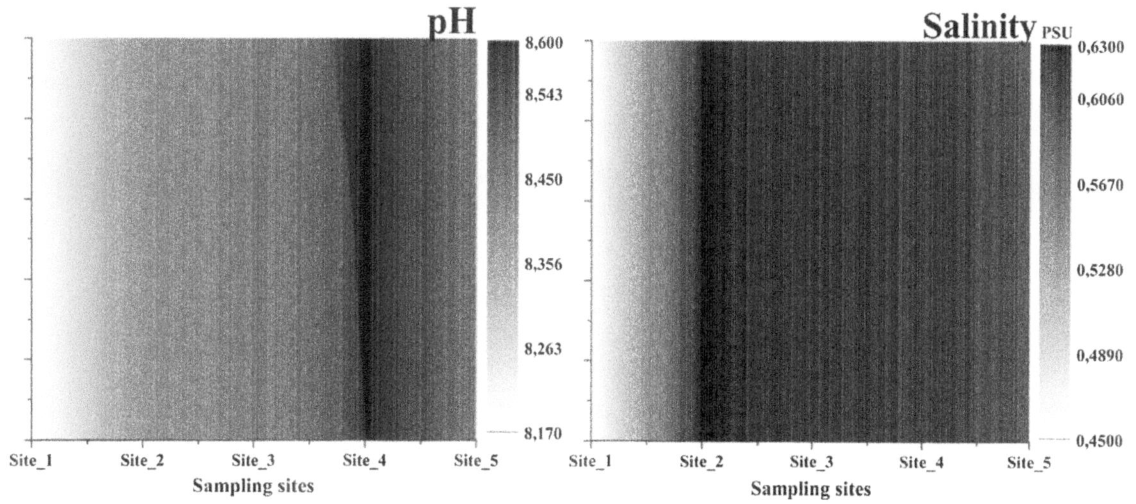

Figure 2 Variations of pH and salinity in water.

was recorded an increasing pattern for salinity 0.45-0.63 PSU, total dissolved solids (TDS) 453-625 ppm (Figure 3) and conductivity 907-1250 μS cm^{-1} (Figure 4) that suggested a strong variation of these starting from Site_2 near industrial area. The redox potential (ORP) was 13.55-28.8 with the highest value between Site_2 and Site_4, around the Heavy Equipment Works (CUG), at present Fortus, that appeared to have the highest influence in variation of this parameters. The lowest value was recorded at Site_5, which suggested once more how urban activities can fast change some parameters of the water.

There were identified and measured in water samples Cr, Pb and Ni (Figure 5). The other analyzed metals (Cu, Cd, Co) were under detection limit of the GF-HR-CS-AAS. The metal that was present in the highest concentration was nickel followed by lead and chromium. Nickel concentration did not exceed significant according to ANOVA ($p > 0.05$, $df = 4$, $F = 1.61$) even the averages were between 4.47-5.9 μg L^{-1}. This result is explained by the absence of an active pollution source with Ni at present. Same explanation was in case of lead ($p > 0.05$, $df = 4$, $F = 0.91$) 1.28-2.1 μg L^{-1} but the

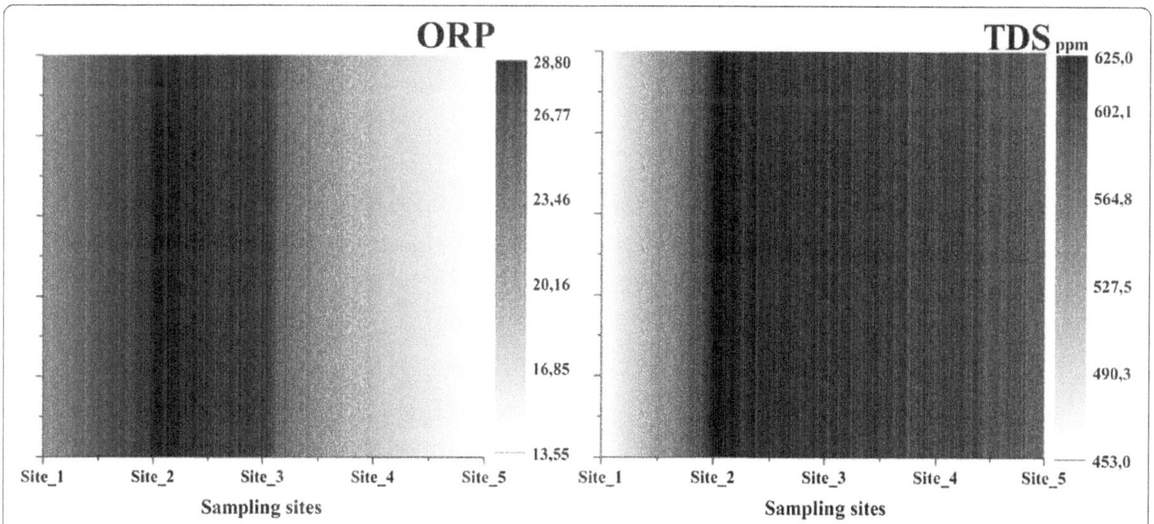

Figure 3 Variations of ORP and TDS in water.

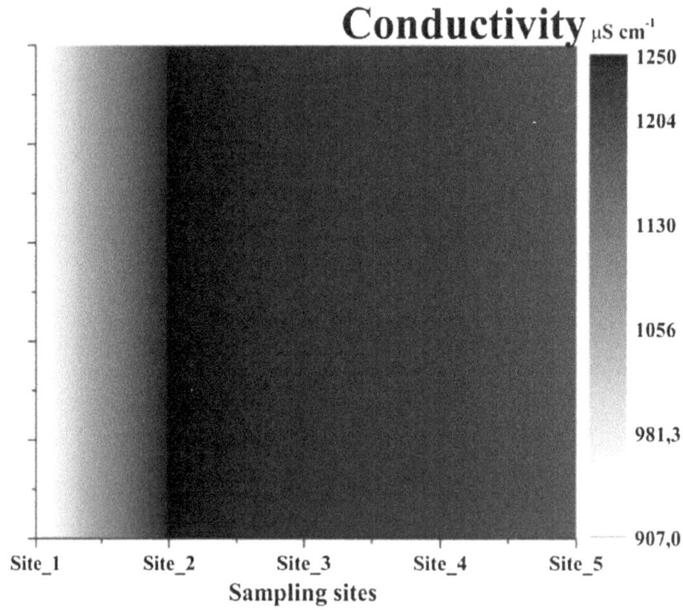

Figure 4 Variations of conductivity in water.

chromium concentration in water had a significant difference (**$p < 0.01$, df = 4, F = 8.89) with averages 0.11-0.54 µg L^{-1}. The highest values were recorded at Site_1, outside the city, in the area with the lowest anthropogenic activity; the water pH may influence the concentration of this metal, even if its value was closer to 8.

Cattail analysis

In samples of *T. latifolia* (L.) tissues, the levels of cadmium were not detectable, but the others analyzed metals were quantified (Figure 6) in this order of the concentration: Cu > Ni > Cr > Pb > Co. Copper concentrations in samples were 1.67-7.17 µg g^{-1} (d.w., $p > 0.05$, df = 3, F = 1.86) with no significant variations between the sampling sites. There were not any significant variations for Ni 1.74-4.4 µg g^{-1} (d.w., $p > 0.05$, df = 3, F = 3.03), Cr 0.26-1.47 µg g^{-1}(d.w., df = 3, F = 1.28) and Co 0.04-0.35 µg g^{-1} (d.w., $p > 0.05$, df = 3, F = 0.75). The only significant difference ($p < 0.001$, df = 3, F = 29.49) was for Pb 0.062-0.86 µg g^{-1} (d.w.).

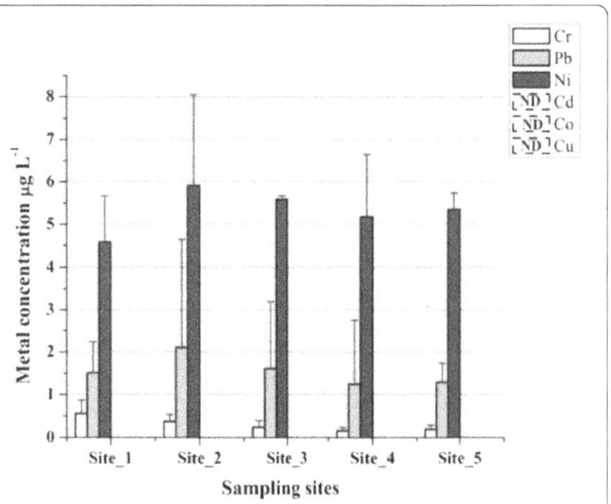

Figure 5 Metal concentrations in water samples (ND-not detectable).

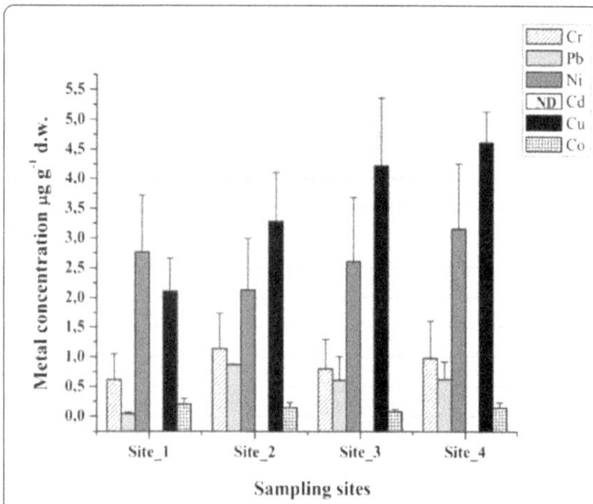

Figure 6 Metal concentrations in leaves from *T. latifolia* (L.) d.w.-dry weight (ND-not detectable).

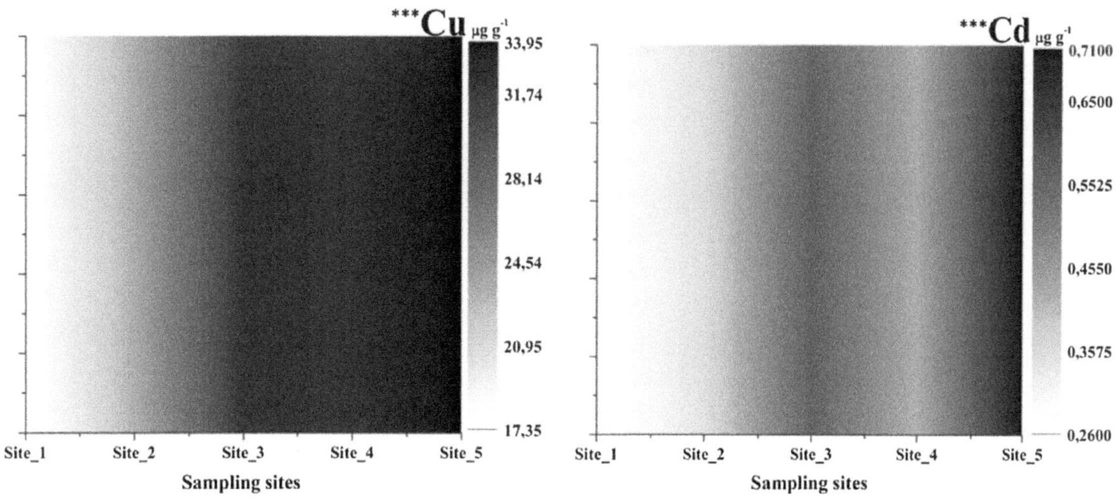

Figure 7 Copper and cadmium concentrations in sediment samples (***- $p < 0.001$, ANOVA Test of variance).

Sediment analysis

The highest variation of the concentrations was in the sediments samples. Copper (17.63–33.95 μg g^{-1}, $p < 0.001$, df = 4, F = 48.05) increased from Site_2 in the industrial area and concentrated to Site_4 and Site_5. The concentrations for cadmium (0.26–0.71 μg g^{-1}, $p < 0.001$, df = 4, F = 225.19) increased from Site_1 (Figure 7) to Site_5 where was the highest concentration. At Site_4 there was recorded a decrease in cadmium because of the sediment mixed with stones.

The lead (14.50–41.70 μg g^{-1}, $p < 0.01$, df = 4, F = 9.3) was concentrated at Site_5 with a slow decrease at Site_4. Downstream of the industrial area there was a significant increase of lead (Figure 8), possibly caused by the intensive traffic as well. In case of nickel (66.5–91.9 μg g^{-1}, $p < 0.01$, df = 4, F = 4.35), the highest concentration was at Site_1 outside the city compared to the sites inside the city. For this metal, the city's activities had no influence. The concentration with the lowest significant value was at Site_4 the area with the most stones in the substrate.

Values for cobalt (4.57–5.72 μg g^{-1}, $p < 0.01$, df = 4, F = 6.86) were highest in the samples outside (Figure 9) the city and they were not increased at the rest of the sampling stations; Site_4 had the lowest amount because

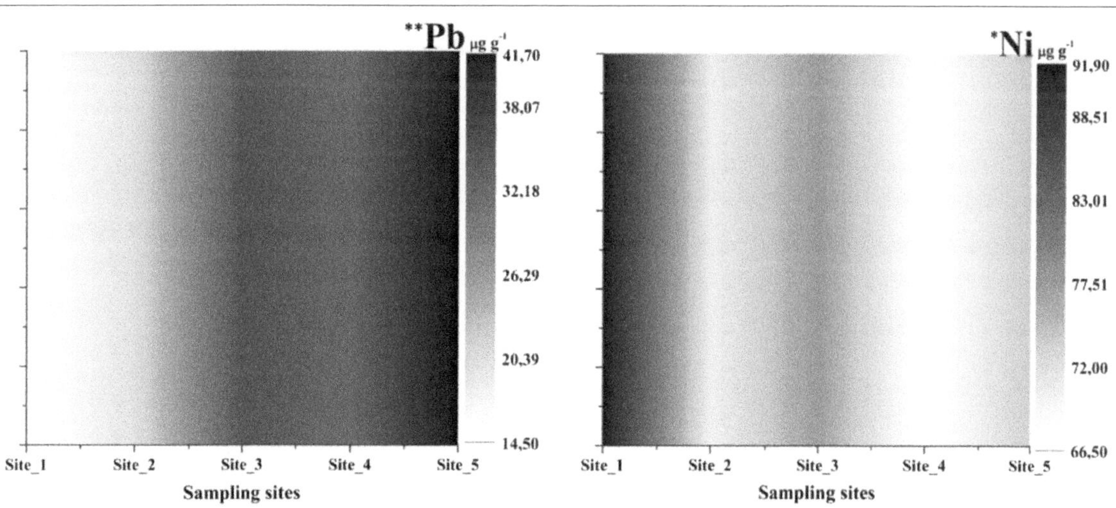

Figure 8 Lead and nickel concentrations in sediment samples (***- $p < 0.001$ and * - $p < 0.05$, ANOVA Test of variance).

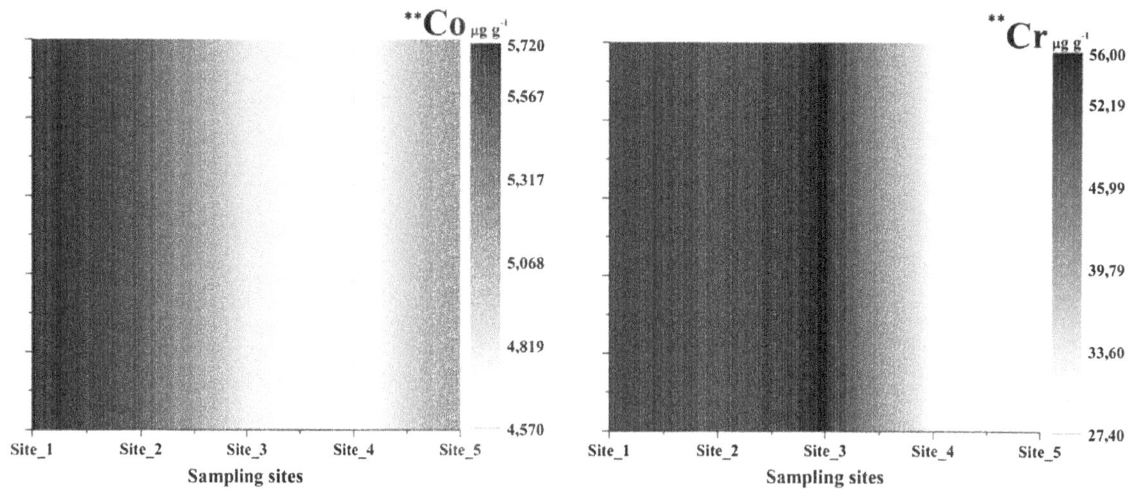

Figure 9 Cobalt and chromium concentrations in sediment samples (**- $p < 0.01$, ANOVA Test of variance).

of the substrate. Chromium (27.4–56 µg g^{-1}, $p < 0.01$, $F = 8.68$) was the only analyzed element with high levels in samples both outside and inside the city.

Discussions

Heavy metal concentration factor

Present study used as a bioindicator for heavy metal pollution *T. latifolia* L. leaves. The level of pollution and transfer capacity were expressed by calculating the metal concentration factor. Sasmaz et al. [13] used the same report to express the metal transfer factor. This factor indicated low capacity of heavy metal absorption in this macrophyte in our study (Table 7). Heavy metal concentration in leaves tissues may depends on multiple variables, like water parameters. Their influence was well studied in toxicological laboratory experiments. The results provided the understanding of the mechanism of toxicity in case of heavy metals from aquatic solutions. The problem in this type of experiment is the reduction of the variables. Between the variable they exists interactions: environment - organism, organism-organism and inside the organism. The studied sites from the Nicolina River have different parameters for water, metal content from sediment and water. They were correlated with the uptake of the studied metals from environment. Copper is an essential micronutrient for plants and it has important role physiological functions of the plant [21]. In this study the copper was uptake in leaves in the highest concentration. This element increased in concentration from Site_1 to Site_4 for sediments but it had not significant differences in cattail leaves.

In Sasmaz et al. [13] the transfer factor was highest for cadmium and lead. In the present study, copper and nickel (considered to be another important micronutrient for plants) had the greatest values and the lowest one was for cobalt, chromium and lead (Table 7).

Heavy metal uptake from water in leaves

Chromium was the only heavy metal from water samples with a significant variation over the studied sites. It was applied the first correlation between the chromium from water and from cattail leaves. It was necessary to demonstrate and to show the uptake capacity of chromium from water by this macrophyte. It had an insignificant negative correlation between water and analyzed biota (Figure 10). In this case chromium from the water was not significantly uptake even if the concentration was higher for this aquatic macrophyte. Lead was the only metal with

Table 7 Metal concentration factor (MCF) in leaves samples from *T. latifolia* L.

Cu	Cd	Pb	Ni	Co	Cr	References
0.77	1.070	0.91	0.74	0.51	0.35	[13]
(0.38-1.47)	(0.3-2.38)	(0.26-2.25)	(0.31-2.10)	(0.18-1.20)	(0.17-0.72)	
0.12	ND	0.018	0.035	0.027	0.02	Present study
(0.103-0.14)		(0.003-0.017)	(0.03-0.047)	(0.015-0.035)	(0.011-0.032)	

ND-not detectable.
MCF was expressed as average of the values interval.

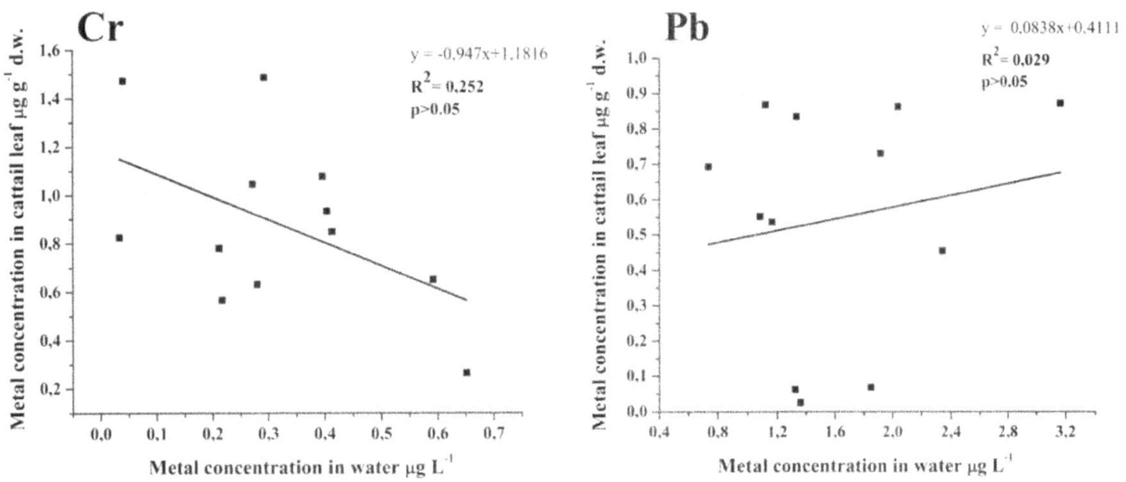

Figure 10 Pearson correlation followed by 2-tailled test for chromium and lead.

different concentrations in leaves from Site_1 to Site_2, but with no significance in water samples. We correlated its concentrations between water and cattail leaves. The lead from water was not the main source for cattail leaves. There was no significant correlation to show chromium and lead uptake by this macrophyte from water.

Heavy metal uptake from sediments in leaves

The main source of lead in cattail samples was not from water. Sediments were the main source of lead in leaves samples and this was revealed by the positive correlation between sediments and leaves concentrations which were different for each sampling site (Figure 11). It uptakes the lead from sediments by roots to leaves. According to the heavy metal concentration factor, this macrophyte did not accumulated lead in leaves (MCF < 1), but the sediments enrichment with lead increased the uptake. The macrophytes from the urban area have more lead in significant concentrations than those located outside the city. Bioremediation processes are necessary inside the city.

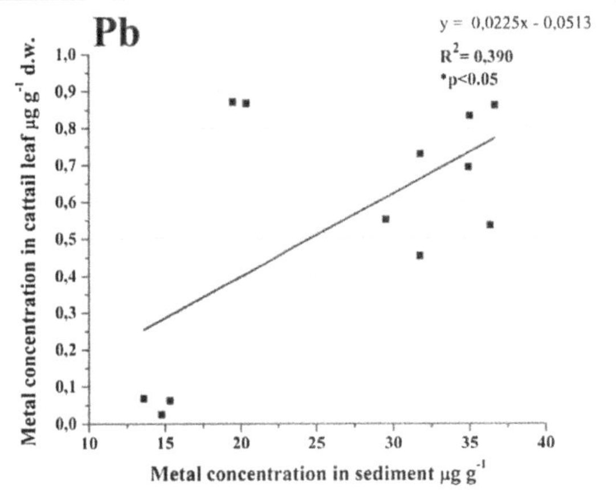

Figure 11 Pearson correlation followed by 2-tailled test for lead in sediment and biota.

Water parameters and heavy metal uptake in biota samples

The water parameters values were different at each sampling site. Prasad et al. [8] explained the importance of these in heavy metal uptake from the environment by macrophytes. The present study showed, using the correlations, the influence of water parameters in the lead uptake by cattail leaves. For the first two parameters (pH and salinity) it was a strong positive correlation. Acidic medium increases the metals uptake into the plants parts [7]. In our study, an increasing of alkalinity was correlated with a higher amount of lead in cattail leaves (Figure 12). This can be possible as an adaptation of this species to an alkaline environment. The salinity was very strongly positively correlated with lead from the sample. The importance of salinity in metal uptake was well studied. Furthermore, it is possible that same species to uptake differently the metal at same salinity because of the interaction between other factors (physical, chemical, biological).

The redox potential represents an important factor in metal uptake from sediments. In our study, this parameter had not a significant role (Figure 13) in metal uptake from sediments to leaves. It had the highest value between Site_2 and Site_3, the industrial area and it did not influence the metal uptake by leaves. The values were positive typical for an oxidative environment. Total dissolved solids (TDS) had a strong influence in metal uptake from

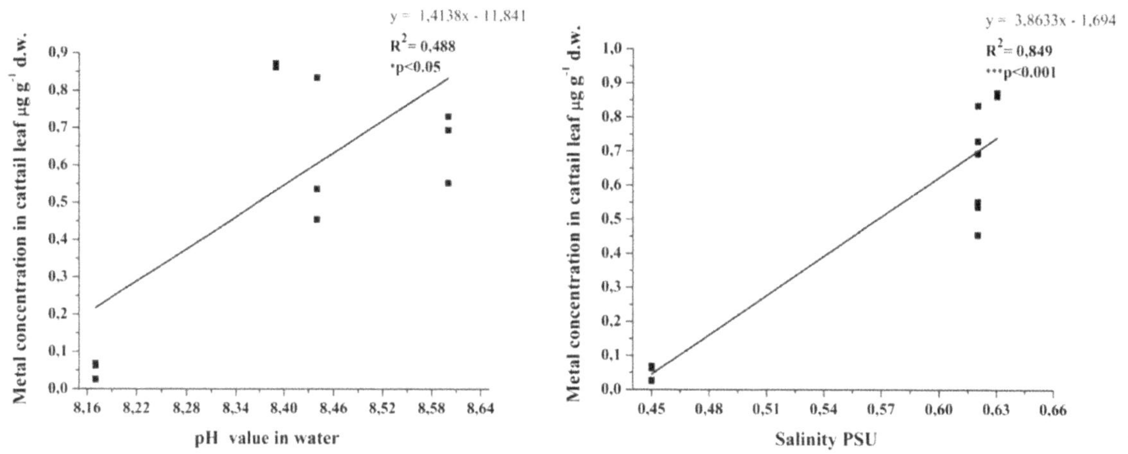

Figure 12 Pearson correlation followed by 2-tailled test between Pb with pH and salinity.

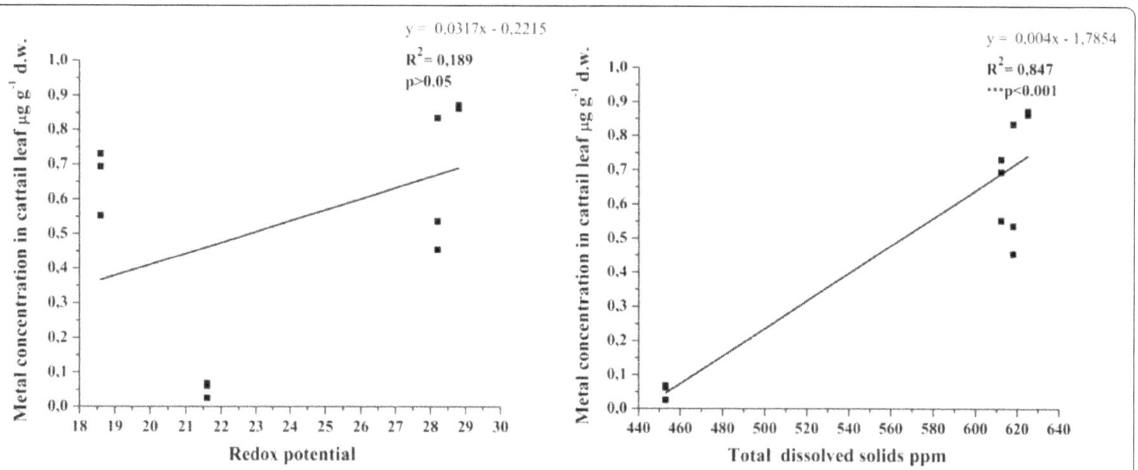

Figure 13 Pearson correlation followed by 2-tailled test between Pb with Redox potential and total dissolved solids.

sediments. It is possible that other compounds dissolved in water body (calcium, magnesium, carbonates, chloride) to increase the metal absorption capacity in leaves biomass even this did not accumulate the metal.

The connection between conductivity and lead in cattail leaf had a strong positive correlation that made the city activity to affect even more the lead uptake from the environment (Figure 14). Though there was a strong relation of heavy metal through biota-sediment-water parameters, the alkalinity of Nicolina River determinates a possible relative inactivation, being less harmful for the plants, concentrating into the sediments. The urban activities had an important role in uptake of the lead by *T. latifolia* L. They modified the water parameters and increased the capacity to absorb the metal from environment into the leaves.

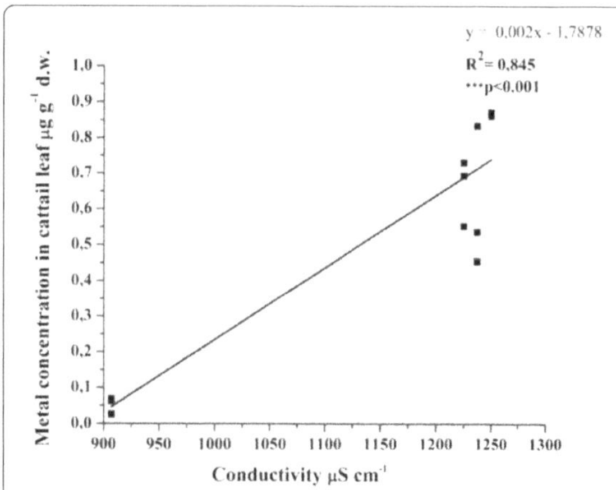

Figure 14 Pearson correlation followed by 2-tailled test between Pb with conductivity.

Conclusions

Urban activities from Iasi City had a direct impact upon water parameters from Nicolina River. These activities like steel and iron industry from the Heavy Equipment Works (CUG), at present Fortus, traffic and wastes increased the salinity, conductivity, TDS, pH and redox potential in the water body. There was not recorded a significant increase of the lead and nickel in water body inside the city, but a significant decrease of the chromium inside the city and possible of other different parameters was noticed. *T. latifolia* L. were used as a bioindicator for the health of this ecosystem and it was noticed that the heavy metals were not accumulated, although the metal uptake was influenced by sediments and water parameters. An increase of Cd, Pb and Cu in the city area was recorded for sediments and a decrease of Co, Cr and Ni. The water alkalinity, combined with other factors can reduce the toxic activity of these metals. *T. latifolia* L. cannot be use in the process of bioremediation in Nicolina River because it didn't accumulated the studied metals.

This study represents a beginning in understanding the action of anthropogenic activities upon the environment at different levels and factors. These interactions will provide new data for future bioremediation experiments and in understanding of the chemical behavior (heavy metals uptake) of different species. There are many of variables in a stream that are influencing the organism's behavior. To understand all the processes the measurement technology must to develop more and more.

Competing interests
The authors declare that they have no competing interests.

Authors' contributions
The first author and the corresponding author did the primary plan of this research. All authors of this research paper have directly participated in the planning, execution, and analysis of this study. All authors read and approved the final manuscript.

Acknowledgements
This study was financial supported by the project Resources pilot center for cross-border preservation of the aquatic biodiversity of Prut River MIS-ETC 1150 Romania – Ukraine – Republic of Moldova. The support of strategic grant POSDRU/159/1.5/S/133391, Project "Doctoral and Post-doctoral programs of excellence for highly qualified human resources training for research in the field of Life sciences, Environment and Earth Science" cofinanced by the European Social Fund within the Sectorial Operational Program Human Resources Development 2007 – 2013 is also acknowledged.

Author details
[1]Department of Biology, "Alexandru Ioan Cuza" University of Iasi, Faculty of Biology, 700505 Iasi, Romania. [2]Department of Environmental Engineering and Management, "Gheorghe Asachi" Technical University of Iasi, 73, "Prof. Dr. D. Mangeron" Street, 700050 Iasi, Romania.

References
1. Welch EB, Jacoby JM. Pollutant effects in freshwater. Appl Limnol, Third Edition. 2004;89–94:271–353.
2. Shekoohiyan S, Ghoochani M, Mohagheghian A, Mahvi AH, Yunesian M, Nazmara S. Determination of lead, cadmium and arsenic in infusion tea cultivated in north of Iran. Iranian J Environ Health Sci Eng. 2012;9:37.
3. Hu X, Sun Y, Ding Z, Zhang Y, Jichun W, Lian H, et al. Lead contamination and transfer in urban environmental compartments analyzed by lead levels and isotopic compositions. Environ Pollut. 2014;187:42–8.
4. Speak AF, Rothwell JJ, Lindley SJ, Smith CL. Metal and nutrient dynamics on an aged intensive green roof. Environ Pollut. 2014;184:33–43.
5. Juckers M, Watmough SA. Impacts of simulated drought on pore water chemistry of peatlands. Environ Pollut. 2014;184:73–80.
6. Gunawardana C, Egodawatta P, Goonetilleke A. Role of particle size and composition in metal absorption by solids deposited on urban road surfaces. Environ Pollut. 2014;184:44–53.
7. Yu K-C, Tsai L-J, Chen S-H, Ho S-T. Chemical binding of heavy metals in anoxic river sediments. Wat Res. 2000;35(17):4086–94.
8. Prasad MNV, Greger M, Smith BN. Aquatic Macrophytes. Metals in the Environment - Analysis by Biodiversity. 2001. p. 259–88.
9. Mohsenzadeh F, Shahrokhi F. Biological removing of Cadmium from contaminated media by fungal biomass of Trichoderma species. J Environ Health Sci Eng. 2014;12:102.
10. Rajaei GE, Aghaie H, Zare K, Aghaie M. Adsorption of Cu(II) and Zn(II) ions from aqueous solutions onto fine powder of *Typha latifolia* L. root: kinetics and isotherm studies. Res Chem Intermed. 2013;39:3579–94.
11. Ye ZH, Baker AJM, Wong MH, Willis AJ. Copper and nickel uptake, accumulation and tolerance in *Typha latifolia* with and without iron plaque on the root surface. New Phytol. 1997;136:481–8.
12. Carranza-Álvarez C, Alonso-Castro AJ, Alfaro-De La Torre MC, García-De La Cruz RF. Accumulation and distribution of heavy metals in *Scirpus americanus* and *Typha latifolia* from an artificial lagoon in San Luis Potosí, México. Water Air Soil Pollut. 2008;188:297–309.
13. Sasmaz A, Obek E, Hasar H. The accumulation of heavy metals in *Typha latifolia* L. grown in a stream carring secondary effluent. Ecol Eng. 2008;33:278–84.
14. Ye ZH, Baker AJM, Wong MH, Willis AJ. Zinc, lead and cadmium tolerance, uptake and accumulation by *Typha latifolia*. New Phytol. 1997;136:468–80.
15. Leto C, Tuttolomondo T, La Bella S, Leone R. Effects of plants species in a horizontal subsurface flow constructed wetland – phytoremedation of treated urban wastewaster with *Cyperus alternifolius* L. and *Typha latifolia* L. in the west of Sicily (Italy). Ecol Eng. 2013;61:282–91.
16. Klink A, Macicoł A, Wisłock A, Krawczyk J. Metal accumulation and distribution in the organs of *Typha latifolia* L.(cattail) and their potential use in bioindication. Limmnologica. 2013;43:164–8.
17. Jamshidi S, Akbarzadeh A, Woo K-S, Valipour A. Wastewater treatment using integrated anaerobic baffled reactor and Bio-rack wetland planted with *Phragmites* sp. and *Typha* sp. J Environ Health Sci Eng. 2014;12:131.
18. Marcovecchio JE, Botté SE, Freije RH. Heavy metals, major metals, trace elements. Handbook of water analysis, second edition. 2007. p. 275–311.
19. Biziuk M, Beyer A, Zukowska J. Preservation and storage of water samples. In: Analytical Measurements in Aquatic Environments. 2010. p. 19–39.
20. Coelho JP, Lillebø AI, Pacheco M, Pereira ME, Pardal MA, Duarte AC. Biota analysis as a source of information on the state of aquatic environments. In: Analytical Measurements in Aquatic Environments. 2010. p. 103–20.
21. Thomas G, Stärk H-J, Wellenreuther G, Dickinson BC, Küpper H. Effects of nanomolar copper on water plants – Comparison of biochemical and biophysical mechanisms of deficiency and sublethal toxicity under environmentally relevant conditions. Aquat Toxicol. 2013;140–141:27–36.

Suitability of electrolyzed oxidizing water for the disinfection of hard surfaces and equipment in radiology

Robert Pintaric[1*], Joze Matela[1] and Stefan Pintaric[2]

Abstract

Background: Hospitals are faced with increasingly resistant strains of micro-organisms. When it comes to disinfection, individual parts of electronic equipment of angiology diagnostics such as patient couches of computer tomography (CT) and magnetic resonance imaging (MRI) scanners prove to be very hard to disinfect. Disinfectants of choice are therefore expected to possess properties such as rapid, residue-free action without any damaging effect on the sensitive electronic equipment. This paper discusses the use of the neutral electrolyzed oxidizing water (EOW) as a biocide for the disinfection of diagnostic rooms and equipment.

Methods: The CT and MRI rooms were aerosolized with EOW using aerosolization device. The presence of micro-organisms before and after the aerosolization was recorded with the help of sedimentation and cyclone air sampling. Total body count (TBC) was evaluated in absolute and log values.

Results: The number of micro-organisms in hospital rooms was low as expected. Nevertheless, a possible TBC reduction between 78.99–92.50% or 50.50–70.60% in log values was recorded.

Conclusions: The research has shown that the use of EOW for the air and hard surface disinfection can considerably reduce the presence of micro-organisms and consequently the possibility of hospital infections. It has also demonstrated that the sedimentation procedure is insufficient for the TBC determination. The use of Biocide aerosolization proved to be efficient and safe in all applied ways. Also, no eventual damage to exposed devices or staff was recorded.

Keywords: Biocide, Electrolyzed oxidizing water (EOW), Disinfection, Micro-organisms

Background

Modern radiological imaging examinations are expected to provide detailed, swift and reliable examination yielding maximum diagnostic data while representing minimum burden on the patient. This is the reason why more and more electronic equipment is built into the diagnostic devices to acquire maximum information on patient's condition in the shortest time possible. Also, with the ever-growing number of diagnostic examinations, the possibility of hard surface contamination with micro-organisms from infected patients is increasing as well. Such surfaces may represent a possible source of infections for other patients and medical staff [1-6]. One of the key factors of a successful disinfection procedure is disinfectant's exposure time. The selection of a disinfectant, however, is not an easy task to do. The basic requirement is rapid, residue-free action. Today, there are altogether 250 substances that are known to have biocidal effect. According to the World Organisation for Animal Health (OIE), a total of 154 are used independently or in combination with other biocides. The highlighted problem becomes so much greater once we take into account the increase of the hospital infections (such as MRSA for instance) and the growing number of patients infected with the infectious disease causing agents [7-16]. Bearing in mind the increasing number of electronic equipment built into diagnostic devices, residue-free surfaces are of crucial importance. The more equipment the greater the possibility of corrosive actions causing damage to the device's vital parts,

* Correspondence: robert.pintaric@gmail.com
[1]Department of Radiology, University Medical Centre Maribor, Maribor, Slovenia
Full list of author information is available at the end of the article

especially when we take into account that the biocides themselves have a corrosive effect. Touch screen command modules of the state-of-the-art angiographic diagnostics, for instance, are extremely sensitive to various cleaning agents and disinfectants containing alcohol and other substances with corrosive effect. Accessibility for cleaning represents an additional problem. Patient couches of computer tomography (CT) and magnetic resonance imaging (MRI) scanners are very hard to access when it comes to cleaning and disinfection [17-19]. Consequently, new approaches to disinfection procedures have been studied. Thanks to its mechanism of action, neutral electrolyzed oxidizing water (EOW) has been considered as a possible biocide of the new generation [20,21]. The principle of the EOW production has been known for some time now. Basically, the alkaline ionized water and acid oxidized ionized water are generated from diluted non-iodised cooking salt (NaCl solution), whereby the alkaline fraction reaches a pH of 11–12, while the acid one has a pH of 1–3. While the alkaline ionized water is considered to have a cleaning effect, the acid one has extremely biocidal effect. Mostly, the effect of the EOW action has been attributed to the pH change only. However, more detailed analysis has revealed that electro-oxidized water works through several mechanisms. Among them, the most important ones for the biocidal effect are the redox potential, generated oxidized and super-oxidized ions, and to a smaller extent the produced chlorides, sodium hypochlorite and residual chlorine. Moreover, EOW is characterized by a marked deficiency of electrons due to which it has a tendency for electro-neutral environment that can be achieved only through the abstraction of electrons from the surrounding environment. If there are any micro-organisms in that environment, EOW abstracts the electrons from their membrane disrupting their balance and thereby causing their death. The production of oxidized and super-oxidized ions classifies EOW among the biocidal agents that give off oxygen. An important characteristic of this group of agents is rapid action and ecologically acceptable breakdown products. From the point of view of weaknesses, the most important ones are violent reaction with any existing organic substances, special storage requirements (special containers with air-vent valves that relieve excess pressure in the container), corossivity and respiratory system irritation as well as causticity. The above-mentioned substances are produced during the electrolysis and are classified among biocidal substances. They are produced in very small quantities. One of the key factors in disinfection is acidity, whereby a pH between 1–3 is very acidic and has biocidal effect as such. Not to forget, however, that low pH values expose surfaces to corrosive acting [22-28]. Thanks to its mechanism of action, EOW has a broad spectrum of activity. It has proved itself as a very good agent in the presence of biofilms. The main substance of the pH is supposed to be hypochioric acid which is in nature produced by white blood cells in their fight against pathogenic microbes (attacking the microbe cell membrane by dissolving protective membrane's biofilm) [29-33]. Numerous articles list wide EOW application possibilities in the fields, for instance plant production [34], pig production (preventive disinfection), poultry and food processing industries [35]. It has shown particularly good results in cold fogging of the rooms and can also be listed in the disinfection program in the event of any epizootic disease outbreak. In humane medicine, it is applied both for the disinfection of the surgical instruments such as endoscopes as well as for the hospital hard surface cleaning.

Methods

In its search for a possible solution, the Radiology Department of the Maribor University Medical Centre (UKC) decided to test the air samples and the samples taken from the test surfaces of the various types of

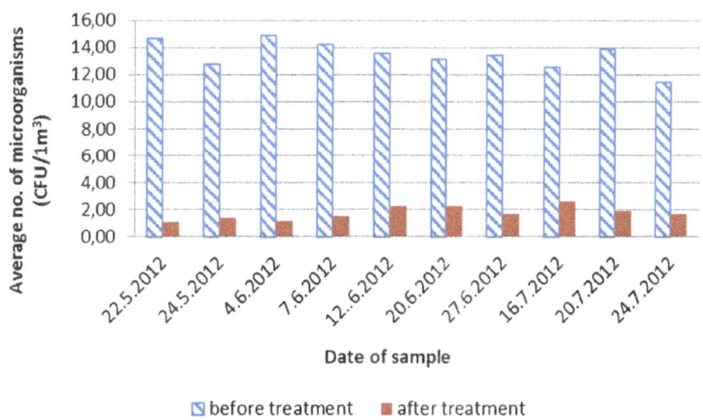

Figure 1 Total number of micro-organisms and the presence of micro-organisms after the EOW aerosolization (absolute values).

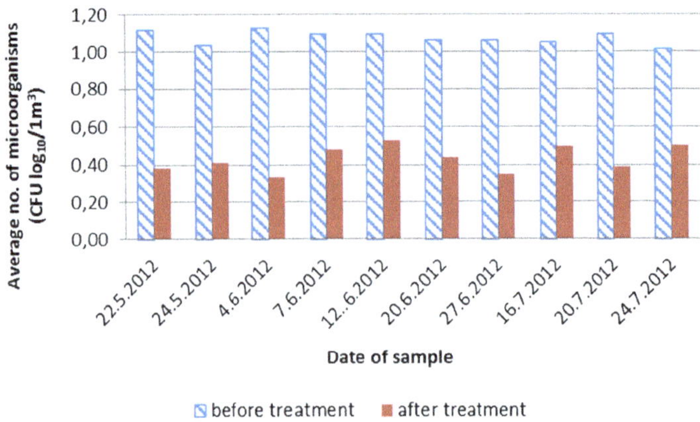

Figure 2 **Total number of micro-organisms and the presence of micro-organisms after the EOW aerosolization (calculated to log_{10}).**

diagnostic equipment in order to establish the actual condition and the scope of the micro-organism presence in the air and their significance for the surface contamination. Ethical Commission of the Republic of Slovenia approved the study under the serial number 110/05/11. Additionally, the possibility of the air aerosolizationwith the EOW was tested. More specifically, the product tested was EOV Steriplant® N produced by OBISAN –Institute for Biotechnological Research and Development from Murska Sobota, Slovenia. The available commercial form of the product contains sodium hypochlorite, chlorate, chlorine dioxide and ozone. Its pH value ranges between 6 and 8 and its redox potential is +800 ± 100 mV. The research involved 6 diagnostic pieces of equipment, thereof two for angiology, two for CT and two for MRI respectively. The purpose of the research was to establish the efficacy of the applied EOW biocidal action on the present bioaerosol. The identification of the micro-organism presence in the air and on surfaces was carried out to establish the level of the contamination in order to be able to determine the importance of the reduction of the micro-organisms present in the air with the EOW aerosolisation. To determine the micro-organism presence, the micro-organism sedimentation method was applied directly on the surface of the prepared medium. The medium was placed horizontally on the surface and fixed vertically. Following the expiry of the one hour exposure time, the plates with the collected micro-organisms were taken to the laboratory. The second air sample collection method involved Coriolis Air Sampler (produced by Coriolis, France) using cyclone technology. Through the whirling motion of the medium and with the help of the centrifugal force, the samples were collected to a bioaerosol and prepared for further treatment. With the air flow rate of 300 liters per minute, altogether 1,200 litres of air were pulled through the liquid collection media during the collection time of 4 minutes. As a liquid medium, the sterile physiological saline was used in which the bioaerosol from the air was collected. All collected samples from the 6 diagnostic rooms were taken while the air ventilation system

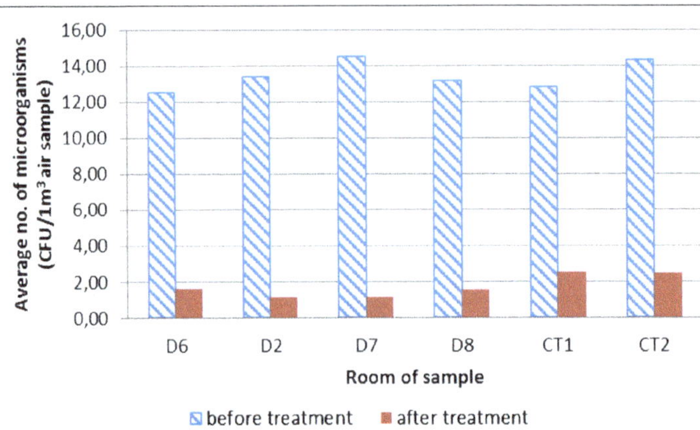

Figure 3 **Total number of micro-organisms in diagnostic rooms (absolute values).**

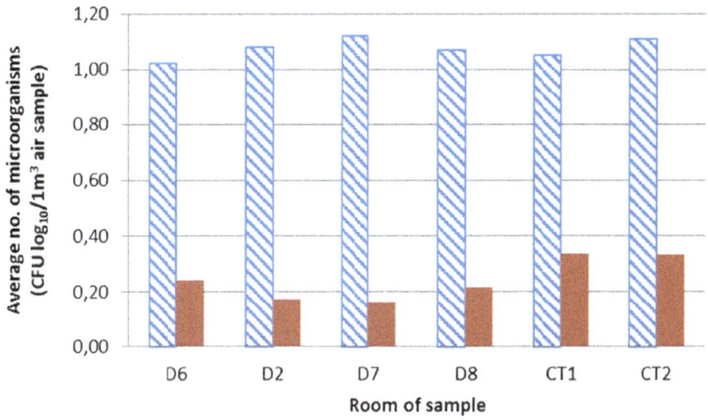

Figure 4 Total number of micro-organisms in diagnostic room (calculated on log_{10}).

was off and they were transported to laboratory for further treatment at the temperature of 4°C. Plates with medium collected according to the sedimentation method were incubated for 48 hours. Following the expiry of that time, the grown colonies were counted (ISO 132697/2002). Air samples collected in the suspension of the physiological saline were first diluted and then sown to a medium. Depending on the cultures grown, further determination was carried out (ISO 4833/2003). What followed was the counting of micro-organisms and the determination of their actual total number.

Results and discussion

The research involved 6 diagnostic rooms, 600 air samples collected in the liquid medium and 50 samplings on exposed mediums. The values of the samples gathered are shown in the tables below. For the sake of greater clarity, they are displayed as graphs. As anticipated, the number of micro-organisms present in the diagnostic room air was low. Clearly, to get a more reliable confirmation of the decrease in the number of micro-organisms it is preferable – from the point of view of the aerosol biocide action efficiency – to ensure as high initial number of micro-organisms as possible. However, this research was determining the reliability of action in actual conditions. As a result, the recorded decreases were smaller than they might have been in experimental conditions. On average, the total average number of micro-organisms in all rooms was between 11.43– 14.87 CFU/m^3 of the sampled air (Figure 1). Expressed in log values it totaled 1.01–1.13 CFU log_{10}/m^3 (Figure 2).

During the air sampling, the two most affected rooms by micro-organisms were the diagnostic room D7 (on average 14.50 CFU/m^3) and CT2 (on average 14.32 CFU/m^3) (Figure 3), relative to log values of 1.11 for D7 and 1.12 CFU log10/m^3 for the room CT 2 (Figure 4).

Figures 1 and 2 display a relatively small presence of micro-organisms during the sampling period. The main

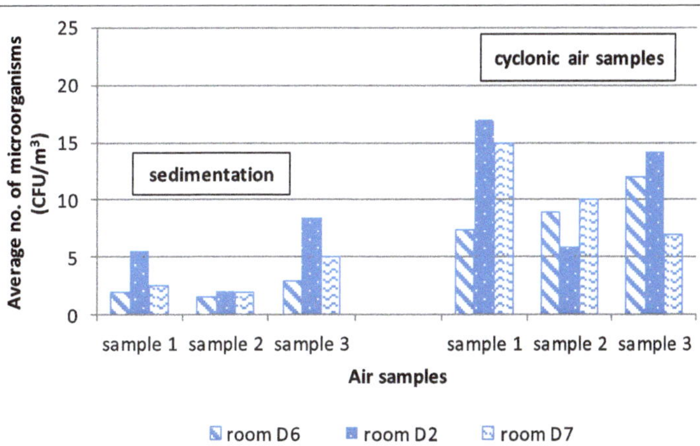

Figure 5 The total number of micro-organisms determined by the sedimentation procedure and cyclone method-based sampling in diagnostic rooms.

reason for that is controlled diagnostic room ventilation through air conditioning systems. A comparison of data for all rooms together before and after the EOW aerosolization shows a 78.99–92.50% decrease in the total number of micro-organisms (Figure 1). Log comparisons display a reduction between 0.71-0.96 $\log_{10}$ CFU/m^3 (Figure 2). A comparison of individual room data before and after the EOW aerosolization shows 80.19–92.14% decrease of the total micro-organism number (Figure 3). Log comparisons display a decrease between 0.51-0.80 $\log_{10}$ CFU/m^3 (Figure 4). The presence of micro-organisms was also determined with the help of the sedimentation procedure on Petri's plates with medium. The results were compared with the cyclone sampling method. It was found that the sedimentation procedure detected 28.57–82.67% less micro-organisms in the air compared to cyclone sampling method as shown in Figure 5.

During the counting the forms of colonies were observed as well. Any suspicious colonies were subject to further determination. However, in none of the cases studied there were no particularly dangerous agents to health.

Conclusions

The results of air sampling in the microbiological burden of the diagnostic rooms showed a fairly uniform load of microorganisms. We believe that the reason of an identified microbial presence in the way of forced air ventilation spaces of the entire hospital (central ventilation system with air prior preparation). Particularly worrisome is the presence of microorganisms in the operating rooms intended for surgery because of possible postoperative complications. Recent studies by other authors highlight the importance of microbial aerosolization in the operating rooms [36] and the importance of burden rooms with micro-organisms for the presence of microorganisms in the respiratory system of health personnel [37]. Recommendations of some authors are that the diagnostic and operational spaces achieve the presence of microorganisms of less than 10 CFU/m^3 airs [38,39]. According to the results of our study it was for 25-45% microorganisms higher than recommended. Biocide aerosol-based on EOW showed a reduction in CFU in the air spaces of test on average values from 1.14 to 2.54 CFU/m^3 or decrease of 80.19 to 92.14%. According to the recommendations of the authors [38,39] we believe that the use of the biocide aerosol Steriplant® N in practical terms in prepared space in which substantially reduce the burden of microorganisms. We believe that this helps to establish a bio-security between operational and diagnostic interventions. Considering the fact that the biocide aerosolization need 6–8 ml of biocide solution/1 m^3 of air can reach very small amounts of disinfectant effects in operation rooms and equipment. Important features of the biocide Steriplant ®N hospital environment is a broad spectrum of activity mainly in the form of resistant microorganisms (metycillin resist with S. aureus, E. coli) uncorrosivity, security for operators disinfection, medical staff and patients, and that does not remain on the surfaces of the biocide residues (not required disposal of residues). We also wish to highlight the importance of the choice of the methodology air sampling for the presence of micro-organisms. We believe that the compulsory cyclone method of air sampling in the liquid medium is appropriate to identify the presence of micro-organisms in relation to the sedimentation process, as we found from 28.57 to 82.67% for the higher levels of microorganisms.

Competing interests

The authors declare that they have no competing interests.

Authors' contributions

All authors participated in conception and design, generation, analysis and interpretation of data also revision of manuscript. All authors read and approved the final manuscript.

Acknowledgements

This research was supported by University Medical Centre Maribor and Institute Obisan.

Author details

[1]Department of Radiology, University Medical Centre Maribor, Maribor, Slovenia. [2]University of Ljubljana, Veterinary faculty, Ljubljana, Slovenia.

References

1. Aubert B. Practical aspects of personal exposure monitoring in hospitals and research laboratories. Radioprotection. 1991;26:481–91.
2. Baffoy-Fayard N, Maugat S, Sapoval M, Cluzel P, Denys A, Sellier N, et al. Potential exposure to hepatitis C virus through accidental blood contact in interventional radiology. J Vasc Interv Radiol. 2003;14:173–9.
3. Balonov MI, Krisyuk EM, Ramel C. Environmental radioactivity, population exposure and related health risks in the east Baltic region. Scand J Work Environ Health. 1999;25:17–32.
4. Buerke B, Mellmann A, Kipp F, Heindel W, Wessling J. Hygienic aspects in radiology: what the radiologist should know. Röfo. 2012;184:1099–109.
5. Chaoui AS, Dahran S, Terrier F, Ducel G. Microbiologic contamination in interventional radiology rooms. Radiology. 1995;197:137.
6. Grabsch EA, Burrell LJ, Padiglione A, O'Keeffe JM, Ballard S, Grayson L. Risk of environmental and healthcare worker contamination with vancomycin-resistant enterococci during outpatient procedures and hemodialysis. Infect Control Hosp Epidemiol. 2006;27:287–93.
7. Chan D, Downing D, Keough CE, Saad WA, Annamalai G, D'Othee BJ, et al. Joint Practice Guideline for Sterile Technique during Vascular and Interventional Radiology Procedures: From the Society of Interventional Radiology, Association of periOperative Registered Nurses, and Association for Radiologic and Imaging Nursing, for the Society of Interventional Radiology (Wael Saad, MD, Chair), Standards of Practice Committee, and Endorsed by the Cardiovascular Interventional Radiological Society of Europe and the Canadian Interventional Radiology Association. J Vasc Interv Radiol. 2012;23:1603–12.
8. Guerini H, Ayral X, Vuillemin V, Morvan G, Thevenin F, Campagna R, et al. Infiltration under ultrasound pathology osteo arthritis: general principles and precautions. J Radiol Diagn Inter. 2012;93:715–20.
9. Zhang E, Burbridge B. Methicillin-resistant staphylococcus aureus: implications for the radiology department. Am J Roentgenol. 2011;197:1155–9.
10. Ramli MF, Hussin AS, Yusoff A. Microbial contamination of dental radiology equipment. Intern Med J. 2009;16:169–73.

11. Bibbolino C, Pittalis S, Schinina V, Rizzi EB, Puro V. Hygiene precautions and the transmission of infections in radiology. Radiol Med. 2009;114:111–20.
12. Astagneau P. Prevention of hepatitis C in clinical practice. Med Mal Infect. 1999;29:345–7.
13. Garcin F, Bergeaud Y, Joly B. Study of the antimicrobial efficacy of ultraviolet rays for the disinfection of radiology cassettes. Pathol Biol. 1998;46:325–9.
14. Cowan RE, Manning AP, Ayliffe GAJ, Axon ATR, Causton JS, Cripps NF, et al. Aldehyde disinfectants and health in endoscopy units - the report of a working party of the british society of gastroenterology endoscopy committee. Gut. 1993;34:1641–5.
15. Meakin NS, Bowman C, Lewis MR, Dancer SJ. Comparison of cleaning efficacy between in-use disinfectant and electrolysed water in an English residential care home. J Hosp Infect. 2012;80:122–7.
16. Wu G, Yu X, Gu Z. Ultrasonically nebulised electrolysed oxidising water: a promising new infection control programme for impressions, metals and gypsum casts used in dental hospitals. J Hosp Infect. 2008;68:348–54.
17. Kim JS, Kim HS, Park JY, Koo HS, Choi CS, Song W, et al. Contamination of X-ray Cassettes with Methicillin-resistant Staphylococcus aureus and Methicillin-resistant Staphylococcus haemolyticus in a Radiology Department. Ann Lab Med. 2012;32:206–9.
18. Cabanis EA, Chouard CH. Good practices for disinfection of endo-vaginal and endorectal ultrasonic probes. Bull Acad Natl Med. 2009;193:2121–6.
19. Rahman SME, Park JH, Oh DH. The bactericidal and fungicidal effects of salicid on pathogenic organisms involved in hospital infections. Afr J Microbiol Res. 2011;5:2773–8.
20. Landa-Solis C, Gonzalez-Espinosa D, Guzman-Soriano B, Snyder M, Reyes-Teran G, Torres K, et al. Microcyn (TM): a novel super-oxidized water with neutral pH and disinfectant activity. J Hosp Infect. 2005;61:291–9.
21. Vorobjeva NV, Vorobjeva LI, Khodjaev EY. The bactericidal effects of electrolyzed oxidizing water on bacterial strains involved in hospital infections. Artif Organs. 2004;28:590–2.
22. Len SV, Hung YC, Chung D, Anderson JL, Erickson MC, Morita K. Effects of storage conditions and pH on chlorine loss in electrolyzed oxidizing (EO) water. J Agric Food Chem. 2002;50:209–12.
23. Cano A, Canizares P, Barrera-Diaz C, Saez C, Rodrigo MA. Use of conductive-diamond electrochemical-oxidation for the disinfection of several actual treated wastewaters. Chem Eng J. 2012;211:463–9.
24. Zeng XP, Zhang M, Wang XD, Chen XY, Su XZ, Tang WW. Effects of Sn content on Ti/RuO2-SnO2-TiO2 anodes used in the generation of electrolyzed oxidizing water. J Electroanal Chem. 2012;677:133–8.
25. Hao JX, Qiu S, Li HY, Chen TP, Liu HJ, Li LT. Roles of hydroxyl radicals in electrolyzed oxidizing water (EOW) for the inactivation of Escherichia coli. Int J Food Microbiol. 2012;155:99–104.
26. Tang WW, Zeng XP, Zhao YS, Ye GQ, Gui WC, Ni YM. Disinfection effect and its mechanism of electrolyzed oxidizing water on spores of bacillus subtilis var. niger. Food Sci Biotechnol. 2011;20:889–95.
27. Zeng XP, Ye GQ, Tang WW, Ouyang T, Tian L, Ni YM, et al. Fungicidal efficiency of electrolyzed oxidizing water on Candida albicans and its biochemical mechanism. J Biosci Bioeng. 2011;112:86–91.
28. Zeng XP, Tang WW, Ye GQ, Ouyang T, Tian L, Ni YM, et al. Studies on disinfection mechanism of electrolyzed oxidizing water on E. coli and staphylococcus aureus. J Food Sci. 2010;75:M253–60.
29. Sun JL, Zhang SK, Chen JY, Han BZ. Efficacy of acidic and basic electrolyzed water in eradicating Staphylococcus aureus biofilm. Can J Microbiol. 2012;58:448–54.
30. Moretro T, Heir E, Nesse LL, Vestby LK, Langsrud S. Control of Salmonella in food related environments by chemical disinfection. Food Res Int. 2012;45:532–44.
31. McCarthy S, Burkhardt W. Efficacy of electrolyzed oxidizing water against Listeria monocytogenes and Morganella morganii on conveyor belt and raw fish surfaces. Food Control. 2012;24:214–9.
32. Ayebah B, Hung YC, Kim C, Frank JF. Efficacy of electrolyzed water in the inactivation of planktonic and biofilm Listeria monocytogenes in the presence of organic matter. J Food Prot. 2006;69:2143–50.
33. Kim C, Hung YC, Brackett RE, Frank JF. Inactivation of Listeria monocytogenes biofilms by electrolyzed oxidizing water. J Food Process Preserv. 2001;25:91–100.
34. Subrota H, Surajit M, Minz P, Shilpa V, Yogesh K, Singh B, et al. Electrolyzed Oxidized Water (EOW): non-thermal approach for decontamination of food borne microorganisms in Food Industry. Food Nutr Sci. 2012;3:760–8.
35. Hung YC, Tilly P, Kim C. Efficacy of Electrolyzed Oxidizing (EO) water and chlorinated ater for inactivation of Escherichia colli 0157:H7 on Strawberries and Broccoli. J Food Qual. 2010;24(12):984–7.
36. Erichsen Andersson A, Petzold M, Bergh I, Karlsson J, Eriksson BI, Nilsson K. Comparison between mixed and laminar airflow systems in operating rooms and the influence of human factors: experiences from a Swedish orthopedic center. Am J Infect Control. 2014;42(6):665–9.
37. Tinley PD, Eddy K, Collier P. Contaminants in human nail dust: an occupational hazard in podiatry. J Foot Ankle Res. 2014;7(1):15.
38. Hansen D, Krabs C, Benner D, Brauksiepe A, Popp W. Laminar air flow provides high air quality in the operating field even during real operating conditions, but personal protection seems to be necessary in operations with tissue combustion. Int J Hygiene Environ Health. 2005;208:455–60.
39. Lidwell OM, Lowbury EJL, Whyte W. Effect of ultraclean air in operating rooms on deep sepsis in the joint after total hip or knee replacement: a randomised study. BMJ. 1982;285:10–4.

Spatiality, seasonality and ecological risks of heavy metals in the vicinity of a degenerate municipal central dumpsite in Enugu, Nigeria

Kanayochukwu C Ajah, Joel Ademiluyi and Chidozie C Nnaji*

Abstract

Background: Improper waste disposal is responsible for the contamination of both surface and ground water resources. Heavy metals leached from improperly disposed solid waste constitute grave environmental and health hazards because of their toxic and persistent nature. There are thousands of open dumps in Nigeria one of which is the Enugu State Waste Management Authority dumpsite.

Method: Forty sampling nodes were systematically established around the Enugu State waste Management Authority central dumpsite located at Ugwuaji, Enugu State, Nigeria. Ten heavy metals (arsenic, cadmium, cobalt, copper, chromium, iron, lead, manganese, nickel and zinc) were sampled at different depths of each node in both rainy and dry seasons.

Result: Iron and lead were the predominant metals in the vicinity of the waste dump with average values of 132.10 mg/kg and 117.52 mg/kg respectively. The order of abundance of the ten heavy metals monitored is Pb > Fe > As > Zn > Cu > Co > Ni > Cd > Cr > Mn. Generally, there was significant correlation (0.25 to 0.74) among all the metals except between cobalt and manganese in the rainy season. In the dry season, all the metals were significantly correlated (0.29 to 0.813) except for copper and lead, copper and arsenic, zinc and arsenic, and cobalt and manganese. The concentrations of most of the heavy metals approached a constant level at a depth of 1 m. On the other hand, the concentrations of arsenic, cobalt and iron continued to decrease even at a depth of 2 m. The pollution loading index values for the soil are 1.706 for rainy season and 2.54 for dry season.

Conclusion: The high pollution loading index represents a significant level of deterioration. It can be concluded that the dumpsite constitute a serious environmental and health hazard.

Keywords: Heavy metals, Solid waste, Health, Rainfall, Pollution

Introduction

One of the most menacing challenges facing developing countries is an ever ballooning quantity of waste generation without commensurate facilities and resources to face this challenge. Inability of waste management authorities to cope with waste generated and consequent indiscriminate disposal of waste has turned many erstwhile beautiful Nigerian cities into mega ghettos. The result is unmitigated pollution of land, air and water which exposes the populace to miasma of health hazards. There is no doubt that a healthy environment has a high correlation with human health. Air pollution usually results from industrial and domestic emissions, water contamination results from industrial effluent discharges, agricultural runoff and sewage disposal; while soil pollution results from uncontrolled solid waste disposal on land. The two major concerns regarding waste disposal on land are: (i) surface and ground water contamination by leachate and (ii) bioaccumulation of toxic heavy metals in soil, uptake of these heavy metals by plants and biomagnifications of these metals up the food chain. Besides, heavy metals accumulation in soil can hamper soil productivity by interfering with soil fauna and flora. Most heavy metals naturally occurring in the earth

* Correspondence: chidozie.nnaji@unn.edu.ng
Department of Civil Engineering, University of Nigeria, Nsukka, Enugu State, Nigeria

crust as trace elements are usually found buried deep in the heart of the earth. However, massive exploitation of natural resources has given rise to a build-up of these toxic elements in the human environment.

Anthropogenic sources of heavy metals include: emissions from vehicle exhaust pipe, tyre wear particles, weathered street surfaces, brake lining wear particles, power plant combustion, metallurgical industry, auto repair shops, chemical plants, weathering of buildings and pavement surfaces, atmospheric deposits, mining, smelting, waste disposal, urban effluents, pesticides, fertilizers, sawdust disposal, herbicides, pharmaceuticals, batteries, fungicides, paints, pigments and dyes, leather tanning, photographic films, fireworks, printer and photocopier toners, cement, candles, rubber, etc. These are commonly used products with which humans come in contact on a daily basis, and which constitute a substantial part of waste at dump sites. Several researchers have found elevated levels of heavy metals in street dusts [1-5] agricultural soils [6-8], cemetery [9] solid waste dumps [10], oil and gas facilities [11] and lake sediments [12]. Chemical and physical affinity of metal ions for various waste materials may reduce their leachability, however, metal ions mobility increases over time as acidic and oxidizing conditions prevail [13]. It has been suggested that soil acidity be used as basis for evaluating soil contamination by several elements [6]. Potential binding ligands include carbonates, chloride, dissolved organic matter, colloidal solids and sulfide.

Heavy metal toxicity is determined by route, pattern and duration of exposure. Routes of exposure to heavy metals include (i) ingestion of soils, contaminated water, vegetables and fruits grown on contaminated soils, and animals that grazed on contaminated areas; (ii) inhalation of soil particles, dust and fumes and (iii) dermal contact [14-16]. Drinking of contaminated water and consumption of agricultural products represent an important source of heavy metals ingestion. Accumulation of heavy metals in agricultural products results from unwholesome practices such as use of domestic and industrial effluent for irrigation, cultivation of plants on waste dumps and surrounding soils, and grazing of animals on grasses growing on contaminated soils. It is common practice in Nigeria and some other developing countries for people to grow their crops on waste dumps and on soils where raw sewage is discharged [17,18]. Currently, there is no official policy to stop these practices or sensitize the masses on the dangerous implications of these practices. Leachability and uptake of heavy metals by plants are soil and plant specific. While leafy vegetables exhibit preferential uptake of cadmium and copper, cigarette leaves can accumulate large amounts of arsenic and cadmium, arsenic and lead. Elevated levels of arsenic (0.5 – 7.5 mg/kg) have been found in rice and vegetables grown in Chenzhou City of Southern China [19]. Several health hazards have been associated with consumption of high doses of heavy metals [20,21]. These health hazards range from mild illnesses such as ulcers, diarrhea, nausea, abdominal pain, gastrointestinal disorders, respiratory disorders, cough, nervous disorder, psychological disturbances to life threatening diseases such as cancers, cardiovascular diseases, asthma, kidney and liver damage, coma and diabetes.

In the light of the aforementioned realities, there is need for a detailed study of heavy metal contamination of the soils in the vicinity of the Enugu municipal dumpsite with a view to ascertain the extent of soil contamination.

Methodology

Description of study area

Enugu state is one of the five Southeastern states of Nigeria, located between latitude 6°.00'N and 7°.00'N and longitude 7°.00'E and 7°.45'E. It falls within the humid tropical rainforest belt of the Southeastern Nigeria. It has two distinct seasons: dry and rainy seasons. The rainy season commences in April and ends in October, followed by the dry season. The annual rainfall ranges between 937.2 mm to 2243.3 mm while the temperature ranges between 20.3°C to 32.16°C [22,23]. The 2006 census put the population of Enugu at 722, 664 [22]. Enugu State Waste Management Authority (ESWAMA) municipal solid waste (MSW) disposal site of approximately 7.878 ha of land space, is located in the southern part of Enugu Metropolis with its geographic position system (GPS) coordinates as: Elevation: 186 m; North: 6°26.27'; and East: 7°32.831'.

The dump site is about 1.6 kilometers away off Enugu-Port Harcourt expressway as shown in Figure 1. The site slopes gently downwards away from its centre in all directions into the environs. The dumpsite is the final disposal ground for all wastes (domestic, construction/demolition, industrial and agricultural) generated in Enugu metropolis. The dumpsite was originally conceived as a landfill but has degenerated to a massive open dump because of poor management, inadequate manpower and lack of requisite technology. The bottom is not lined for leachate containment, and no compaction is undertaken. There is no perimeter fencing, hence scavengers and stray animals roam the dumpsite unrestricted. ESWAMA is supposed to be a waste management authority but what it essentially does is to undertake waste collection within Enugu metropolis and disposal of collected waste at the central dumpsite. The waste does not undergo any level of treatment or processing before disposal. There is no formal sorting for material recovery and recycling. Informal material

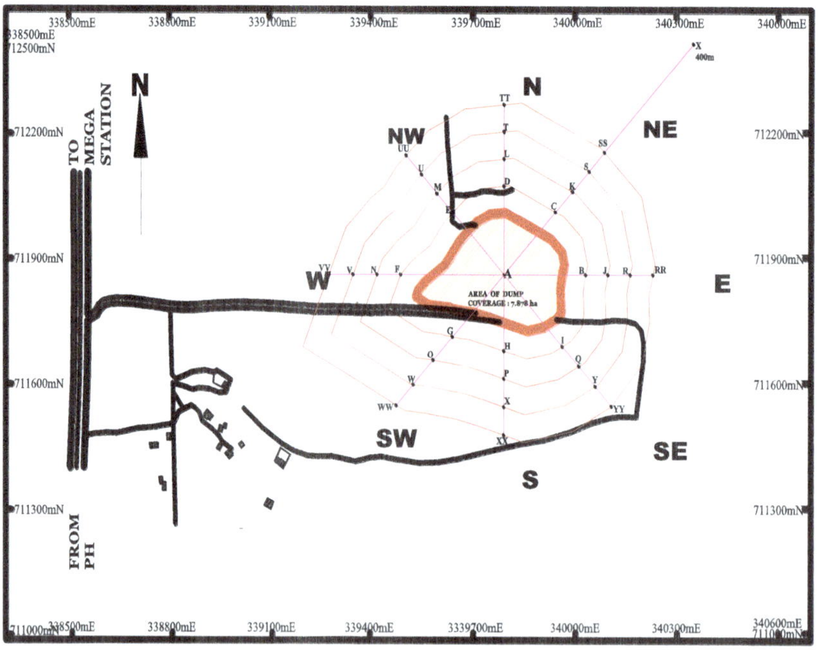

Figure 1 Map showing Enugu state waste management authority waste dump and environs.

recovery is undertaken by scavengers who sometimes set newly deposited heaps of waste ablaze in a bid to recover valuable metal waste. According to [24,25], the dump site lies on the massive, dark coloured Enugu shale formation predominantly made up of shales, clays, silts and limestones. It is overlain by the Mamu formation and underlain by the Awgu shale formation. This shale formation is made up of porous clays and impermeable shale units. Nevertheless, the weathered top soils are permeable, but are not of great thicknesses; hence they cannot yield appreciable quantities of water to boreholes. As a result of the aforementioned hydrogeologic characteristics of Enugu Metropolis and environ, shallow dug wells are the only sources of groundwater supply.

Sample collection

For the purposes of data collection, the area was divided into eight equal segments of 45° each. Concentric loops were then introduced at equal distances of 20 m from each other starting from the boundary of the dump site. In order to determine the number of loops required before sampling could commence in earnest, trial soil samples were collected at nodes (formed by the intersection of the concentric loops and 45° radial lines) equally spaced at 20 m intervals from the boundary of the dumpsite, along the radial line AE. When two nodes on two successive loops showed no significant difference in pollutant concentration, additional loops were no longer necessary. Hence, concentric loops equally spaced at 20 m beginning from the boundary of the dumpsite were established and detailed sampling commenced. Soil samples were collected at the centre (A) of the dumpsite and at the nodes formed by the intersection of the loops with the 45° radial lines. Soil samples were collected at the nodes by means of auger bits at depths of 0.5 m, 1 m, 1.5 m and 2 m. This implies that for each node, samples were collected at four sampling depths. Hence there are 164 sampling points for contaminated soil. In order to obtain the background levels of heavy metals in the soil, soil samples were obtained from point X located 400 m away from the boundary of the dump site (see Figure 1). Soil samples collected were bagged in transparent polythene bags and then sent to the laboratory for heavy metals analyses. The samples were oven dried and then ground to a fine texture using pestle and mortar in the laboratory. The finely ground soil samples were sieved and 1 g was used for digestion. Supra pure-merck nitric acid and hydrogen peroxide (30%) were used for the digestion in an open vessel. Soil sample were analysed for each heavy metal using a calibrated atomic absorption spectrophotometer (AA320N). For the purpose of this research, two periods were selected, viz: dry season (October – March) and wet season (April – September). During these two periods, soil samples were collected and analysed in the laboratory.

This approach produced results that are more representative of the actual field situation in the dump site. The metals monitored are iron, copper, lead, zinc, arsenic, cobalt, nickel, chromium, cadmium and manganese.

Undisturbed soil samples were also collected at depths of 0 to 1 m and 1 – 2.5 m in four (4) randomly selected locations for physical characterization. Based on the American Association of State Highway and Transport Association of State Highway and Transport Officials (AASHTO) classification of soil, the soil type of the study area is reddish, sandy and silty clay A-2-6 which is locally called lateritic soil. The soil has the following parameters: percentage passing No 200 sieve (26.8%), liquid limit (26.2), plastic limit (9.5), plasticity index (16.7), moisture content (12.5%), bulk density (2.21 g/cm^3), dry density, (1.98 g/cm^3), specific gravity (2.41) and porosity (0.36). Result of soil characterization by [26] within this vicinity showed that the soil contains 55% gravel, 13% sand, 18% silt, 14% clay.

Data analyses

Laboratory results were further subjected to statistical analyses, in order to facilitate interpretation. Using Microsoft Excel, the data was subjected to descriptive statistical analyses. Correlations between pairs of metals were also obtained. Geostatistical methods were employed to obtain the spatial variation of the various heavy metals in the dumpsite and environs.

Since the metals were sampled at only finite and discrete number of points, it was necessary to estimate metal concentration at other points where samples were not taken. The semivariogram ($\gamma_{(k)}$) function was adopted. It is defined as follows [27,28]:

$$\gamma_{(k)} = \frac{1}{2n(k)} \sum_{i=1}^{n(k)} [Z(x_i) - Z(X_{i+k})]^2 \quad (1)$$

Where $\gamma_{(k)}$ is the square of the difference between a soil property (metals in this case) at a point x_i and the same soil property at another point located at a distance x_{i+k}, and *n(k)* is the number of pairs of observations separated by a lag distance of k. Three-dimensional contour maps of heavy metals distribution were drawn by the Krigin method of point interpolation using Surfer 11.

Risk assessments were performed using already established indices such as the pollution index, geoaccumulation index and ecological risk index. Pollution index was calculated as the ratio of the mean concentration of each heavy metal to the baseline or background concentration. It is defined as follows [7]:

$$PI = \frac{C_i}{S_i} \quad (2)$$

Where C_i is the average concentration of individual metal in the dumpsite and S_i is the baseline concentration. PI values < 1 indicate low level of pollution, $1 \le PI \le 2$ indicate moderate level of pollution, $2 \le PI \le 5$ indicate high level of pollution, while $PI \ge 5$ indicate extreme pollution level.

Another index, the geoaccumulation pollution index was also used to assess the degree of soil contamination by metals. The geoaccumulation index (I_{geo}) is defined as [7,29]:

$$I_{geo} = Log_2\left(\frac{C_i}{1.5S_i}\right) \quad (3)$$

$I_{geo} < 0$ indicates pristine or uncontaminated state, $0 \le I_{geo} \le 1$ indicates uncontaminated to moderately contaminated state, $1 \le I_{geo} \le 2$ indicates moderately contaminated state, $2 \le I_{geo} \le 3$ indicates moderately to heavily contaminated state, $3 \le I_{geo} \le 4$ indicates heavily contaminated state, $4 \le I_{geo} \le 5$ indicates heavily to extremely contaminated state, and $I_{geo} > 5$ indicates extremely contaminated state.

Since PI values give the pollution status of the site with respect to individual metal, overall pollution status of the site was determined using the pollution loading index (PLI) calculated as follows, for *n* number of metals [29].

$$PLI = \left(\prod_{i=1}^{n} PI_i\right)^{\frac{1}{n}} \quad (4)$$

PI has been defined by Equation 2.

Ecological risk index (*ERI*) was used to assess the level of risk posed by the heavy metals using the heavy metal toxic factors of [30]. *ERI* is defined as follows [19]:

$$ERI = \sum_{i=1}^{n} T_i \frac{C_i}{B_i} \quad (5)$$

Where C_i has been previously defined, T_i is heavy metal toxic factor for a given metal, B_i is the guideline value for the metal and *n* is the number of metals. Toxic response factors used are: Cd(30), Cu(5), Cr(2), Zn(1), AS(10), Co(5) and Ni(5) in mg/Kg [31]. Heavy metals guideline values of the Department of Petroleum Resources were used, and they are as follows: Cu(56), Zn (140), Pb(85), Cd(0.8), Ni (35), Cr (100), Co (20) and As (29) in mg/Kg [32]. *ERI* are classified as follows: low contamination ($ERI \le 50$), moderate contamination ($50 \le ERI \le 100$), considerable contamination ($100 \le ERI \le 200$) and high contamination ($ERI > 200$). Finally, an attempt was made at source identification by hierarchical cluster analysis using the Statistical Package for Social Sciences (SPSS 16.0).

Results and discussion

Heavy metals concentration in dumpsite soil

Results obtained from field studies indicate very clearly the preponderance of heavy metals in dumpsite soil. Table 1 shows that iron and lead were the predominant metals in the vicinity of the waste dump with average values of 132.10 mg/kg and 117.52 mg/kg respectively. The order of abundance of the ten heavy metals monitored is Pb > Fe > As > Zn > Cu > Co > Ni > Cd > Cr > Mn. Many previous researchers have found that the concentration of iron and lead in soil were higher than the concentration of other metals. The order of abundance of these heavy metals displayed slight seasonal variation as shown below.

Pb > Fe > As > Co > Zn > Ni > Cu > Cd > Cr > Mn (rainy season).

Pb > Fe > As > Cu > Zn > Co > Ni > Cd > Cr > Mn (dry season).

A summary of the order of abundance of anthropogenic heavy metals in the soil as obtained by various researchers has been presented in Table 2.

High level of iron and lead were found in agricultural soils in Bulgaria, alluvial and dune soils in Japan, flood plains in the Netherlands, around gas plants in Niger Delta, Nigeria, irrigated soils in Egypt, waste dumps in India and Nigeria, roadside dust in china, Botswana, Nigeria and Iran [1-6,10,11,33,34,36,37]. Lead accumulation can be attributed to low mobility and strong association to soil constituents such as organic matter, minerals of clay fraction, and oxides of iron and manganese [36].

To buttress this point, Table 3 below shows significant correlations of 0.68 between lead and iron, and 0.43 between lead and manganese. Lead (Pb) exists in many forms in the natural sources [42]. Its concentration in the human environment increased with the introduction of leaded gasoline in the 1920s. Lead accumulation in the surrounding soil is facilitated by the presence of large proportion of organic matter in disposed waste. Generally, there was significant correlation among all the metals except between cobalt and manganese in the rainy season. In the dry season, all the metals were significantly correlated except for copper and lead, copper and arsenic, zinc and arsenic, and cobalt and manganese. The most significant correlation was 0.813 between copper and zinc (rainy season), 0.74 between nickel and iron, and 0.7 between chromium and iron. Significant correlation between the metals might be attributed to commonality of source and their common tendency to persist in the environment.

In almost all cases, concentration of heavy metals peaked at the dump site but gradually tailed to the environs. Figures 2 and 3 show that there was a gradual attenuation of lead in both lateral and vertical directions. This is evidenced by the undulating nature of the curves and by the closeness of the concentration lines for different depths. This can be attributed to the effect of leaching by infiltrating water. Besides, during heavy rainfall, runoff from the dumpsite spreads to the surrounding soil, thereby redistributing the heavy metals. The same phenomenon applies to copper and zinc as depicted by the curves. For most of the metals especially lead, cobalt, cadmium and iron, the vertical variation of metal concentration becomes almost insignificant at a distance of about 80 m from the dumpsite. This suggests persistence, and that the preferred direction of transport is downward. Moreover, the spatial variation of heavy metals in a given catchment area decreases with depth. This is easily visualized from Figures 2 and 4. Curves of heavy metals variation at 0.5 m depth are much more pronounced than those of 2 m depth. It has been observed that it is this persistence and low mobility of heavy metals in the environment, even under high precipitation, that aggravates the risk posed by heavy metals [43].

Table 1 Seasonal descriptive statistics of heavy metals

	Rainy season							Dry season						
Heavy metal	Mean	S.D.	Variance	Kurtosis	Skewness	Min	Max	Mean	S.D.	Variance	Kurtosis	Skewness	Min	Max
Copper	25.17	8.92	79.60	-0.76	0.18	7.50	45.00	87.77	72.96	5322.71	-0.03	0.81	7.50	311.00
Zinc	43.37	11.71	137.21	1.09	0.47	12.50	85.00	76.37	62.56	3914.28s	8.47	2.55	12.50	431.75
Lead	138.48	57.99	3362.76	0.18	0.74	42.50	357.50	125.72	61.10	3732.78	-0.21	0.48	18.00	324.25
Arsenic	96.44	62.46	3901.73	-0.54	0.43	0.00	247.50	90.63	60.99	3720.22	-0.72	0.39	0.00	245.00
Chromium	11.40	10.47	109.57	17.90	3.58	2.50	80.00	18.34	21.76	473.54	16.55	3.48	2.50	162.50
Nickel	34.19	41.37	1711.12	11.36	3.13	0.00	242.50	25.49	21.11	445.83	0.81	1.17	0.00	92.00
Cadmium	20.15	24.92	621.26	17.72	3.45	0.00	192.50	21.55	22.87	523.14	23.19	3.63	0.00	192.50
Iron	113.79	132.24	17486.78	8.85	2.76	2.50	706.00	121.26	104.39	10896.94	6.22	1.88	2.50	677.50
Cobolt	51.65	63.54	4087.48	15.00	3.18	2.50	475.00	45.23	46.45	2157.72	3.42	1.90	2.00	232.50
Manganese	6.44	14.12	199.34	21.88	4.45	0.00	97.50	12.28	12.81	163.97	7.91	2.18	0.00	85.00

Table 2 Order of heavy metal anthropogenic-induced abundance in the soil

Source	Location	Order of abundance	Reference
Agricultural soil	Chelopech, Bulgaria	Fe > Cu > Zn > Pb > Cr > As > Ni > Co > Cd > Hg	[6]
Agricultural soil	China	Zn > Cr > Pb > Cu > Ni > As > Cd > Hg	[7]
Agricultural soil	Xiamen, China	Mn > Zn > Pb > Cr > As > Cu > Ni > Cd > Hg	[8]
Alluvial soil	Japan	Zn > Cu > Pb > Ni > Cd	[33]
Cemetery	Kigali, Rwanda	Cr > Zn > Pb > As > Cu > Al > Fe	[9]
Dune soil	Japan	Zn > Cu > Pb > Ni > Cd	[33]
Flood plain	Biesboch, Netherlands	Zn > Pb > Cu > Cd	[34]
Gas plant	Niger Delta, Nigeria	Fe > Mn > Zn > V > Cr > Cu > Pb > Ni > Cd > Hg > As	[11]
Industrial areas	Gujarat, India	Ba > V > Cr > Sr > Cu > Zn > Ni > Co	[35]
Irrigated soil	Bahr El-Baker, Egypt	Cd > Cu > Zn > Cr > Ni > Pb	[36]
Jute mill waste dump	Assam, India	Fe > Zn > Pb > Cu > As > Cd > Cr > Ni	[37]
Lake sediment	Dongting, China	Zn > Cr > Cu > Pb > As > Cd > Hg	[12]
Metal mining and smelting site	Baiyin, China	Cr > Zn > Pb > Cu > As > Cd	[38]
Metal scrap dump	Delta State, Nigeria	Fe > Zn > Cr > Cu > Pb > Co > Ni > Cd	[39]
Oilfield	Niger Delta, Nigeria	Fe > Mn > Zn > V > Cr > Pb > Cu > Ni > Cd > Hg > As	[11]
Pipeline	Niger Delta, Nigeria	Fe > Ni > Mn > Zn > V > Cr > Pb > Cu > Cd > Hg > As	[11]
Red soil	Japan	Zn > Ni > Cu > Pb > Cd	[33]
Roadside	Botwana	Fe > Al > Ni > Mn > Pb > Zn > Cu > Co	[1]
Roadside	Urumqi, China	Cd > Zn > Cu > Pb > Be > Ni > Mn > Cr > Co	[2]
Roadside dust	Ilorin, Nigeria	Fe > Mn > Pb > Cr > Zn > Cu	[3]
Solid waste dump	Ibadan, Nigeria	Pb > Cr > Ni > Co > Cd	[10]
Street dust	Tehran, Iran	Fe > Mn > Zn > Pb > Cu > Ni > Cr > Cd > Li	[5]
Street dust	Cairo, Egypt	Zn > Pb > V > Cr > Ni > Co > Ag > As > Cd	[4]
Top soil	Fuyang, China	Zn > Cu > Pb > Ni > Cd	[40]
Urban road dust	China	Zn > Pb > Cu > Cr > Ni > Cd	[7]
Urban soil	China	Pb > Zn > Cu > Ni > Cr > Cd	[7]
Urban soil	China	Zn > Pb > Cu > Cd	[41]
Urban soil	Poznań, Polland	Zn > Pb > Cu > Cd	[28]
Volcanic soil	Japan	Zn > Cu > Pb > Ni > Cd	[33]
Solid waste dump	Enugu, Nigeria	Pb > Fe > As > Zn > Cu > Co > Ni > Cd > Cr > Mn	This study

Table 3 Seasonal correlation of heavy metals

	Rainy season										Dry season									
	Cu	*Zn*	*Pb*	*As*	*Cr*	*Ni*	*Cd*	*Fe*	*Co*	*Mn*	*Cu*	*Zn*	*Pb*	*As*	*Cr*	*Ni*	*Cd*	*Fe*	*Co*	*Mn*
Cu	1										1									
Zn	0.606	1									0.813	1								
Pb	0.542	0.59	1								0.189	0.37	1							
As	0.376	0.47	0.66	1							0.070	0.198	0.65	1						
Cr	0.372	0.56	0.61	0.68	1						0.457	0.63	0.52	0.43	1					
Ni	0.286	0.54	0.57	0.56	0.47	1					0.237	0.43	0.63	0.53	0.53	1				
Cd	0.299	0.54	0.59	0.61	0.66	0.61	1				0.291	0.4	0.52	0.52	0.5	0.42	1			
Fe	0.448	0.68	0.55	0.54	0.7	0.74	0.52	1			0.321	0.43	0.47	0.44	0.68	0.44	0.39	1		
Co	0.470	0.45	0.53	0.55	0.63	0.37	0.46	0.5	1		0.060	0.29	0.66	0.58	0.53	0.51	0.58	0.62	1	
Mn	0.250	0.37	0.43	0.33	0.26	0.32	0.54	0.31	0.055	1	0.602	0.37	0.37	0.33	0.43	0.43	0.57	0.3	0.145	1

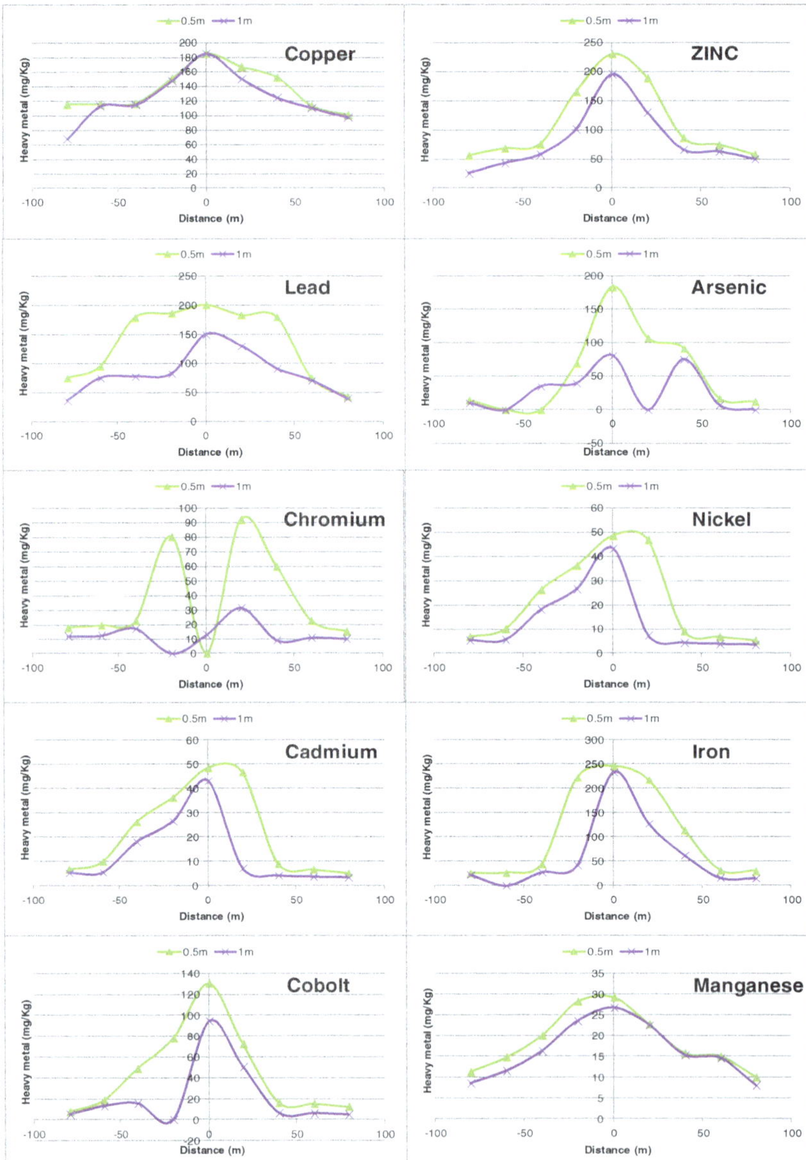

Figure 2 Spatial distribution of heavy metals in dry season.

From Figures 2, 3 and 5, it can easily be deduced that cobalt, cadmium, nickel and chromium are the most persistent of all the heavy metals studied. Their very high concentrations within the dumpsite as well as the comparatively low concentration at lower soil depths suggest a tendency to persistence and accumulation within the dumpsite. The problem of heavy metal accumulation in dumpsites is a matter of serious concern particularly in developing countries where farmers prefer to cultivate vegetables in waste dumps because of their perceived fertility. Vegetables grown on such soils are usually very leafy and attractive to consumers. Paw paw fruits and maize cultivated around the dumpsite are commonly sold in Enugu Urban market [44]. Elevated levels of Cd and Pb have been reported in vegetables cultivated in urban waste dumps of Kumasi, Ghana [16]. However, consumption of vegetables cultivated in heavy metals polluted soils has been reported to reduce life expectancy by 9 to 10 years [45]. Leafy vegetables exhibit preferential uptake of cadmium and lead from the soil

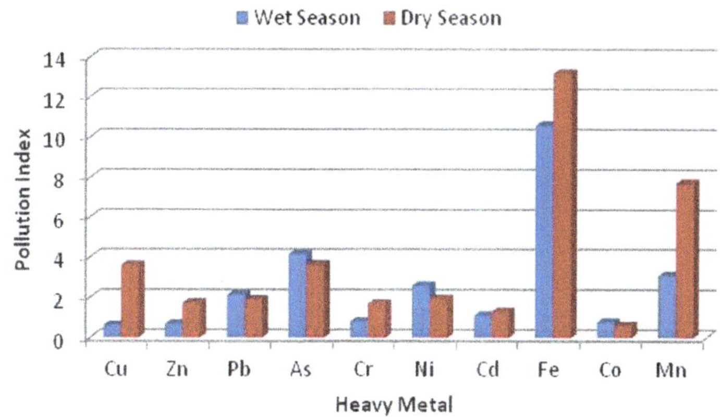

Figure 3 Seasonal variation of pollution index.

[46]. The order of soil to plant transfer is Cd > Cu > Zn > Pb > As. Figure 5 also shows that heavy metal accumulation in dumpsite soil is more pronounced in the dry season. This can be expected since leaching which is the major mechanism of pollutant transport in the soil hardly occurs during the dry season. With the exception of copper and lead, all the other metals had high concentration at the core of the dumpsite in the dry season.

The leachability/mobility of heavy metals is usually inhibited by their affinity for certain substances in the soil such as clay, organic matter, hydrous oxides, etc. The pronounced variability in the spatial and lateral behaviours of the heavy metals can be attributed to the difference in their physicochemical characteristics. Heavy metal binding capacities is site specific and parameters relevant to binding at one site may be insignificant at another [13]. Another very crucial factor responsible for the high level of heavy metals accumulation in the waste dump is that the conditions prevailing in the dumpsite are not optimal for proper waste stabilization. The result is that organic fraction of disposed waste decomposes at a very slow rate.

Geoaccumulation (I_{geo}) and Pollution Indices (PI)

Geoaccumulation and pollution indices are used to assess the risks associated with heavy metals in the environment. From the pollution indices of the various heavy metals depicted in Figure 3, there is a moderate to extreme level of heavy metal pollution in the study area. Iron and manganese have PI values of 13.2 (dry season), 10.6 (rainy season) and 7.7 (dry season), 3.1 (rainy season) respectively. Apart from the rainy season PI value for manganese, the other PI values indicate extreme levels of soil pollution by these metals. Copper, arsenic, and nickel have PI values which indicate high level of pollution ($2 \leq PI \leq 5$). These heavy metals are most likely from sawdust and timber products disposed on the dumpsite [47]. The most commonly used wood preservatives are the copper chromium arsenic (CCA) salts. Though these metals have low mobility under normal conditions, under acidic conditions their mobility increases [48]. Salts of chromium, copper and arsenic can easily enter the human environment through improper disposal of sawdust. These metals are usually held tightly within the wood matrices but can get liberated during sawing. Moreover, sawdust has large surface areas which can facilitate desorption of these salts.

Zinc, cadmium and chromium have PI values between 1 and 2 which indicates moderate level of pollution. Only cobalt has a PI value less than 1 in both dry and rainy seasons. This implies that cobalt pollution in the dumpsite currently stands at a very low level. It can be seen from Figure 3 that the dry season PI values computed for most of the metals were much higher than rainy season PI values. This can be attributed to the fact that heavy metals tend to accumulate near the top soil during the dry season [49]. However, with the onset of rainy season, the metals are mobilized and dispersed by leachates. The pollution index gives the pollution status of the soil with respect to individual metals. Hence a composite value is needed to ascertain the overall status of the soil. The pollution loading index (PLI) meets that requirement. The PLI values for the soil are 1.706 for rainy season and 2.54 for dry season. PLI value greater than 1 signifies deterioration. It seems that conditions that favour heavy metals mobility prevail in the rainy season. A substantial degree of heavy metals attenuation via plant uptake occurs in the rainy season when plants and grasses are growing. As dry season approaches, grasses and remains of plant roots and shoots wither and are re-integrated into the soil giving rise to a cyclic sequence of up-take and deposition.

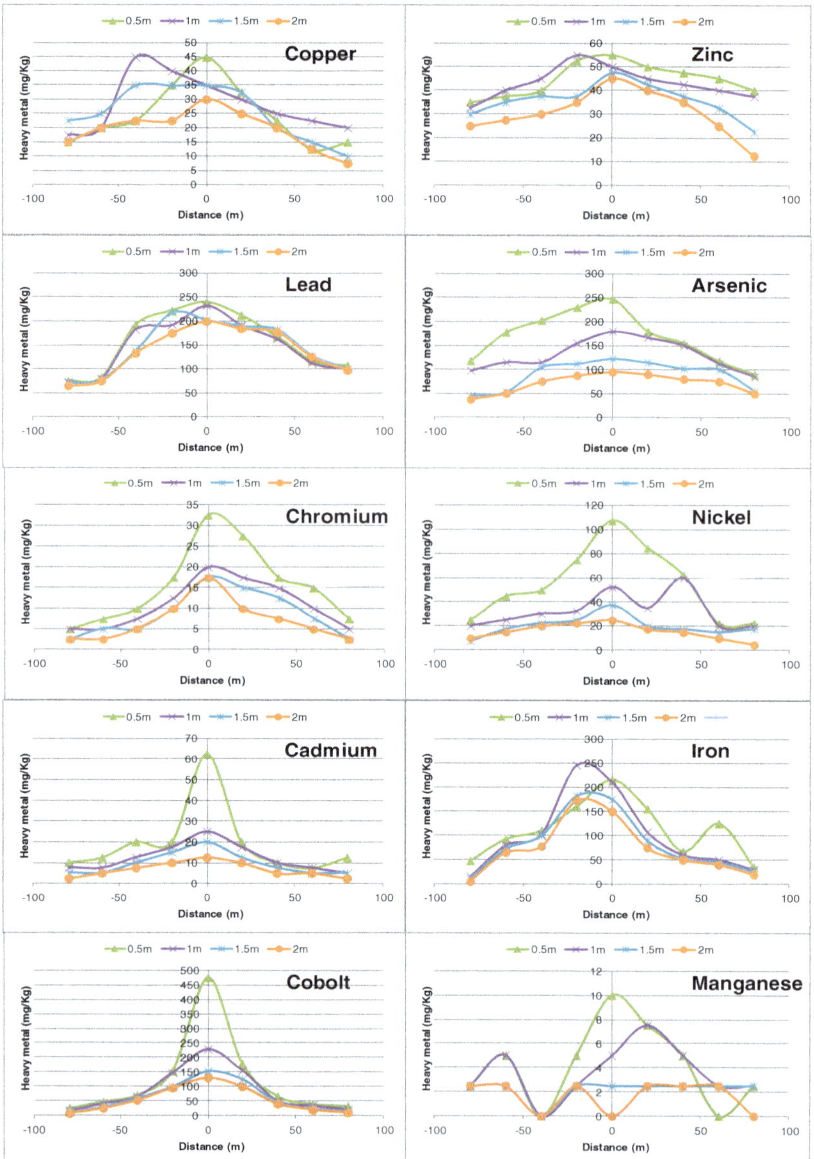

Figure 4 Spatial distribution of heavy metals in rainy season.

The values of I_{geo} obtained for the individual metals (Figure 6) serve to further buttress the results of the PI values. Iron, manganese, copper and arsenic have the highest I_{geo} values, while cobalt, chromium, cadmium and zinc have I_{geo} values less than zero. From the I_{geo} values, it can be deduced that the soil is currently uncontaminated with respect to cobalt, cadmium, chromium and zinc; moderately to heavily contaminated with respect to iron and manganese; and moderately contaminated with respect to copper, lead, arsenic and nickel. From Figure 7, it appears that a substantial concentration of heavy metals is confined within the first 1 m of soil depth. This suggests that the mobility of heavy metals is affected by the concentration in the top soil. The concentrations of most of the heavy metals, specifically, chromium, manganese, copper, nickel, cadmium and zinc approached a constant level at a depth of 1 m. On the other hand, the concentrations of arsenic, cobalt and iron continued to decrease even at a depth of 2 m. This phenomenon confirms the suggestion that

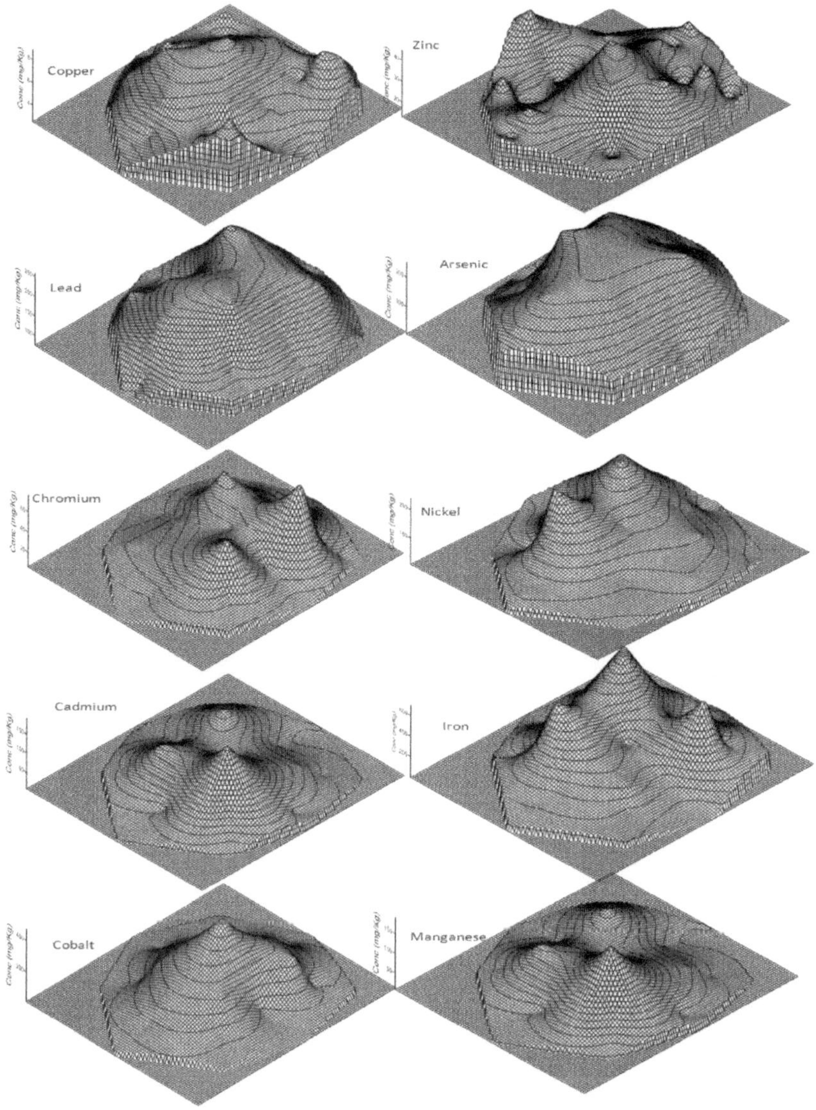

Figure 5 Three dimensional maps of heavy metal distribution in study area.

individual heavy metals, move at different rates in the soil [50]. It also suggests that individual heavy metals move in plumes. Hence the plumes or copper, lead, chromium, nickel, manganese, cadmium, and zinc are lagging behind the plume of arsenic, iron and cobalt. The rate of movement of this plume is dependent on the loading of the heavy metals on the top soil and other site characteristics. It can further be deduced that the mobility of arsenic, cobalt and iron is most favoured by condition prevailing in this site. It is also likely that these heavy metals will breakthrough to groundwater faster than other metals.

Figure 7 also shows that copper is very reluctant to move and therefore has a tendency to accumulate in soil. The concentration of copper dropped from 330 mg/kg to less than 50 mg/kg in just 0.5 m of soil depth, and afterwards dropped no further. Zinc and cadmium also follow the same pattern to a smaller degree. Another reason for the high disparity between heavy metal concentration in the top soil and that in the soil below is that many of the heavy metals are still bound to waste materials in the waste dump. It is however, expected that as biological processes in the dumpsite progress, these heavy metals will be released from their parent

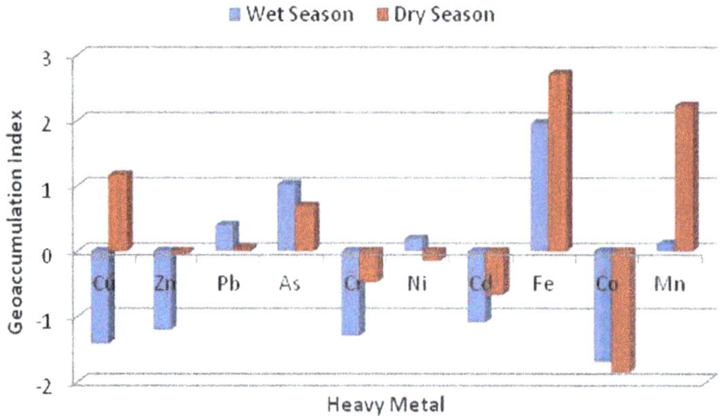

Figure 6 Seasonal variation of geoaccumulation index.

sources into the soil [51]. When these metals are mobilized, they become more available for leaching and plant uptake, thereby increasing their environmental risk. This implies that waste dumpsites without impermeable linings as is common in developing countries should undergo remediation in order to reduce associated long term risks [52]. The high concentration of iron in the dumpsite as well as other locations investigated by various researchers is understandable. Iron is the second most abundant metal in the earth crust and has a wide range of domestic and industrial applications. Its relatively high activity makes it susceptible to corrosion. When iron corrodes, it forms a flaky and porous oxide so that particles from the parent material are easily detached and deposited in the environment. Iron is a very essential mineral and is a basic component of blood. However, excess intake of iron beyond the recommended dietary limits can cause health problems.

Other metals such as arsenic, cobalt, cadmium, chromium and nickel are extensively used in the industries either as raw materials, stabilizers, preservatives, catalysts or inhibitors. They form a major component of very common materials such as paints, pigments, ink, batteries, fungicides, pesticides, fertilizers, dyes, printer and photocopier toner, adhesives, paper etc. All these products and many more are disposed at dumpsites. Though arsenic is a component of most plants, its biological function has not been determined and the risk of arsenic transfer from plant to man is very low as plants cannot survive high doses of the metal. Table 4 shows that the ecological risk posed by heavy metals in the study location is high. About 91% of this risk is contributed by cadmium, whereas the risk posed by the other heavy metals is very low. The decreasing order of risk is: Cd > Co > Pb > Ni > Cu > Zn > Cr. There is therefore a need to discontinue waste disposal at this site and immediately embark on remediation measures in order to reduce environmental impact.

Sources of cadmium at the dumpsite include cigarette butts, sewage, fertilizers, batteries, pigments, plastics and

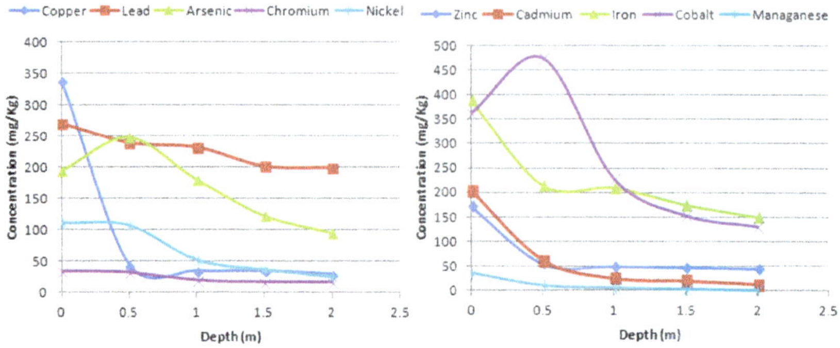

Figure 7 Attenuation of heavy metals with soil depth.

Table 4 Ecological risk indices

	Copper	Zinc	Lead	Chromium	Nickel	Cadmium	Cobalt	Total
Rainy season	0.90	0.14	2.31	0.15	1.37	*201.52*	15.19	221.58
Dry season	3.13	0.25	2.10	0.24	1.02	*215.53*	13.30	235.58
Level of contamination	Low	Low	Low	Low	Low	*High*	Low	High

paints. The global adult tobacco survey estimated that 5.6% (4.7 million) of Nigerians smoke cigarette at an average daily consumption rate of 8 sticks [53]. This translates to 37.6 million cigarette stubs disposed at dumpsites on a daily basis or 14 billion cigarette butts annually. Other heavy metals contained in cigarette are lead and arsenic which are easily leached into the soil from the highly porous butts. It has been estimated that the lead, arsenic and cadmium contents of cigarette ranged from 0.02– 6.75 μg/g, 0.02– 0.71 μg/g [54] and 0.4 – 2.3 μg/g [55] respectively. However, only 10 to 20% of these heavy metals are inhaled by the smoker, while the rest is discharged into the environment [56]. Anthropogenic release of cadmium into the environment can also be attributed to the rise in use of nickel-cadmium rechargeable batteries in phones, torches, laptops, radio sets and other electronic gadgets. In Nigeria, most of these wastes are co-disposed with other low risk wastes in municipal waste dumps. Other metals associated with electronic wastes are: zinc used as screen coating; copper used as circuit board solder; lead used in cathode ray tubes, solders and batteries/accumulators; chromium used as metal coating; and nickel.

An attempt at systematic source identification was made using hierarchical cluster analysis. It appears that cluster analysis was not very successful in delineating the heavy metals into sources of origin. This is partly because most waste materials contain a diversity of metals and non metals. Hence, these metals are found to co-exist with one another as a result of their varied and complementary industrial applications. However, a very careful examination of the clusters revealed groupings in terms of metal toxicity and essentiality to living things. Using hierarchical cluster analysis (Figure 8), the heavy metals can be grouped into four classes. Cluster 1 consists of cadmium, manganese, chromium, nickel and cobalt. All these apart from cadmium are essential minerals which, however, pose high risks when consumed in large doses. The major sources of these metals at the dumpsite are: paints, fertilizers, battery, photographic films, match, demolition waste, brake lining, etc. Cluster 2 consists of zinc and copper which are medium risk essential minerals possibly from batteries, printing ink, photocopier toner, fertilizers, cigarette butts, wood preservatives, copper wire, roofing sheets, cosmetics and pharmaceuticals. Cluster 3 consists of lead and arsenic which are confirmed carcinogens. The major sources of these metals are cigarette butts, paints, pigments, dyes, pharmaceuticals, battery and preservatives at the dumpsite. The only metal in cluster 4 is iron which can be classified as a low risk essential mineral.

Conclusion

The status of soil in the dumpsite and environs has been heavily compromised due to indiscriminate disposal of untreated waste. Unfortunately, this dumpsite is the final resting place for all waste generated within the municipality. These heavy metals accumulate in plants and are subsequently transmitted to humans. They are also leached into groundwater by rainfall. In order to check groundwater contamination from this site, the dump should be converted to a constructed landfill with impermeable lining. This lining will serve as a barrier between leachate and groundwater.

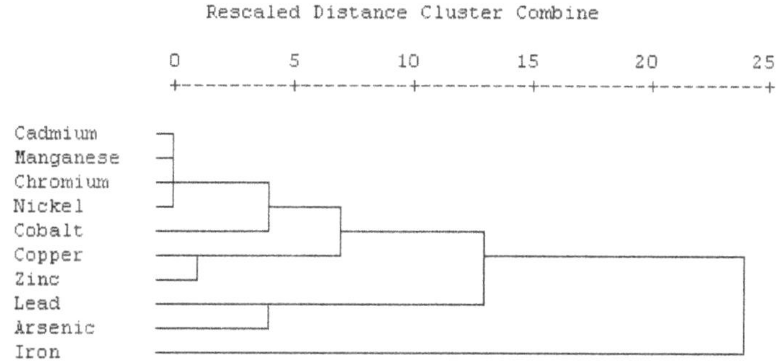

Figure 8 Hierarchical clusters of heavy metals.

Competing interests

The authors declare that they have no competing interests.

Authors' contributions

KCA was involved in research design, soil sample collection and laboratory analyses. JA was involved in research conceptualization, design and supervision. CCN was involved in research design and carried out mathematical and statistical analyses of results as well as the drafting of the manuscript. All authors read and approved the final manuscript.

Authors' information

Kanayochukwu Charles Ajah has a Ph.D in Water resources and Environmental Engineering. He was also a former commissioner for Water Resources in Enugu State, Nigeria.

Joel Ademiluyi is a professor of Water Resources and Environmetal Engineering in the Department of Civil Engineering, University of Nigeria, Nsukka. He has authored many publications and has supervised several postgraduate students.

Chidozie Charles Nnaji is a lecturer in the Department of Civil Engineering University of Nigeria, Nsukka. He has a Ph.D in Water resources and Environmental Engineering. He has authored about twenty five peer reviewed articles in water supply, hydrology, waste management and water/wastewater treatment.

Acknowledgements

We thank Okechukwu Ukpabi for providing the software (Surfer 11) that we used for geospatial plots.

References

1. Mnolawa KB, Likuku AS, Gaboutloeloe GK. Assessment of heavy metals pollution in soils along major roadside areas of Botswana. Afr J Environ Sci Technol. 2011;5(3):186–96.
2. Wei B, Jiang F. Heavy metals induced ecological risk in the City of Urumqi, NW China. Environ Monit Assess. 2010;160:33–45.
3. Baba AA, Adekola FA, Lawal A. Trace metals concentration in roadside dust of Ilorin Town. Centrepoint (Science Edition). 2009;16:57–64.
4. Abdel-Latif NM, Saleh IA. Heavy metals contamination in roadside dust along major roads and correlation with urbanization activities in Cairo, Egypt. J Am Sci. 2012;8(6):379–89.
5. Salmamanzadeh M, Saeedi M, Nabibidhendi G. Heavy metals pollution in street dusts of Tehran and their ecological risk. J Environ Stud. 2012;38(61):4–6.
6. Dinev N, Banov M, Nikova I. Monitoring and risk assessment of contaminated soils. Gen Appl Plant Physiol. 2008;34(3–4):389–96.
7. Wei B, Yang L. A review of heavy metal contamination in urban soils, urban road dust and agricultural soils from China. Michrochem J. 2010;94:99–107.
8. Qiu H. Studies on the potential ecological risk and homology correlation of heavy metals in the soil surface. J Agr Sci. 2010;2(2):194–201.
9. Amuno SA. Potential ecological risk of heavy metal distribution in cemetary soils. Water Air Soil Poll. 2013;224(2):1–12.
10. Adelekan BA, Alawode AO. Contribution of municipal refuse dumps to heavy metal concentration in soil profile and groundwater in Ibadan, Nigeria. J Appl Biosci. 2001;40:2727-37.
11. Iwegbue CMA, Egbozue FE, Opuene K. Preliminary assessment of heavy metals levels of soils of an oilfield in the Niger Delta, Nigeria. Int J Environ Sci Tech. 2006;3(2):167–72.
12. Li F, Huang J, Zeng G, Yuan X, Li X, Liang J, et al. Spatial risk assessment and sources identification of heavy metals in surface sediments from Dongting Lake, Middle China. J Geochem Explor. 2013;132:75–83.
13. Ward ML, Bitton G, Townsend T. Heavy metal binding capacity (HMBC) of municipal soild waste landfill leachate. Chemosphere. 2005;60:206–15.
14. Kurt-Karakus PB. Determination of heavy metals in indoor dust from Istanbul, Turkey: estimation of the health risk. Environ Int. 2012;50:47–55.
15. Tchounwou PB, Yedjou CG, Patlolla AK, Sutton DJ. Heavy metal toxicity and the environment. Mol Clin Environ Toxicol Exp Supplementum. 2012;101:133–64.
16. Odai SN, Mensah E, Sipitey D, Ryo S, Awuah E. Heavy metals uptake by vegetables cultivated on urban waste dumpsites: a case study of Kumasi, Ghana. Res J Environ Toxicol. 2008;2:92–9.
17. Khana MU, Malika RN, Muhammad S, Ullah F, Qadird A. Health risk assessment of consumption of heavy metals in market food crops from Sialkot and Gujranwala Districts, Pakistan. Hum Ecol Risk Assess. 2015;21(2):327–37.
18. Magaji JY. Effects of waste dump on the quality of plants cultivated around Mpape dumpsite FCT Abuja, Nigeria. Ethiopian J Environ Stud Manage. 2012;5(4):567–73.
19. Liao X, Chen T, Xie H, Liu Y. Soil As contamination and its risk assessment in the areas near the industrial districts of Chenzhou City, Southern China. Environ Int. 2005;31:791–8.
20. Mahmood A, Malik RN. Human health risk assessment of heavy metals via consumption of contaminated vegetables collected from different irrigation sources in Lahore, Pakistan. Arabian J Chem. 2014;7:91–9.
21. Jarup L. Hazards of heavy metal contamination. B Med Bull. 2003;68(1):167–82.
22. Ogbuene EB. Impact of temperature and rainfall disparity on human comfort index in Enugu urban environment, Enugu State, Nigeria. J Environ Issues Agric Dev Ctries. 2012;4(1):92–103.
23. Enete IC, Alabi MO. Characteristics of urban heat island in Enugu during rainy season. Ethiop J Environ Stud Manage. 2012;5(4):391–6.
24. Simpson A. The geology of parts of Onitsha, Owerri and Benue Provinces. Bull Geol Survey Nigeria. 1954;24:1–85.
25. Reymont RA. Aspects of the geology of Nigeria. Ibadan: Ibadan University Press; 1965. p. 145.
26. Aguwa IJ. Study of compressive strengths of laterite-cement mixes as a building material. AU JT. 2009;13(2):114–20.
27. Hani A. Spatial distribution and risk assessment of As, Hg, Co and Cr in Kaveh Industrial City, using geostatistic and GIS. Int J Environ Earth Sci. 2010;1(1):38–43.
28. Grzebisz W, Ciesla L, Komisarek J, Potarzycki J. Geochemical assessment of heavy metals pollution of urban soils. Pol J Eviron Stud. 2002;11(5):493–9.
29. Rout S, Kumar A, Sarkar PK, Mishra MK, Ravi PM. Application of chemometric methods for assessment of heavy metal pollution and source apportionment in Riparian zone soil of Ulhas River estuary India. Int J Environ Sci. 2013;3(5):1485–96.
30. Hakanson L. An ecological risk index for aquatic pollution control—a sediment ecological approach. Water Res. 1980;14:975–1001.
31. Yan X, Gao D, Zhang F, Zeng C, Xiang W, Zhang M. Relationship between heavy metal contamination in roadside topsoil and distance to road edge based on field observation in Qingbai-Tibet Plateau, China. Int J Environ Res Publ Health. 2013;10(3):762–75.
32. Department of Petroleum Resources. Environmental guidelines and standards for the petroleum industry in Nigeria, Ministry of Petroleum Resources, Lagos. 1991. p. 35–76.
33. Yanai J, Yamada K, Yamada H, Nagano Y, Kosaki T. Risk assessment of heavy metal-contaminated soils with reference to ageing effect. Pedologist. 2011;54:278–84.
34. Hobbelen PHF, Koolhas JE, van Gestel CAM. Risk assessment of heavy metal pollution for detritivores in flood plain soils in Biesboch, the Netherlands, taking bioavailability into account. Environ Pollut. 2004;129:409–19.
35. Krishna AK, Govil PK. Soil contamination due to heavy metal leaching from and industrial area of Surat, Gujarat, Western India. Environ Monit Assess. 2007;124:263–75.
36. Omran SE, El-Razeek A. Mapping and screening risk assessment of heavy metals concentrations in soils of Bahr El-baker region Egypt. J Soil Sci Environ Manage. 2012;6(7):182–95.
37. Bora PK, Chetry S, Sharma DK, Saikia PM. Distribution pattern of some heavy metals in the soils of Silghat region of Assam (India), influenced by jute mill soild waste. J Chem. 2013;2013:1–7.
38. Li Y, Wang Y, Gou X, Su Y, Wang G. Risk assessment of heavy metals in soils and vegetables around non-ferrous metals mining and smelting sites, Baiyin, China. J Environ Sci. 2006;18:1124–34.
39. Akpoveta OU, Osakwe SA, Okoh BE, Otuya BO. Physicochemical characteristics of some heavy metals in soils around metal scrap dumps in some parts of Delta State, Nigeria. J Appl Sci Envi Manage. 2010;14(4):57–60.
40. Zhang XY, Lin FF, Wong MTF, Feng L, Wang K. Identification of heavy metal sources from anthroopgenic activities and pollution assessment of Fayang County, China. Environ Monit Assess. 2009;154:439–49.

41. Sun Y, Zhou Q, Xie X, Liu R. Spatial sources and risk assessment of heavy metals contamination of urban soils in typical regions of Shenyang, china. J Hazard Mater. 2010;174:455–62.
42. Tangahu BV, Abdullah SRS, Basri H, Idris M, Anuar N, Mukhlisin M. A review on heavy metals (As, Pb, and Hg) uptake by plants through Phytoremediation. Int J Chem Eng. 2011;2011:1–31. doi:10.1155/2011/939161.
43. Mench M, Didier V, Löffler M, Gomez A, Masson P. A mimicked in-situ remediation study of metal-contaminated soils with emphasis on cadmium and lead. J Environ Qual. 1994;23:58–63.
44. Ogbuene EB, Igwebuike EH, Agusiegbe UM. The impact of open solid waste dump sites on soil quality: a case study of Ugwuaji in Enugu. Br J Adv Acad Res. 2013;2(1):43–53.
45. Lăcătuşu R, Răuţă C, Cârstea S, Ghelase I. Soil-plant-man relationships in heavy metal polluted areas in Romania. Appl Geochem. 1996;11(1–2):105–7.
46. Chang CY, Yu HY, Chen JJ, Li FB, Zhang HH, Liu CP. Accumulation of heavy metals in leaf vegetables from agricultural soils and associated potential health risks in the Pearl River Delta, South China. Environ Monit Assess. 2014;186(3):1547–60.
47. Majid NM, Islam MM, Riasmi Y. Heavy metal uptake and translocation by Jatropha curcas L. in sawdust sludge contaminated soils. Aust J Crop Sci. 2012;6(5):891–8.
48. Fadiran AO, Ababu TT, Mtshali JS. Assessment of mobility and bioavailability of heavy metals in sewage sludge from Swaziland through speciation analysis. Am J Environ Protect. 2014;3(4):198–208.
49. Etim EU, Adie GU. Assessment of toxic heavy metal loading in topsoil samples within the vicinity of a limestone quarry in South Western Nigeria. Afr J Environ Sci Technol. 2012;6(8):322–30.
50. Shaheen SM, Derbalah AS, Moghanm FS. Removal of heavy metals from aqueous solution by zeolite in competitive sorption system. Int J Environ Sci Dev. 2012;3(4):362–7.
51. Hu Y, Liu X, Bai J, Shih K, Zeng EY, Cheng H. Assessing heavy metal pollution in the surface soils of a region that had undergone three decades of intense industrialization and urbanization. Environ Sci Pollut Res. 2013;20:6150–9.
52. Amadi AN, Olasehinde P, Okosun EA, Okoye NO, Okunlola IA, Alkali YB, et al. A comparative study on the impact of avu and ihie dumpsites on soil quality in Southeastern Nigeria. Am J Chem. 2012;2(1):17–23.
53. Kale Y, Olarewaju I, Usoro A, Ilori E, Ogbonna N, Ramanandraibe N, et al. Global adult tobacco survey: country report 2012. Abuja: Federal Minisrty of Health; 2012.
54. Lazarević K, Nikolić D, Stošić L, Milutinović S, Videnović J, Bogdanović D. Determination of lead and arsenic in tobacco and cigarettes: an important issue of public health. Cent Eur J Public Health. 2012;20(1):62–6.
55. Nnorom IC, Osibanjo O, Oji-Nnorom CG. Cadmium determination in cigarettes available in Nigeria. Afr J Biotechnol. 2005;4(10):1128–32.
56. Jung MC, Thornton I, Chon HT. Arsenic, cadmium, copper, lead, and zinc concentrations in cigarettes produced in Korea and the United Kingdom. Environ Technol. 1998;23(2):237–41.

Evaluating soil metallic pollution and consequent human health hazards in the vicinity of an industrialized zone, case study of Mubarakeh steel complex, Iran

Zohreh Ghaemi[1], Abdolreza Karbassi[2*], Faramarz Moattar[1], Amirhesam Hassani[1] and Nematollah Khorasani[1]

Abstract

Background: Being established in 1988 in the vicinity of Isfahan city, Mubarakeh Steel complex has imposed adverse environmental and health effects within the area. The study area is covered by lots of farms through which major crops like wheat and rice are provided.

Methods: Considering the imposed pollution load of the complex, the current study has monitored the concentration of metals Fe, Al, Cd, Cr, Ni, Pb, Cu, Zn, Mn, Co, Mo, As in 14 soil samples within the study area. Furthermore, human health hazards of mentioned metals due to consumption of domestic rice and wheat have also been evaluated through different scenarios. In order to evaluate the mobility of metals in soil samples the sequential chemical analysis is performed.

Results: Regarding the accumulation of metals in loose phases the order of metals bioavailability risk level is estimated to be as follows:
Co > Cd > Mo > Ba > As > Pb > Mn > Cu > V > Zn > Cr > Ni

Discussion: An index approach is also considered to evaluate the severity of metal contamination. Regarding geochemical accumulation index, only cadmium is detected to be in a moderately contaminated status while other metals declare an unpolluted condition. Index of pollution pays more attention to mobility potential of metals and accordingly detects metals Co, Mn, As, Pb, Cd, Ba and Mo to be in a moderately contaminated level. On the other hand, enrichment factor declares all toxic metals except for Co, Ba and V to be enriched.

Conclusions: Considering human health hazard assessment, except for Fe, Ba, Cu and Zn, all metals intakes in different scenarios are considered as hazardous while their CDI values are much more than the respective oral reference doses.

Keywords: Metal pollution, Soil, Mobility, Mubarakeh steel complex, Isfahan

Introduction

Metal contaminated sites contain a potentially hazardous risk for human beings and the environment. The bioavailability of such pollution is sophisticatedly used as an indicator of potential risk [1, 2]. Metals may exist in various species in the environment, where they may be transformed from one form into another or exist in different forms simultaneously. Depending on environmental conditions, the chemical speciation of metals changes widely. Such differences in chemical speciation play a key role in forming the environmental fate, bioaccessibility and environmental risk of the metals.

Knowledge on metals bulk concentrations alone may not be sufficient enough to evaluate the adverse effects of contaminated soils while toxic metals are present in different chemical forms in soil (easily exchangeable ions, metal carbonates, oxides, sulfides, organometallic compounds, ions in crystal lattices of minerals, etc.), which determine their mobilization capacity and bioavailability [3–5].

Knowledge of metal's speciation may help to evaluate the metal tendency to remain in soil or sediments and how easily it may be released into the water phase.

* Correspondence: akarbasi@ut.ac.ir
[2]Graduate Faculty of Environment, University of Tehran, P.O. Box 14155-6135 Tehran, Iran
Full list of author information is available at the end of the article

Sequential extraction procedures are among the most widely used methods through which several extractants are used consecutively to separate the portion of phases from the bulk metallic concentration in a soil sample.

A vast variety of extraction processes providing information about the strength of bonds between metal species and soil fractions have been used by different researchers [2, 6–8]. However, none has been fully accepted as a universal method to be applied for all types of soils metallic pollution studies. Such lack of integrity may result in an erroneous diagnosis in soils. The study of potential mobility involves summing up all reactions that are capable of mobilising metals [9].

Being established in 1988 in the vicinity of Mubarakeh county, Mubarakeh Steel complex has imposed adverse environmental and health effects within the area. A remarkable increase in the number of reported disease cases in Mubarakeh and Zarrinshahr in recent years may be attributed to the mentioned complex activities. The study area is covered by lots of farms through which major crops of Isfahan province are provided. The study area within Iran is demonstrated in Fig. 1.

Considering the imposed pollution load of the complex, the current study has monitored the concentration of metals iron, aluminum, cadmium, chromium, nickel, lead, copper, zinc, manganese, cobalt, molybdenum and arsenic in soil samples within the study area.

The current study presents not only the bulk concentration of eight metals (Fe, Al, Cd, Cr, Ni, Pb, Cu, Zn, Mn, Co, Mo, As) in superficial soil samples of Mubarakeh steel complex vicinity, but also the chemical partitioning of mentioned elements. The latter findings create a clear view of metals potential mobility and consequently the tendency to be absorbed by plants or animals within the bioaccessibility phenomenon. For this study, a modified sequential extraction procedure has been considered [10, 11].

Materials and methods

Soil samples were collected from 14 stations in the vicinity of Mubarakeh steel complex during the summer of 2012 using a Peterson grab sampler (Fig. 2). Spatial details of sampling locations are indicated in Table 1.

Soil samples, which were brown to grey in color, were air-dried and passed through a 63-μm mesh (equivalent to a No. 230 sieve, ASTM E-11). Being powdered using an agate mortar and pestle, about 0.5 g of the sample was placed in a Teflon beaker containing 10 mL aqua regia.

The mixture was heated until most of the liquid had evaporated, and allowed to cool before 5 mL of hydrogen fluoride (HF) were added. The samples were further cooled to room temperature before being filtered. The filtrates were transferred to 50 mL volumetric flasks and brought to volume with 1 N HCl [10]. Slightly modified from the old procedure, chemical partitioning was conducted in three sequential steps: (1) acetic acid 25 % v/v,

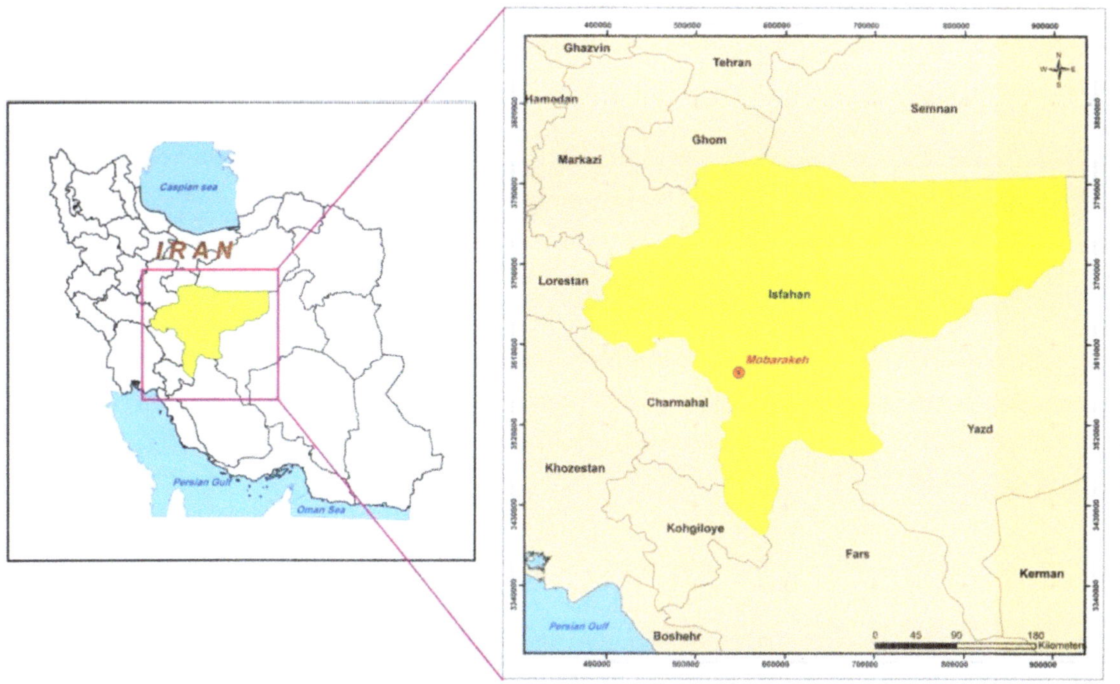

Fig. 1 Study area within Iran and Isfahan province

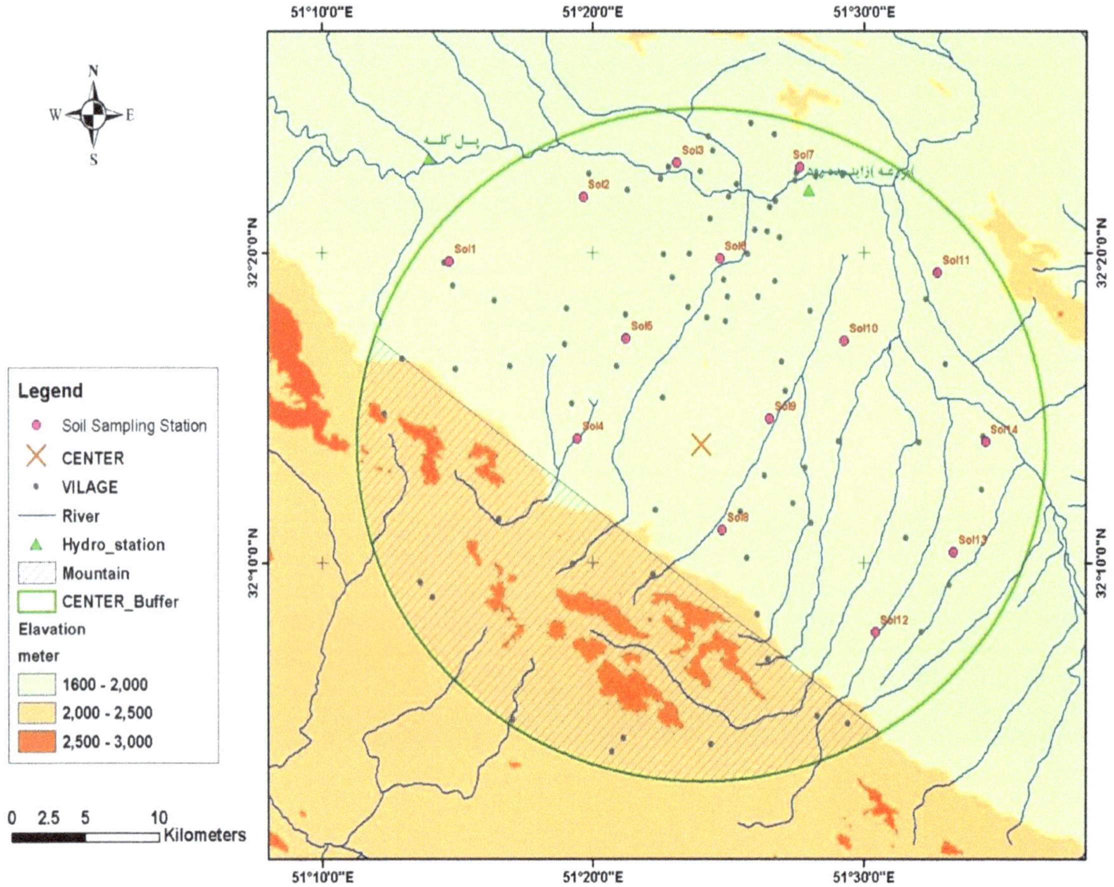

Fig. 2 Layout of soil sampling stations within the study area

Table 1 Spatial characteristics of soil sampling stations

Station	UTM X	UTM Y
1	51.24535	32.32831
2	51.32745	32.36294
3	51.38493	32.3814
4	51.32361	32.23317
5	51.35387	32.28718
6	51.41157	32.33025
7	51.46045	32.37887
8	51.4129	32.18419
9	51.44207	32.24389
10	51.48821	32.28587
11	51.54518	32.32231
12	51.50707	32.12949
13	51.55509	32.17231
14	51.57471	32.23179

(2) acetic acid 25 % v/v-0.1 M hydroxylamine hydrochloride and (3) 30 % H202 "extraction with 1 M ammonium acetate" [11]. To digest rice and wheat samples, 15 milliliters of the mixture HNO_3:H_2SO_4:$HClO_4$ 1:1:5 was added to 1 gram of powdered rice/wheat and heated to 80° centigrade. The mixtures were further cooled and filtered before injection process [12].

The analysis of metals in solutions was carried out by an inductively coupled plasma atomic emission spectrometer. Certified reference material (CRM 320) was used to check the accuracy of the analytical procedures. Replicate analysis of this CRM showed an acceptable accuracy, with recovery rates for metals between 92 % and

Table 2 Details of rice consumption scenarios within the study area

Scenario No.	1	2	3	4	5	6
Body weight (kg)	70	70	70	15	15	15
Daily rice consumption (gr)	100	250	400	100	250	400

Table 3 Details of wheat consumption scenarios within the study area

Scenario No.	1	2	3	4	5	6
Body weight (kg)	70	70	70	15	15	15
Daily wheat consumption (gr)	150	300	450	150	300	450

105 %. Furthermore, two samples were analyzed in triplicate to determine the precision of the analytical processes. The average values of the variation coefficients were estimated to be less than 10 % which may be considered acceptable for such studies [13].

To have an estimate of background status, according to soil samples collected from the vicinity of Mubarakeh steel, metals concentrations in shale have been considered. Such assumption is normally used as background values in sediment studies [13–16].

In order to determine the value of metal concentrations in different sedimentary phases, the modified sequential chemical partitioning method was considered [11].

To evaluate the severity of metallic pollution within the study area, geochemical accumulation index, enrichment factor and index of pollution were taken into consideration.

An index approach was used to assess the severity of metal contamination in the vicinity of Mubarakeh steel complex. Accordingly, the geochemical accumulation index was calculated using:

$$\text{Igeo} = \text{Log2}\left[\text{Cn}/(1.5 * \text{Bn})\right] \quad (1)$$

Where Igeo stands for geochemical accumulation index, Cn is the bulk metal concentration and Bn is the average metal concentration in shale [17, 18].

The enrichment factor (EF) values was calculated for metals using:

$$\text{EF} = \left[(\text{Cn}/\text{CFe})\ \text{sample}\right] / \left[(\text{Cn}/\text{CFe})\text{crust}\right] \quad (2)$$

Where (Cn/CFe) sample indicates the ratio of the concentration of a specific element (Cn) to that of Fe (CFe) in soil sample and (Cn/CFe) crust is the same ratio in an unpolluted reference sample [19].

Finally, index of pollution which is a modification of Igeo is referred by the following formula:

$$\text{IPOLL} = \text{Log2}\left[\text{Bc}/\text{Lp}\right] \quad (3)$$

The study area is a major agricultural site in the province and crops like wheat and rice are widely cultivated within the region. In order to evaluate the probable crops metal uptake, metals concentration in eight different rice and 15 different wheat samples were measured.

To evaluate the hazard level threatening local habitants due to consumption of rice and wheat products, nutritional pattern and physiological characteristics of residents should be taken into consideration. Accordingly six different scenarios are defined (Tables 2 and 3).

Table 4 Bulk concentration of metals (mg/kg, dry mass) in soil samples within the study area

Station	Co	Mn	As	Ni	Pb	Cr	Cd	Cu	Ba	Mo	Zn	V	Fe %	Al %
S1	1.80	391.98	6.39	49.63	6.84	53.66	0.98	27.46	94.31	0.69	70.85	25.27	1.89	0.10
S2	2.31	455.58	6.67	47.35	2.84	38.22	0.92	33.08	95.64	0.45	67.03	25.64	1.37	0.10
S3	5.88	419.01	6.28	45.91	7.58	40.77	0.84	72.39	68.33	0.69	87.91	31.49	1.45	0.11
S4	3.90	501.45	8.56	64.20	20.84	47.45	4.34	70.18	98.77	0.35	95.72	27.34	1.61	0.11
S5	3.66	603.02	9.99	80.00	8.62	59.70	1.24	59.07	98.87	0.49	102.81	25.78	2.19	0.12
S6	4.90	560.10	8.43	65.06	8.42	47.19	1.08	44.01	87.62	0.47	77.03	24.55	1.64	0.13
S7	2.37	465.56	7.30	65.21	10.61	45.64	1.14	35.89	100.81	0.61	80.71	22.70	1.85	0.13
S8	2.43	445.69	8.64	66.53	7.55	43.88	0.98	31.68	71.48	0.76	73.95	23.26	1.58	0.12
S9	2.18	341.01	7.34	59.28	6.41	46.01	4.77	38.51	88.40	0.24	68.30	19.04	1.43	0.12
S10	3.03	421.85	7.14	59.58	7.93	42.74	1.01	29.38	73.71	0.28	70.09	18.26	1.46	0.10
S11	1.73	414.25	8.42	58.69	10.77	42.94	1.06	36.40	93.12	0.41	87.59	21.18	1.50	0.12
S12	1.88	466.20	8.88	69.48	9.55	47.47	1.10	32.02	75.65	0.72	79.21	20.92	1.67	0.13
S13	1.00	398.80	9.01	70.65	8.11	47.77	1.07	31.34	68.14	0.64	81.15	16.91	1.70	0.13
S14	2.04	341.36	11.20	55.94	8.49	37.43	0.91	39.63	68.66	0.31	74.13	20.28	1.34	0.11
Max	5.88	603.02	11.20	80.00	20.84	59.70	4.77	72.39	100.81	0.76	102.81	31.49	2.19	0.13
Min	1.00	341.01	6.28	45.91	2.84	37.43	0.84	27.46	68.14	0.24	67.03	16.91	1.34	0.10
SD	1.35	73.93	1.41	9.52	3.94	5.82	1.29	14.85	12.83	0.18	10.58	3.96	0.23	0.01
Mean	2.79	444.70	8.16	61.25	8.90	45.78	1.53	41.50	84.54	0.51	79.75	23.04	1.62	0.12
Shale values	19	850	13	68	20	90	0.3	45	498	2.6	95	130	4.70	8.2

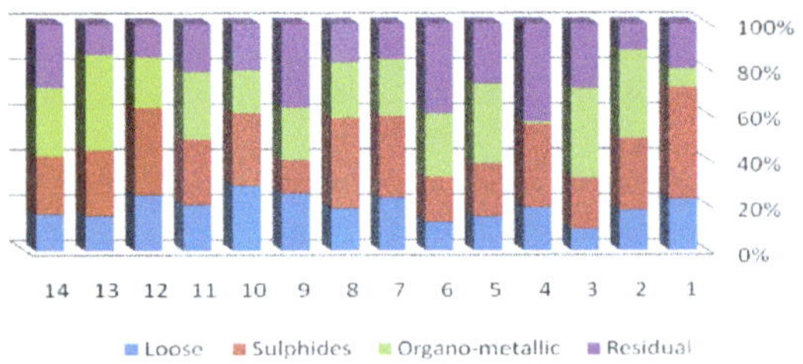

Fig. 3 Chemical partitioning of Cobalt in soil samples

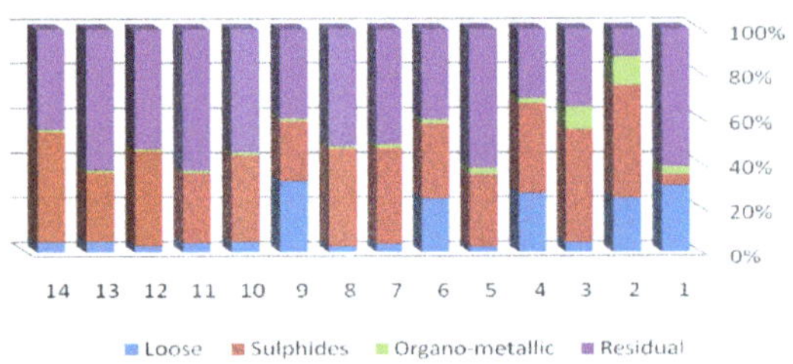

Fig. 4 Chemical partitioning of Manganese in soil samples

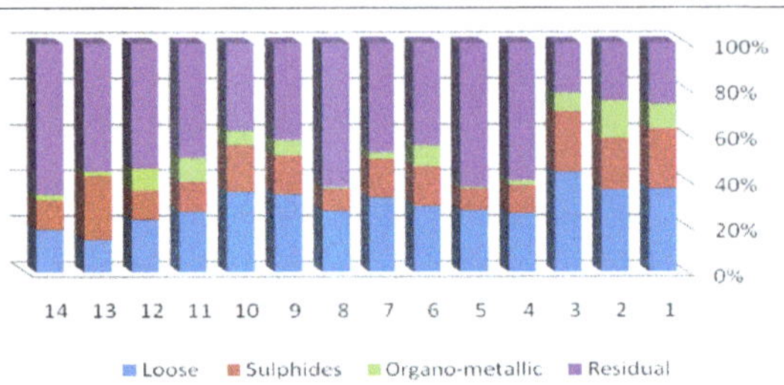

Fig. 5 Chemical partitioning of Arsenic in soil samples

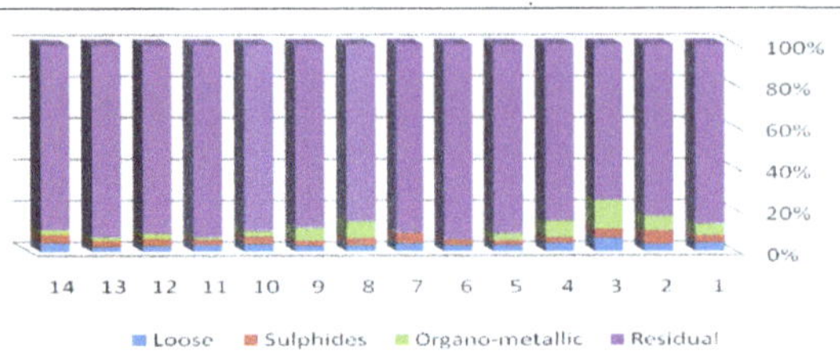

Fig. 6 Chemical partitioning of Nickel in soil samples

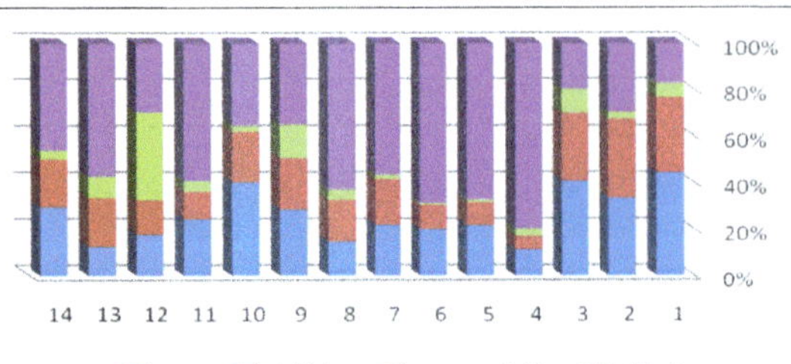

Fig. 7 Chemical partitioning of Lead in soil samples

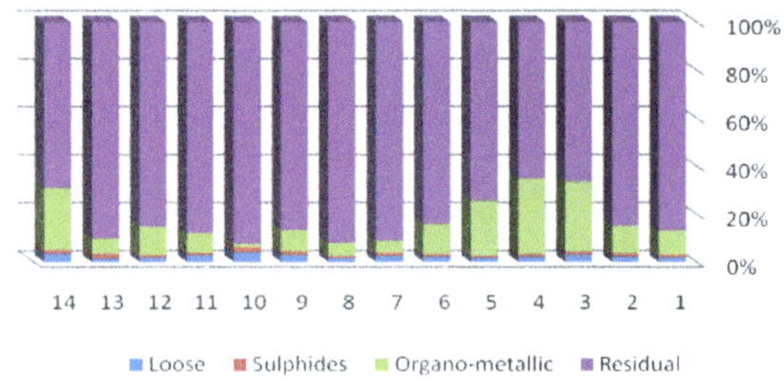

Fig. 8 Chemical partitioning of Chromium in soil samples

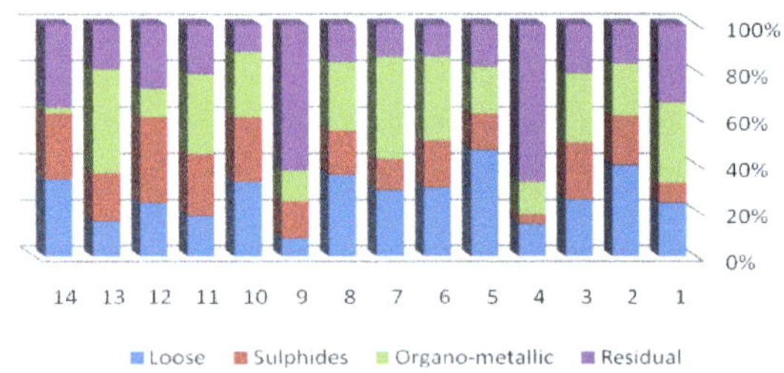

Fig. 9 Chemical partitioning of Cadmium in soil samples

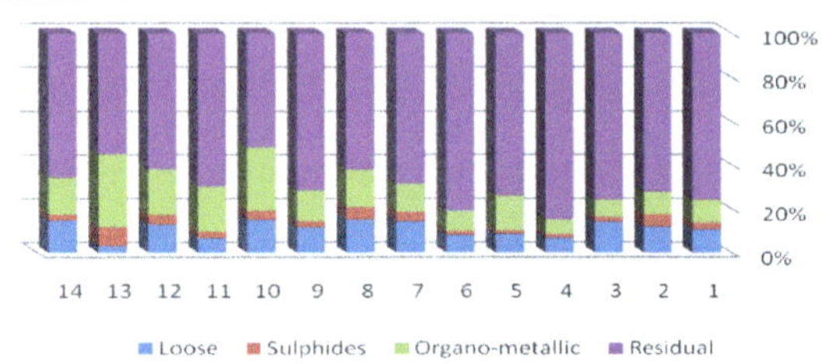

Fig. 10 Chemical partitioning of Copper in soil samples

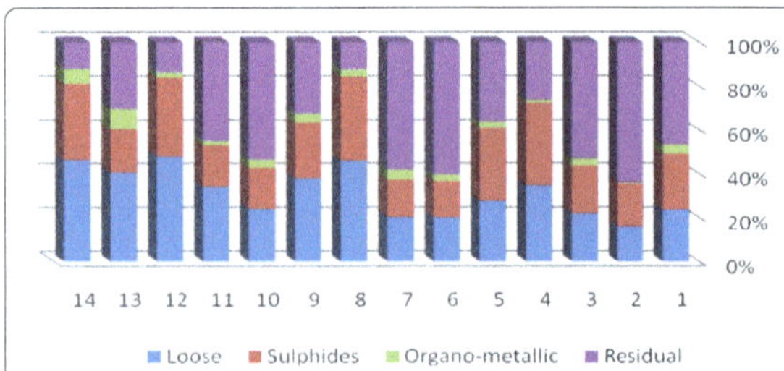

Fig. 11 Chemical partitioning of Barium in soil samples

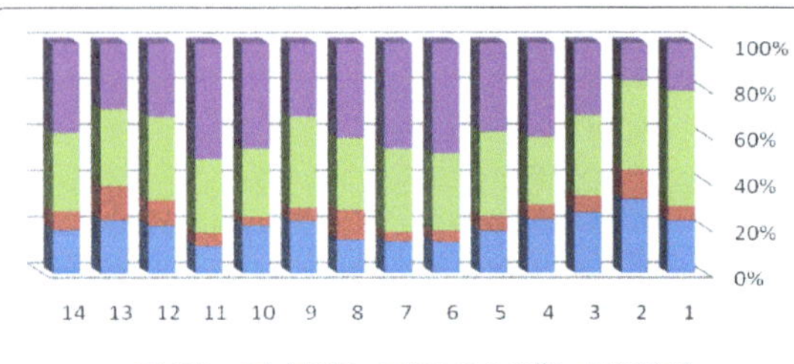

Fig. 12 Chemical partitioning of Molybdenum in soil samples

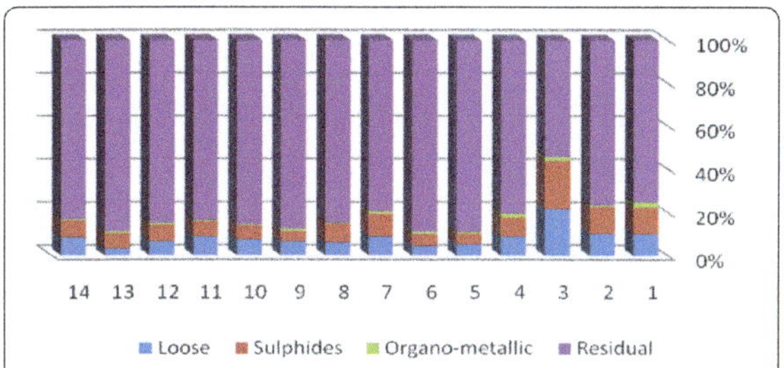

Fig. 13 Chemical partitioning of Zinc in soil samples

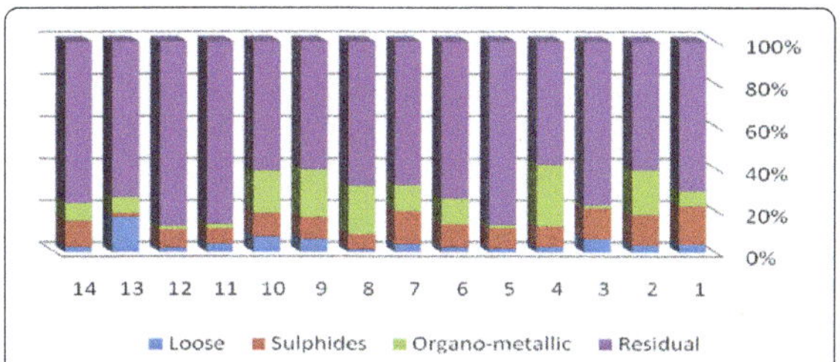

Fig. 14 Chemical partitioning of Vanadium in soil samples

Chronic daily intakes of different metals within the framework of defined scenarios are compared with respective chronic oral reference doses to assess the existent hazards. Details for exposure assessment and hazard analysis are fully described within the literature [20].

Results

Total concentration of mentioned metals in soil samples collected from the vicinity of Mubarakeh steel complex are shown in Table 4.

In comparison with average shale values, all metals show lower concentrations except for Cd. Average cadmium concentration within the study area is more than five times higher than that of shale which indicate an intensified enrichment. On the other hand, although the concentration of other metals is lower than that of shale, such condition should not be considered as a low-risk and safe one. Potential mobility of existing metallic concentration in soil should be regarded before any judgment.

The results of chemical partitioning for metals are demonstrated in Figs. 3, 4, 5, 6, 7, 8, 9, 10, 11, 12, 13 and 14.

The percent of metals concentration bound to different phases are grouped in a descending order as follows:

Loose ions :

Ba (31.53) > As (29.17) > Cd (26.73) > Pb (25.82) > Mo (20.37) > Co (19.21) > Mn (12.23) > Cu (10.98) > Zn (8.27) > V (4.68) > Ni (3.53) > Cr (2.48)

Sulfide ions :

Mn (36.97) > Co (30.51) > Ba (25.88) > Cd (20.26) > Pb (19.22) > As (17.48) > V (10.92) > Zn (8.96) > Mo (7.74) > Cu (3.67) > Ni (3.36) > Cr (1.25)

Organic ions :

Table 5 Percentile of anthropogenic portion in bulk metallic concentration of soil samples

Station	Anthropogenic portion of metallic pollution (%)													
	Al	Co	Mn	As	Ni	Pb	Cr	Cd	Cu	Ba	Fe	Mo	Zn	V
1	11.54	72.31	34.58	66.14	11.80	74.41	12.01	59.90	21.86	47.99	0.78	71.34	22.27	26.47
2	17.93	79.47	78.68	67.46	15.31	63.25	13.78	75.13	25.09	32.48	0.77	75.19	21.15	35.46
3	5.74	64.45	58.75	70.40	22.32	72.17	30.21	71.34	21.77	42.31	2.29	61.82	41.24	20.26
4	11.87	51.15	62.07	35.99	13.22	18.23	31.37	29.26	13.76	66.41	0.40	53.43	17.48	37.59
5	4.12	66.29	34.02	33.28	7.82	29.40	22.99	73.88	23.44	57.60	0.21	55.32	9.83	11.79
6	5.04	54.36	53.67	50.04	5.26	28.05	14.31	77.69	17.19	35.70	0.32	46.77	10.00	23.14
7	5.44	75.91	43.47	47.32	8.14	39.16	8.00	77.62	28.30	37.74	0.73	48.67	18.58	28.94
8	7.75	74.68	42.77	33.19	13.19	33.31	7.20	75.75	34.16	78.91	0.47	53.02	13.56	28.67
9	7.68	56.89	53.93	52.16	10.37	58.51	12.13	33.73	25.59	60.73	0.32	61.23	11.07	35.70
10	3.64	71.54	40.39	55.79	8.89	58.11	6.77	79.60	43.46	41.90	0.75	48.65	12.85	35.08
11	2.03	71.01	33.00	45.29	6.24	36.63	10.91	71.00	27.29	49.42	0.33	44.50	14.76	12.15
12	6.64	76.99	41.71	40.87	7.80	63.31	13.47	65.22	34.30	77.72	0.71	61.16	13.48	11.47
13	9.94	77.84	33.28	39.72	6.18	38.57	8.84	72.83	40.69	62.64	0.19	64.24	10.13	23.88
14	3.04	64.97	49.61	30.54	9.44	48.62	27.87	58.02	30.79	79.14	0.51	54.80	15.25	21.32
Max	17.93	79.47	78.68	70.40	22.32	74.41	31.37	79.60	43.46	79.14	2.29	75.19	41.24	37.59
Min	2.03	51.15	33.00	30.54	5.26	18.23	6.77	29.26	13.76	32.48	0.19	44.50	9.83	11.47
SD	4.30	9.08	13.23	13.31	4.54	17.75	8.66	15.91	8.40	16.38	0.52	9.13	8.16	9.11
Mean	7.31	68.42	47.14	47.73	10.43	47.27	15.70	65.78	27.69	55.05	0.63	57.15	16.55	25.14

Table 6 Mean values of various pollution indices in soil samples

Index	Al	Co	Mn	As	Ni	Pb	Cr	Cd	Cu	Ba	Fe	Mo	Zn	V
Igeo	−6.75	−3.50	−1.54	−1.28	−0.75	−2.00	−0.36	1.94	−0.57	−3.10	−2.14	−3.04	−1.19	−3.10
Ipoll	0.11	1.72	0.97	0.99	0.16	1.01	0.25	1.66	0.48	1.26	0.01	1.26	0.27	0.43
EF	0.04	0.44	1.45	17.05	2.38	2.03	1.42	48.67	2.60	0.64	1.00	1.04	3.31	0.45

Mo (35.39) > Co (26.30) > Cd (26.10) > Cu (16.12) > Cr (13.72) > V (12.33) > Pb (7.48) > As (6.38) > Ni (4.65) > Ba (3.75) > Mn (3.18) > Zn (1.15)

Residual ions :

Ni (88.41) > Cr (82.55) > Zn (81.61) > V (72.07) > Cu (69.23) > Mn (47.62) > Pb (47.48) > As (46.97) > Ba (38.84) > Mo (36.50) > Cd (26.91) Co (23.98)

In order to have an overall estimate of metals mobility potential, the results of the sum of loose, sulfide and organic ions are grouped as the anthropogenic portion of metals are shown in Table 5.

As was explained in methodology, IPOLL, Bc, and Lp refers to pollution intensity, bulk concentration, and lithogenous portion, respectively. Average indices

Table 7 concentration of metals in different rice samples from the study area (mg/kg dry weight)

ID	Al	Co	Mn	As	Ni	Pb	Cr	Cd	Cu	Ba	Fe	Mo	Zn	V
Rice 1	463.15	0.47	16.86	1.79	6.61	1.04	10.41	0.29	3.88	4.43	9.74	2.64	28.72	2.46
Rice 2	214.05	0.44	15.91	0.62	6.63	0.86	8.46	0.32	6.06	4.24	16.37	1.61	32.32	3.35
Rice 3	211.00	0.37	14.81	1.24	5.03	1.22	7.16	0.40	4.01	4.95	8.89	1.77	22.84	3.01
Rice 4	227.10	0.44	15.42	1.14	9.94	1.51	9.25	0.34	4.57	4.52	9.63	0.85	31.79	3.96
Rice 5	480.00	0.51	16.32	1.26	7.17	1.33	9.81	0.29	5.02	5.42	10.31	1.74	29.79	3.87
Rice 6	250.25	0.49	18.64	1.57	6.07	0.64	9.03	0.35	5.70	4.13	8.26	1.52	31.77	2.99
Rice 7	528.10	0.47	13.11	1.52	6.83	3.34	11.83	0.35	3.80	4.71	21.44	1.59	35.45	3.27
Rice 8	572.25	0.42	22.92	1.47	5.93	0.42	9.91	0.26	8.21	5.58	31.63	1.89	32.93	6.46
Mean	368.24	0.45	16.75	1.33	6.78	1.30	9.48	0.33	5.16	4.75	14.53	1.70	30.70	3.67
St.Dev	156.30	0.05	2.96	0.35	1.44	0.90	1.38	0.05	1.49	0.53	8.28	0.49	3.76	1.23

Table 8 concentration of metals in different wheat samples from the study area (mg/kg dry weight)

ID	Al	Co	Mn	As	Ni	Pb	Cr	Cd	Cu	Ba	Fe	Mo	Zn	V
Wheat 1	294.85	0.46	52.17	1.11	5.89	1.23	8.55	1.26	9.23	5.26	11.29	1.93	38.55	6.61
Wheat 2	226.75	0.44	14.84	1.00	6.39	0.34	8.09	0.25	7.80	6.12	16.08	1.42	30.96	6.86
Wheat 3	329.35	0.53	53.54	1.95	6.87	1.09	9.37	0.25	10.67	7.34	13.81	1.81	19.85	8.91
Wheat 4	394.35	0.44	48.11	0.94	4.86	0.91	8.33	0.33	7.79	5.46	12.76	1.76	49.51	6.67
Wheat 5	493.70	0.46	53.86	3.11	6.77	1.07	10.42	1.16	7.90	8.00	14.38	1.55	28.56	7.29
Wheat 6	623.70	0.38	26.92	1.26	5.79	1.02	10.12	0.33	6.08	5.25	105.74	1.92	27.49	4.17
Wheat 7	344.15	0.47	61.94	1.13	6.92	0.49	9.80	0.27	11.38	7.40	17.49	1.86	49.32	7.92
Wheat 8	173.45	0.49	62.96	1.79	6.10	0.83	7.17	0.28	10.36	7.12	33.50	1.61	39.40	8.91
Wheat 9	148.70	0.54	70.96	1.98	10.18	1.92	7.51	0.38	11.50	7.87	18.96	1.39	41.68	8.84
Wheat 10	480.65	0.45	43.56	0.51	5.36	0.41	8.99	0.25	6.41	9.11	24.76	1.69	26.33	6.71
Wheat 11	230.25	0.71	83.25	2.29	7.48	1.23	7.76	0.25	12.81	10.22	27.59	1.47	54.04	11.05
Wheat 12	82.10	0.47	46.19	2.45	7.72	2.80	6.72	0.30	13.13	6.28	14.94	1.38	53.83	6.84
Wheat 13	185.30	0.48	63.82	1.94	7.35	1.19	10.22	0.29	8.42	12.26	10.21	1.86	46.50	8.21
Wheat 14	398.95	0.47	32.56	1.34	6.46	0.69	9.58	0.25	6.32	6.95	8.36	1.72	27.70	4.48
Wheat 15	499.10	0.43	54.17	1.15	5.87	0.43	9.05	0.26	8.14	5.13	20.83	2.02	41.91	8.11
Mean	327.02	0.48	51.26	1.60	6.67	1.04	8.78	0.41	9.20	7.32	23.38	1.69	38.37	7.44
St.Dev	154.67	0.07	17.33	0.69	1.26	0.64	1.16	0.33	2.32	2.00	23.79	0.21	10.99	1.74

Table 9 Chronic daily intakes of metals through different scenarios due to rice consumption

ID	Mean concentration ppb	Scenario 1 mg/kg-day	Scenario 2 mg/kg-day	Scenario 3 mg/kg-day	Scenario 4 mg/kg-day	Scenario 5 mg/kg-day	Scenario 6 mg/kg-day	Oral RfD mg/kg-day
Al	368.24	5.26E-01	1.32E + 00	2.10E + 00	2.45E + 00	6.14E + 00	9.82E + 00	1.00E + 00
Co	0.45	6.43E-04	1.61E-03	2.57E-03	3.00E-03	7.50E-03	1.20E-02	3.00E-04
Mn	16.75	2.39E-02	5.98E-02	9.57E-02	1.12E-01	2.79E-01	4.47E-01	1.40E-01
As	1.33	1.90E-03	4.75E-03	7.60E-03	8.87E-03	2.22E-02	3.55E-02	3.00E-04
Ni	6.78	9.69E-03	2.42E-02	3.87E-02	4.52E-02	1.13E-01	1.81E-01	2.00E-02
Cr	9.48	1.35E-02	3.39E-02	5.42E-02	6.32E-02	1.58E-01	2.53E-01	3.00E-03
Cd	0.33	4.71E-04	1.18E-03	1.89E-03	2.20E-03	5.50E-03	8.80E-03	1.00E-03
Cu	5.16	7.37E-03	1.84E-02	2.95E-02	3.44E-02	8.60E-02	1.38E-01	4.00E-02
Ba	4.75	6.79E-03	1.70E-02	2.71E-02	3.17E-02	7.92E-02	1.27E-01	2.00E-01
Fe	14.53	2.08E-02	5.19E-02	8.30E-02	9.69E-02	2.42E-01	3.87E-01	7.00E-01
Mo	1.7	2.43E-03	6.07E-03	9.71E-03	1.13E-02	2.83E-02	4.53E-02	5.00E-03
Zn	30.7	4.39E-02	1.10E-01	1.75E-01	2.05E-01	5.12E-01	8.19E-01	3.00E-01
V	3.67	5.24E-03	1.31E-02	2.10E-02	2.45E-02	6.12E-02	9.79E-02	7.00E-05

values for each metal in different stations are shown in Table 6.

The result of metal concentration in agricultural crops (wheat and rice), are shown in Tables 7 and 8.

According to defined scenarios in part of material and methods, respective chronic oral reference doses to assess the existent hazards are shown in Tables 9 and 10. Details for exposure assessment and hazard analysis are fully described within the literature [20].

As it is seen except for Fe, Ba, Cu and Zn, all metals intakes in different scenarios are considered to be hazardous while their CDI values are much more than the respective oral reference doses.

Discussion

Evaluating the metallic pollution of soil and the potential mobility of metal species in the vicinity of Mubarakeh steel complex is considered in this study. Fourteen soil samples were collected and analyzed in summer 2012.

Bioavailability and health risks linked to toxic metals are tightly related to the mobility of metal species. aqueous organisms and plants are more vulnerable towards free ions and labile complexes [3, 21–23]. Accordingly, it may be concluded from the chemical partitioning data that there are significant differences in the distribution of the metals studied. Cobalt, Cd, As, Mo and Pb are introduced as the most risky metals since they present the

Table 10 Chronic daily intakes of metals through different scenarios due to wheat consumption

ID	Mean concentration ppb	Scenario 1 mg/kg-day	Scenario 2 mg/kg-day	Scenario 3 mg/kg-day	Scenario 4 mg/kg-day	Scenario 5 mg/kg-day	Scenario 6 mg/kg-day	Oral RfD mg/kg-day
Al	327.02	7.01E-01	1.40E + 00	2.10E + 00	3.27E + 00	6.54E + 00	9.81E + 00	1.00E + 00
Co	0.48	1.03E-03	2.06E-03	3.09E-03	4.80E-03	9.60E-03	1.44E-02	3.00E-04
Mn	51.26	1.10E-01	2.20E-01	3.30E-01	5.13E-01	1.03E + 00	1.54E + 00	1.40E-01
As	1.6	3.43E-03	6.86E-03	1.03E-02	1.60E-02	3.20E-02	4.80E-02	3.00E-04
Ni	6.67	1.43E-02	2.86E-02	4.29E-02	6.67E-02	1.33E-01	2.00E-01	2.00E-02
Cr	8.78	1.88E-02	3.76E-02	5.64E-02	8.78E-02	1.76E-01	2.63E-01	3.00E-03
Cd	0.41	8.79E-04	1.76E-03	2.64E-03	4.10E-03	8.20E-03	1.23E-02	1.00E-03
Cu	9.2	1.97E-02	3.94E-02	5.91E-02	9.20E-02	1.84E-01	2.76E-01	4.00E-02
Ba	7.32	1.57E-02	3.14E-02	4.71E-02	7.32E-02	1.46E-01	2.20E-01	2.00E-01
Fe	23.38	5.01E-02	1.00E-01	1.50E-01	2.34E-01	4.68E-01	7.01E-01	7.00E-01
Mo	1.69	3.62E-03	7.24E-03	1.09E-02	1.69E-02	3.38E-02	5.07E-02	5.00E-03
Zn	38.37	8.22E-02	1.64E-01	2.47E-01	3.84E-01	7.67E-01	1.15E + 00	3.00E-01
V	7.44	1.59E-02	3.19E-02	4.78E-02	7.44E-02	1.49E-01	2.23E-01	7.00E-05

highest percentages in loose, sulfide and organic fractions and the lowest in residual form. Accordingly, exchange of mentioned metals may be expected between the soil and water column.

Sum of loose, sulfide and organic phases in bulk metallic concentration is considered as manipulated contamination. The higher the anthropogenic portion of a metal is, the higher the mobility risk would be occurred. Generally, the mean anthropogenic portions of the metals, as a percent of their bulk concentrations, obey the following pattern:Co > Cd > Mo > Ba > As > Pb > Mn > Cu > V > Zn > Cr > Ni.

Conclusions

Considering index approach, Igeo deals with bulk concentration and is constructed upon the principle of comparison with shale values. As it is expected, only cadmium is detected to be in a moderately contaminated status regarding this index while other metals declare an unpolluted condition. Index of pollution pays more attention to mobility potential of metals and accordingly detects metals Co, Mn, As, Pb, Cd, Ba and Mo to be in a moderately contaminated level. On the other hand, enrichment factor which compares the bulk concentrations with earth crust values declares all toxic metals except for Co, Ba and V to be enriched.

Considering human health hazard assessment, all toxic metals intakes in different scenarios are considered to be hazardous. The status is much more severe for scenarios dealt with children eating more portions. It must be noted that current hazard levels are calculated as single exposures and for more realistic conditions cumulative exposures should be taken into consideration. In other words, a variety of ingredients (containing rice, wheat, water, etc.) exists in diurnal diet of residents within the study area and the overall hazard would exceed the above-mentioned levels.

Competing interests

The authors declare that they have no competing interests.

Authors' contributions

All authors read and approved the final manuscript.

Acknowledgements

Authors want to appreciate kind cooperation of Mubarakeh steel complex and department of environment of Isfahan Province.

Author details

[1]Department of Environmental Science, Graduate School of the Environment and Energy, Science and Research Branch, Islamic Azad University, Tehran, Iran. [2]Graduate Faculty of Environment, University of Tehran, P.O. Box 14155-6135 Tehran, Iran.

References

1. Adriano DC, Wenzel WW, Vangronsveld J, Bolan NS. Role of assisted natural remediation in environmental cleanup. Geoderma. 2004;122:121–42.
2. Martínez-Sánchez MJ, Navarro MC, Pérez-Sirvent C, Marimón J, Vidal J, García-Lorenzo ML, et al. Assessment of the mobility of metals in a mining-impacted coastal area (Spain, Western Mediterranean). J Geochem Explor. 2008;96:171–82.
3. Nasrabadi T, Nabi Bidhendi GR, Karbassi AR, Mehrdadi N. Partitioning of metals in sediments of the Haraz River (Southern Caspian Sea basin). Environ Earth Sci. 2010;59:1111–7.
4. Weisz M, Polyak K, Hlavay J. Fractionation of elements in sediment samples collected in rivers and harbors at lake Balaton and its catchment area. Microchem J. 2000;67:207–17.
5. Yu K-C, Tsai L-J, Chen S-H, Ho S-T. Correlation analyses binding behavior of heavy metals with sediment matrices. Water Res. 2001;35(10):2417–28.
6. Tessier A, Campbell PGC, Bisson M. Sequential extraction procedure for the speciation of particulate trace metals. Anal Chem. 1979;51:844–51.
7. Kersten M, Förstner U. Chemical fractionation of heavy metals in anoxic estuarine and coastal sediments. Water Sci Technol. 1986;18:121–30.
8. Ure AM, Quevauviller PH, Muntau H, Griepink B. Speciation of heavy metals in soils and sediments. An account of the improvement and harmonization of extraction techniques undertaken under the auspices of the BCR of the Commission of the European Communities. Int J Environ Anal Chem. 1993;51:135–51.
9. Vidal J, Pérez-Sirvent C, Martínez-Sánchez MJ, Navarro MC. Origin and behaviour of heavy metals in agricultural Calcaric Fluvisols in semiarid conditions. Geoderma. 2004;121:257–70.
10. Karbassi AR, Monavari SM, Nabi Bidhendi GR, Nouri J, Nematpour K. Metal pollution assessment of sediment and water in the Shur River. Environ Monit Assess. 2008;147:107–16.
11. Chester R, Hughes RM. A chemical technique for the separation of ferro-manganese minerals, carbonate minerals and adsorbed trace elements from pelagic Sediment. Chem Geol. 1967;2:249–62.
12. Allen SE, Grimshaw HM, Rowland AP. Chemical analysis. In: Moore PD, Chapman SB, editors. Methods in plant ecology. Oxford, London: Blackwell, Scientific Publication; 1986. p. 285–344.
13. Nasrabadi T, Nabi Bidhendi GR, Karbassi AR, Mehrdadi N. Evaluating the efficiency of sediment metal pollution indices in interpreting the pollution of Haraz River sediments, southern Caspian Sea basin. Environ Monit Assess. 2010;171(1–4):395–410.
14. Lopez-Sanchez JF, Rubio R, Samitier C, Rauret G. Trace metal partitioning in marine sediments and sludges deposited off the coast of Barcelona (Spain). Water Res. 1996;30(1):153–9.
15. Jones B, Turki A. Distribution and speciation of heavy metals in surficial sediments from the Tees estuary, northeast England. Mar Pollut Bull. 1997;34(10):768–79.
16. Datta DK, Subramanian V. Distribution and fractionation of heavy metals in the surface sediments of the Ganges–Brahmaputra–Meghna river system in the Bengal basin. Environ Geol. 1998;36(1–2):93–101.
17. Gonzalez-Macias C, Schifter I, Lluch-cota DB, Mendez-Rodriguez L, Hernandez-Vazquez S. Distribution, enrichment and accumulation of heavy metals in coastal sediments of Salina Cruz Bay, Mexico. Environ Monit Assess. 2006;118:211–30.
18. Forstner U, Ahlf W, Calmano W, Kersten M. Sediment criteria development-contributions of environmental geochemistry to water quality management. In: D Helling, P Rothe, U Forstner, P. Stoffers editors. Sediments and environmental geochemistry. Berlin: Springer; 1990. pp 311–338.
19. Pekey H. Heavy metal pollution assessment in sediments of the Izmit Bay, Turkey. Environ Monit Assess. 2006;123:219–31.
20. Risk Assessment Information System (RAIS). USEPA (Electronic data base). 2009. http://rais.ornl.gov/.
21. Ibrahim Korfali S, Davies BE. Speciation of metals in sediment and water in a river underlain by limestone: role of carbonate species for purification capacity of rivers. Adv Environ Res. 2004;8:599–612.
22. Murakami M, Fujita M, Furumai H, Kasuga I, Kurisu F. Sorption behavior of heavy metal species by soakaway sediment receiving urban road runoff from residential and heavily trafficked areas. J Hazard Mater. 2009;164:707–12.
23. Degryse F, Smolders E, Merckx R. Labile Cd complexes increase Cd availability to plants. Environ Sci Technol. 2006;40:830–6.

Applicability of models to estimate traffic noise for urban roads

Ricardo A. Melo*, Roberto L. Pimentel, Diego M. Lacerda and Wekisley M. Silva

Abstract

Background: Traffic noise is a highly relevant environmental impact in cities. Models to estimate traffic noise, in turn, can be useful tools to guide mitigation measures. In this paper, the applicability of models to estimate noise levels produced by a continuous flow of vehicles on urban roads is investigated. The aim is to identify which models are more appropriate to estimate traffic noise in urban areas since several models available were conceived to estimate noise from highway traffic.

Results: First, measurements of traffic noise, vehicle count and speed were carried out in five arterial urban roads of a brazilian city. Together with geometric measurements of width of lanes and distance from noise meter to lanes, these data were input in several models to estimate traffic noise. The predicted noise levels were then compared to the respective measured counterparts for each road investigated. In addition, a chart showing mean differences in noise between estimations and measurements is presented, to evaluate the overall performance of the models. Measured Leq values varied from 69 to 79 dB(A) for traffic flows varying from 1618 to 5220 vehicles/h. Mean noise level differences between estimations and measurements for all urban roads investigated ranged from −3.5 to 5.5 dB(A).

Conclusions: According to the results, deficiencies of some models are discussed while other models are identified as applicable to noise estimations on urban roads in a condition of continuous flow. Key issues to apply such models to urban roads are highlighted.

Keywords: Traffic noise, Models, Urban roads

Background

Traffic noise has increased and nowadays is a relevant environmental impact in brazilian cities, because the increasing of number of vehicles. The total vehicle fleet increased 118 % from the year 2000 to 2010, whereas motorcycle fleet grew 309 % during the same period [1, 2].

In a review on the subject [3], several aspects of the problem were discussed and it was mentioned that the noise index mostly employed on noise-annoyance relationships is the equivalent sound pressure level L_{eq}.

The A-weighted equivalent sound pressure level ($L_{eq}(A)$) or, alternatively, the percentile levels L_{10} or L_{90}, are estimated by traffic noise prediction models. The main advantage of models is to estimate noise levels on a much reduced time and cost than by carrying out measurements. Also, it is the sole alternative when planning traffic routes. Due to its peculiar characteristics, noise from traffic in urban roads (city traffic) might potentially differ from that observed in highways.

The aim of this paper is to investigate the adequacy of some models to estimate urban traffic noise, taking as a case study five urban arterial roads of a medium-sized city, in which a continuous traffic flow was observed. The focus is to seek for a combined effect of significant traffic flow and non-congested traffic, so as to represent a critical condition in terms of urban traffic noise. The noise produced in such conditions could be, in principle, estimated by models presented in the literature and based on highway traffic. However, some key issues typical of urban roads such as short distances between road and receiver, traffic composition and speed lower than those observed in highways may interfere. Bearing this in mind, eight traffic noise models were selected so as estimations from these models could be compared to measured values: Golmohammadi et al. [4], Kinsler et al.

* Correspondence: ricardo@ct.ufpb.br
Department of Civil and Environmental Engineering, Federal University of Paraíba, Campus I, Cidade Universitária, 58051-900 João Pessoa, Brazil

[5], Birkan et al. [6], CoRTN [7, 8], Tansatcha et al. [9], RLS-90 [10], Calixto et al. [11] and Paz and Zannin [12].

Features of traffic noise models

The selected traffic noise models are briefly described in this Section; the reader can refer to the respective original works to check the expressions of each model.

Golmohammadi et al.

Golmohammadi et al. [4] conceived a model based on parameters including traffic flow and speed, vehicle types and road dimensions, the latter including section length, width and gradient of road, and height of buildings around the road. Measurements were taken at a distance of 3.0 m from the roadside edge, that it is usually compatible with the space available along urban roads. As for the traffic, a condition of free flow in straight road segments of dual carriageways was considered.

Kinsler et al.

The model presented by Kinsler et al. [5] considers a straight, two-lane road of infinite length, zero grade and negligible truck traffic, and takes the flow of vehicles and speed as input. The equivalent continuous A-weighted sound pressure level (L_{eq}) in dB(A) is evaluated for a reference distance of 15 m between the evaluation point and centerline of the nearest lane, but it is necessary a correction term for distance greater than 15 m.

Regarding the speed, changes are taken into account, based on a ratio of the input speed and a reference speed of 88 km/h, which is higher than the usual speed on urban roads.

Birkan et al.

This model was employed by these authors to estimate traffic noise on urban roads [6]. The sound pressure level in the vicinity of a street segment, L_{eq}, is estimated taking into account the flow of vehicles and speed as input parameters. No explicit reference is made to traffic composition. The noise level is corrected through a term that contains the distance of the sound receptor from road edge plus one third of the width of a lane. A basic correction factor that depends on pavement type is also included.

CoRTN

This model is based on an hourly basic noise level L_{10}, in dB(A), for a given hourly traffic flow at a mean speed of 75 Km/h. The L_{10} is further adjusted to take into account type of vehicles, gradient, road surface and speed.

Regarding the type of surface of the pavement, for impervious bituminous road surfaces, 1 dB(A) should be subtracted from the basic noise level when the traffic speed is below75 Km/h. On the contrary, if traffic speed is equal or greater than 75 Km/h a correction applies, being a function of the texture depth of the road surface [7].

In sequence, further corrections are considered to take into account, as appropriate, the effects of distance from the source line, the nature of the ground surface, and screening from any intervening obstacles.

On sites where the ground surface between the edge of the nearside carriageway and the reception point is totally or partially of an absorbent nature, (e.g. grassland) a correction for ground absorption is obtained from a chart provided [7], which depends on height and distance, and the proportion of absorbing ground.

Recently, updates of the CoRTN model were proposed [8]. Recommendations applicable to this investigation involved adopting the dual source line approach for all dual carriageways, irrespective of the number of lanes per carriageway or the separation of horizontal or vertical alignments. It is worth mentioning that a provision for calculating the noise from separate carriageways was already presented as an option in the CoRTN original model. Also, it was recommended that the heavy vehicle category is redefined as vehicles with unladen weight greater than 3500 kg, instead of the originally adopted unladen weight of 1525 kg.

Finally, since the CoRTN model is based on L_{10} values, a conversion to L_{eq} is needed so as to compare these estimates with those from the other models.

Tansatcha et al.

Tansatcha et al. [9] considered some vehicle classes: automobile, truck, bus and motorcycle. To start, the noise level for a single vehicle is calculated. Such a noise is considered to be produced in a 10-s time interval. Then, the 1 h equivalent sound pressure level for vehicle class i is calculated, as a function of the hourly flow of that vehicle type, and including corrections for ground absorption and distance. Regarding the latter, the reference distance considered is 15 m and the distance of the reception point is taken from the center line of the traffic lane.

By combining the contribution of vehicle classes (herein, automobiles, motorcycles, buses and light trucks were considered), a total hourly equivalent sound level on a single roadway (or lane), namely $L_{eq(1h),j}$ in dB(A), is calculated as the logarithm sum of the contributions of each vehicle type. Finally, the total equivalent sound level in 1 h, $L_{eq(1h)}$, in dBA, is obtained in a similar way by the logarithm sum of the contribution of all lanes.

RLS-90

In Germany, a model for road traffic noise estimation is in use, identified as RLS-90 [10], being applicable for a range of traffic flow from 10 to 10,000 veh/h. This model has flexibility in the sense that it considers several

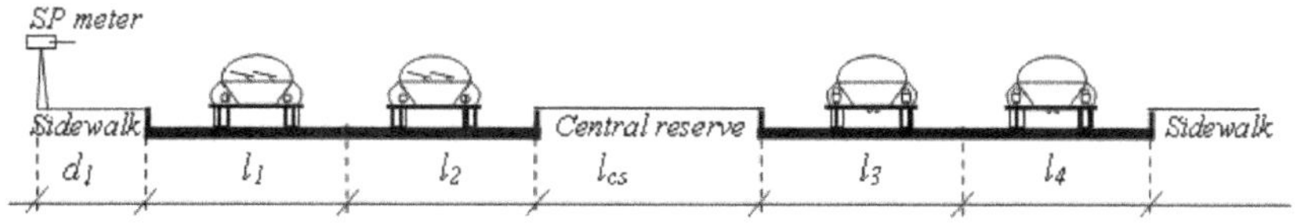

Fig. 1 Typical cross section of the sites (not to scale). (Legend: d_1: distance between sound pressure level meter (SP meter) and edge of the closest lane; l_i: width of ith lane (i: 1 to 6); l_{cs}: width of central reserve)

correction terms for a wide range of traffic and site conditions. It starts from the A-weighted mean noise level at a distance of 25 m from the centerline of the road and for the following conditions: (*i*) speed of 100 Km/h; (*ii*) non-grooved asphalt road surface; (*iii*) road gradient less than 5 %; and (*iv*) free field propagation. Inputs in this expression are the traffic flow (veh/h) and percentage of trucks with mass above 2800 kg.

In sequence, corrections for speed, road surface type, gradient and absorption characteristics of adjacent building surfaces are added. The correction for speed considers a combination of speeds of cars and trucks. Finally, spreading and air absorption are considered through a correction factor as a function of distance between the receiver and the sound source.

Calixto et al.

A model to predict traffic noise from roads inside urban settings was developed by Calixto et al. [11]. The noise emission levels were defined in terms of L_{eq}, L_{10} and L_{90} [dB(A)]. As their work also bore in mind to verify the applicability of the RLS-90 model to brazilian road conditions, they adopted the same reference distance of 25 m. They ended up with simple and straightforward expressions to obtain noise emission levels (L_{eq}, L_{10} and L_{90}), as a function of the traffic flow and percentage of heavy vehicles. It compared well with the evaluation made by the RLS-90 model.

Paz and Zannin

Paz and Zannin [12] proposed linear models based on daytime measurements in urban highways. The range of distances from the road in which measurements were taken was from 15 to 25 m, at a height of 1.20 m. Vehicle flow and traffic composition were the model entries. The concept of class intervals was introduced, that is, different expressions were proposed according to the range of values of noise being estimated. Furthermore, the authors presented expressions based on measured and mean values, the latter being based on adjusted data. Herein, the model selected was identified by Paz and Zannin as Model 18 [12], in which L_{eq} values were estimated based on mean values, class intervals and the entries were the light and total vehicle flows.

Method

Site selection

The investigated sites are located in João Pessoa, a medium-sized city of about 723 thousands inhabitants in the northeast of Brazil. In João Pessoa, the vehicle fleet increased about twice in the last decade and is predominantly composed by cars and motorcycles; these vehicles are about 97 % of total vehicle fleet.

The urban arterial roads studied were five avenues of high traffic volume and relevance in the city (between parentheses the abbreviation used in the following paragraphs): José Américo de Almeida (JA), Rui Carneiro (RC), Epitácio Pessoa (EP), Hilton Souto Maior (HM), and D. Pedro II (PII).

All roads had a central reserve and two lanes in each direction, except PII Avenue, with three lanes per direction. The chosen sites to measure noise levels in each avenue had no surrounding buildings or obstacles, being adequate for the application of several noise prediction models. The roads were straight segments, had flat gradients and asphalt mixture surface course. In Fig. 1, a typical cross section of the sites is shown and the relevant dimensions are shown in Table 1. Table 2, in turn, provides information on the ground condition, to apply corrections on calculations, as appropriate. This information was employed to apply corrections due to ground effects for the CoRTN and Tansatcha models.

Measurements of traffic noise

The traffic noise levels were obtained using a class 1 01 dB sound pressure meter model SIP95. Following the procedures recommended in the Brazilian code NBR 10151 [13], the meter was placed 1.2 m above ground, at the sidewalk. The distance from the road varied (see Fig. 1 and Table 1 for the values), due to peculiarities of

Table 1 Relevant dimensions (in meters) of all sites

Urban road	l_1	l_2	l_3	l_4	l_5	l_6	l_{cs}	d_1
JA	3.45	3.45	3.46	3.47	*	*	6.00	1.80
RC	3.50	3.50	3.50	3.50	*	*	1.75	6.90
EP	3.71	3.60	3.60	3.65	*	*	5.45	4.15
HM	3.40	3.50	3.60	3.20	*	*	7.00	9.50
PII	3.50	3.50	3.50	3.50	3.50	3.50	1.00	2.00

Legend- d_1, l_1 to l_6 and l_{cs}: see legend of Fig. 1

Table 2 Features of the ground in all sites

Urban road	l_1	l_2	l_3	l_4	l_5	l_6	l_{cs}	l_s
JA	Hard	Hard	Hard	Hard	*	*	Soft	Soft
RC	Hard	Hard	Hard	Hard	*	*	Hard	Hard
EP	Hard	Hard	Hard	Hard	*	*	50 % hard/50 % soft	Hard
HM	Hard	Hard	Hard	Hard	*	*	Soft	Soft
PII	Hard	Hard	Hard	Hard	Hard	Hard	Hard	Hard

Legend- l_1 to l_6 and l_{cs}: see legend of Fig. 1; l_s: width of sidewalk in which the sound level meter was placed

the sites. The meter was set in fast mode and the microphone was positioned perpendicular to the lane axis. Sites were always in dry condition and absent of other noise sources; temperatures were around 28 °C and the wind was not of attention. The Brazilian code [13] specifies that measurements should be long enough for the noise to be properly characterized, and measurements can be continuous or in intervals.

Measurements in each site were made within a period of 1 h in week days, either during mornings or afternoons, in which there is a combined effect of significant vehicle flow and non-congested traffic. Four records of traffic noise lasting five minutes each was acquired, each representing a quarter of an hour. In order to consider noise fluctuations within the hour, the four acquisitions were separated by intervals of 10 min. As can be seen in Table 3, noise fluctuations within the hour were small and the value of $L_{eq(1h)}$ was obtained by grouping together all measured values.

Traffic count and determination of speed

A handy video camera Sony model DCR-DVD 610 was used to record the flow of vehicles during 1 h in each site. Later on, in the office, vehicle counting was made from video images. Bearing in mind that the videos also displayed the time together with images, they were also employed to obtain the speed of vehicles. So, the speed of selected vehicles was calculated based upon the time interval that a vehicle took to go through a 20-m long segment, identified in the video by two traffic sign cones. This calculation considered that the speed of a given vehicle remained unchanged between the sign cones. An average of the individual speeds of the selected vehicles was carried out for each lane, carriageway, or for the overall traffic, as appropriate.

Table 3 Sound pressure levels measured at the sites, dB(A)

Urban road	$L_{eq,\ 15\ min}$				$L_{eq(1h)}$	$L_{10(1h)}$	L_{10}-L_{eq}
	1st	2nd	3rd	4th			
PII	81.4	77.8	77.0	77.6	78.6	79.1	0.5
JA	72.8	73.2	72.4	73.0	72.9	74.1	1.2
RC	69.9	71.2	70.2	70.0	70.3	72.4	2.1
EP	70.0	73.3	73.0	74.8	73.5	77.6	4.1
HM	69.2	67.8	66.3	71.1	69.0	71.9	2.9

Results and discussion

Sound pressure levels

In Table 3, a summary of measured equivalent continuous A-weighted sound pressure levels ($L_{eq(1h)}$) and L_{10} are presented. The difference between L_{10} and L_{eq} for each site was specifically employed for the conversion of estimations using the L_{10}-based CoRTN model to L_{eq}, so as to compare with other models.

Speed, vehicle type and flow

These data are shown in Table 4, in terms of flow of vehicles (per lane, per vehicle type and total), and mean speed per vehicle type.

The results presented in Table 4 show that the highest flow of vehicles was on PII Avenue, with 5220 veh/h, followed by RC Avenue, with 3031 veh/h. These avenues link populated neighborhoods to downtown, in which commercial centers, public administration and public services are present. In the other three avenues, a flow of vehicles about 1700 veh/h can be observed.

Furthermore, it can also be seen that automobile, motorcycle and utility vehicles were predominant, corresponding to about 96 % of the traffic volume. Also, it may be observed that motorcycles are a non-neglibible part of the total flow, reaching 24 % of traffic volume in one of the roads. Presence of motorcycles is a trend that is expected to increase since sales of motorcycles increased about 300 % in the last 10 years.

For speed, the values were in the broad range from 46 to 83 km/h, considering the traffic flow per lane. However, most values were between 60 and 70 km/h.

Determination of noise level by the models

Estimations considered the flow of vehicles per lane, per direction and total, as applicable to each model.

It was considered that a tolerable difference between estimated and measured values can be up to 1.5 dB. This is equivalent to a difference of 1 dB to take into account the accuracy of the sound pressure meter, plus an estimating error of ± 0.5 dB, which is a negligible change of sound pressure level perceptible by a human being.

Table 4 Summary of traffic data for all sites

Urban road	JA		RC		EP		HM		PII	
Lane	*Q*	*v*	*Q*	*v*	*Q*	*v*	*Q*	*v*	*Q*	*v*
1	537	61.4	912	45.7	312	61.0	611	70.2	1043	50.5
2	459	74.4	524	61.4	543	63.3	220	82.8	1255	60.4
3	304	65.1	759	64.3	500	59.8	399	76.1	875	68.0
4	318	64.7	836	61.3	406	59.8	427	76.1	602	67.9
5	*	*	*	*	*	*	*	*	891	68.1
6	*	*	*	*	*	*	*	*	554	60.3
Total	1618	*	3031	*	1761	*	1657	*	5220	*
	q	%	*q*	%	*q*	%	*q*	%	*q*	%
q_{aut}	1146	70.8	2258	74.5	1250	71.0	906	54.7	3439	65.9
q_{uti}	229	14.2	343	11.3	230	13.1	244	14.7	605	11.6
q_{mot}	205	12.7	345	11.4	189	10.7	399	24.1	987	18.9
q_{bus}	16	1.0	43	1.4	60	3.4	27	1.6	73	1.4
q_{tru}	22	1.4	42	1.4	32	1.8	81	4.9	116	2.2

Notes: 1) Flow of vehicles (*Q*, veh/h); mean speed (*v*, Km/h); 2) Flow of vehicle type *i*, *q* (*aut* = automobiles; *uti* = utility vehicles; *mot* = motorcycles; *bus* = buses; *tru* = trucks)

Figures 2, 3, 4, 5 and 6 present estimated values of $L_{eq}(A)$ by the aforementioned models, together with the measured values.

It is not expected that a given model always provides estimation within the predefined margin of tolerance from the measured value. A significant number of variables and specific road conditions of a location may impair estimations. However, general trends can be observed, and from these some findings are highlighted:

- There is a tendency presented by the Kinsler et al. [5] and Calixto et al. [11] models in underestimating noise levels. It should be noted that in Kinsler et al. [12], no correction of noise levels for distances less than 15 m is adopted whereas in Calixto et al. [11] model, the reference distance is 25 m and no correction is considered for distance. As for the latter, the estimations agreed well with those from the RLS-90 model for a distance of 25 m [11]. It is, thus, worth mentioning that models to estimate noise in urban areas require correction terms for shorter distances than those adopted by such models, as observed in the sites in which measurements were taken. Therefore, this may be appointed as a reason why these two models underestimated the noise levels;
- Sound pressure levels estimated by Birkan et al. [6] and Tansatcha et al. [9] models were higher than others on all sites. With regard to Tansatcha et al. [9] model, a time interval of 10 s was defined to evaluate the noise level for each vehicle, and this limits the flow to 360 veh/h. This implies that this model would overestimate noise levels for vehicle flows per lane above such values, as it occurred in several lanes of the investigated sites. With regard to the model by Birkan et al. [6], the reason why it

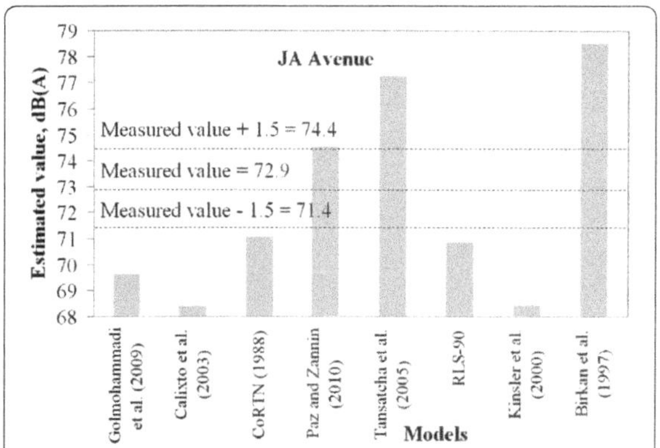

Fig. 2 Measured L_{eq} interval and estimated L_{eq} by models for JA avenue

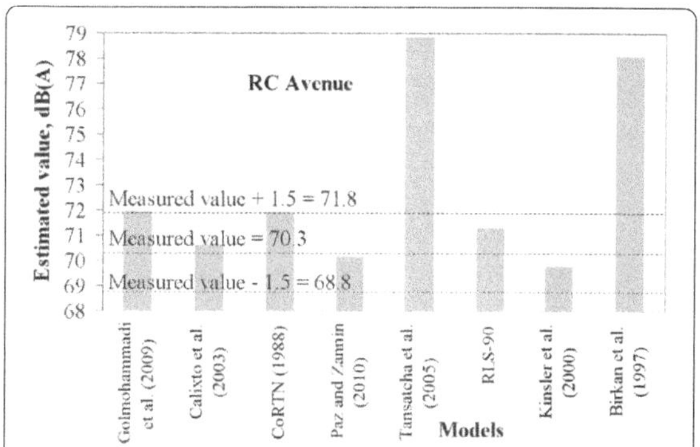

Fig. 3 Measured L_{eq} interval and estimated L_{eq} by models for RC avenue

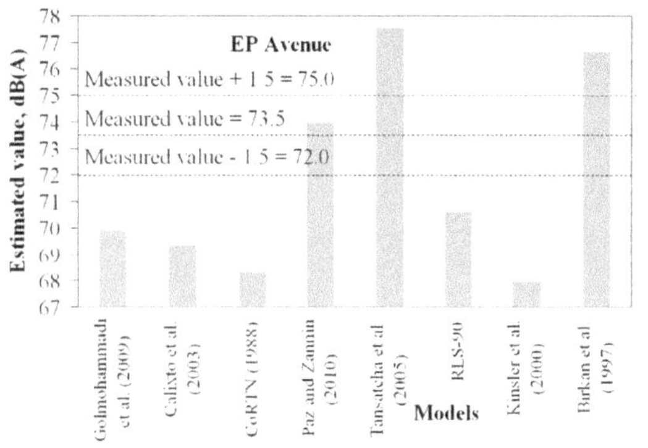

Fig. 4 Measured L_{eq} interval and estimated L_{eq} by models for EP avenue

overestimated the noise is not clear since the information describing the model is limited. One point to call attention is that the traffic composition (that is, the percentage of heavy vehicles) is not taken into account explicitly in the expression of that model. Therefore, the model was possibly adjusted to a specific traffic composition that may differ from those observed in the measurement sites.

- Results for the PII avenue (Fig. 6) shows that a combination of very high traffic volume and a very short distance from the sound level meter to the road edge (due to restrictions on site) led to an underestimation of the traffic noise by the majority of the models that presented good estimates for the other sites.

Figure 7 provides a synthesis of the results for the five avenues, in terms of the mean difference between each estimation and respective measured value. The models of Golmohammadi et al. [4], CoRTN [7], RLS-90 [10] and Paz and Zannin [12] presented a good performance, the latter being within the specified range of the experimental values.

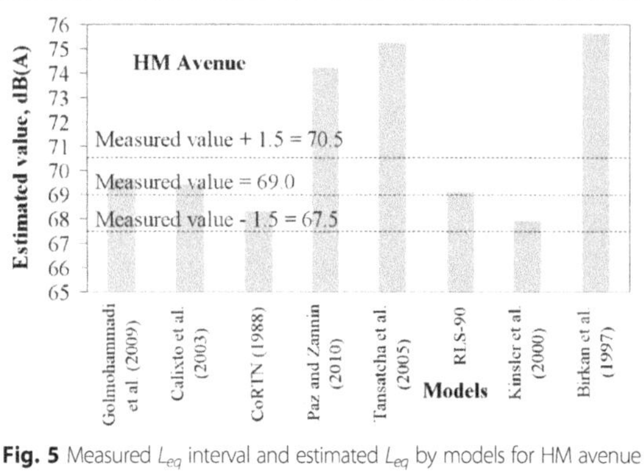

Fig. 5 Measured L_{eq} interval and estimated L_{eq} by models for HM avenue

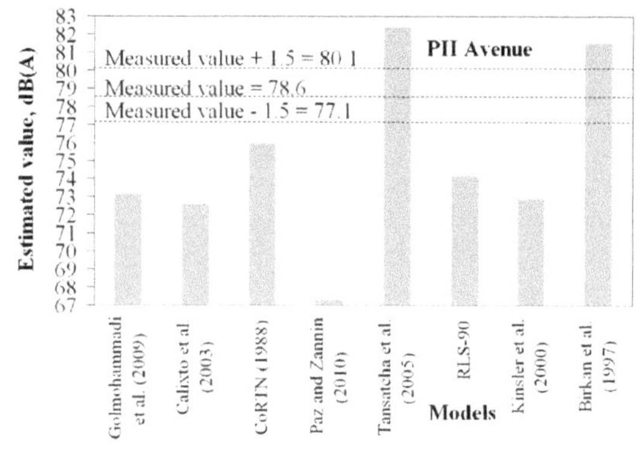

Fig. 6 Measured L_{eq} interval and estimated L_{eq} by models for PII avenue

Conclusions

The aim of this paper was to investigate the adequacy of some noise level models in estimating urban traffic noise in roads of continuous traffic flow. The following models were chosen: Golmohammadi et al. [4], Kinsler et al. [5], Birkan et al. [6], CoRTN [7], Tansatcha et al. [9], RLS-90 [10], Calixto et al. [11] and Paz and Zannin [12]. Measurements of in situ noise levels, flow of vehicles, speed, and road layout were carried out for five urban arterial roads. In sequence, this database was used as input of the models. Then, measured and estimated noise levels were compared to analyze the applicability of the models in estimating the urban traffic noise.

The CoRTN [7], Golmohammadi et al. [4], RLS-90 [10] and Paz and Zannin [12] models showed the best performance, having the lowest mean difference to the measured noise levels. These best performances can be related to some features of urban roads covered by these models, such as flexibility in defining traffic composition, corrections of spreading or else reference distances compatible to urban settings and compatible ranges of

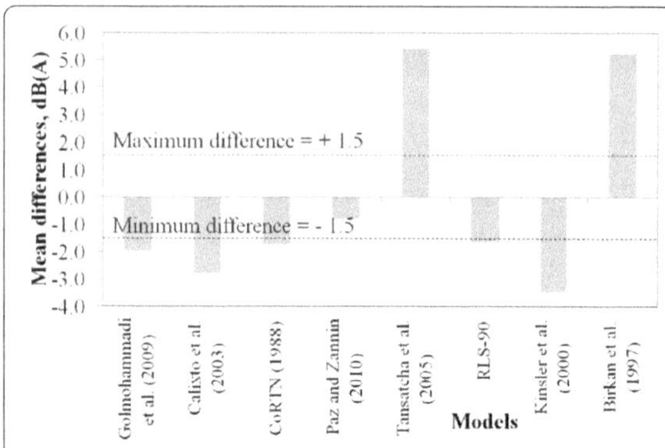

Fig. 7 Summary of mean noise level differences between estimations and measurements for all urban roads

speed and flow. Such models resulted potentially suitable to estimate noise from continuous traffic flow in urban arterial roads with similar traffic features and road layout of the roads investigated here.

Although Calixto et al. [11] model was also developed from measurements in urban roads, the predicted noise levels were not so good. This may be attributed to the absence of corrections for distance, associated to a reference distance of 25 m adopted by this model (to make it intentionally compatible with the RLS-90 model), leading to underestimations when applying this model to the short distances observed at the sites. Kinsler et al. [5] presented the same problem, in the sense that it does not support corrections for distances below 15 m. Finally, for the model from Tansatcha et al. [9], it is apparent that the overestimation of the estimations was related to an upper limit on the flow of vehicles, this being inherently associated to the way the model was conceived. The flows on the investigated sites were much higher than such a limit; this way, when a high flow is input into the model, it results in overestimation.

Competing interests
The authors declare that they have no competing interests.

Authors' contributions
Messrs. DML and WMS took part in the experimental campaign, processing data and estimating noise by using the models. Drs. RAM and RLP analysed the data and wrote the manuscript. All authors have read and approved the final manuscript.

Authors' information
Drs. R.A. Melo and R.L. Pimentel currently work at Federal University of Paraíba. Dr Melo expertise is in transportation engineering and Dr Pimentel is in vibration engineering and acoustics. Messrs. D.M. Lacerda and W.M. Silva were university students who took part in this research project.

Acknowledgements
The authors acknowledge the financial support from CNPq – Brazil in carrying out this research project.

References
1. ANFAVEA- Brazilian Automotive Industry Association. Brazilian automotive industry yearbook 2012. São Paulo: ANFAVEA- Brazilian Automotive Industry Association; 2012. [http://www.anfavea.com.br/anuario.html] (in portuguese).
2. ABRACICLO- Brazilian Industry Association of Motorcycles, Mopeds, Motor Scooters, Bicycles and similar. Motorcycles - Fleet in circulation. 2014. [http://www.abraciclo.com.br/images/stories/dados_setor/motocicletas/frota/2014-4%20frota%20motocicletas.pdf] (in portuguese).
3. Ouis D. Annoyance from road traffic noise: a review. J Environ Psychol. 2001;21:101–20.
4. Golmohammadi R, Abbaspour M, Nassiri P, Mahjub H. A compact model for predicting road traffic noise. Iran J Environ Health Sci Eng. 2009;6:181–6.
5. Kinsler LE, Frey AR, Coppens AB, Sanders JV. Fundamentals of acoustics (4ed.). New York: John Wiley & Sons Inc; 2000.
6. Birkan S, Çilli A, Çetýn AF, Tümay A, Çelenk E. Ankara city traffic impact assessment study. In ESRI International User Conference; San Diego, California; 1997. [http://gis.library.esri.com/cgi-bin/koha/opac-detail.pl?biblionumber=72830&query_desc=au%2Cwrdl%3A%20Birkan%20S]
7. Department of Transport. CoRTN Calculation of Road Traffic Noise. London: Her Majesty's Stationery Office (HMSO); 1988.
8. Department for Transport, The Highways Agency. Design manual for roads and bridges, Vol 11, Section 3, Part 7, HD 213/11 – Revision 1. 2011.
9. Tansatcha M, Pamanikabud P, Brown AL, Affum JK. Motorway noise modeling based on perpendicular propagation analysis of traffic noise. Appl Acoust. 2005;66:1135–50.
10. Der Bundesminister für Verkehr. RLS-90 Richtlinien für den Lärmschutz an Straßen. 1990.
11. Calixto A, Diniz FB, Zannin PHT. The statistical modeling of road traffic noise in an urban setting. Cities. 2003;20(1):23–9.
12. Paz EC, Zannin PHT. Urban daytime traffic noise prediction models. Environ Monit Assess. 2010;163:515–29.
13. ABNT- Associação Brasileira de Normas Técnicas. NBR 10151 – Acústica – Avaliação do ruído em áreas habitadas, visando o conforto da comunidade – Procedimento. Rio de Janeiro: ABNT- Associação Brasileira de Normas Técnicas; 2000. in portuguese.

Assessment and selection of the best treatment alternative for infectious waste by modified Sustainability Assessment of Technologies methodology

Ata Rafiee[1,2], Kamyar Yaghmaeian[1,2], Mohammad Hoseini[3], Saeid Parmy[2], Amirhosein Mahvi[1,2], Masud Yunesian[2,4], Mehran Khaefi[5] and Ramin Nabizadeh[2,4*]

Abstract

Background: Improper treatment of infectious waste can cause numerous adverse environmental and health effects such as transmission of diseases through health personnel and other susceptible groups,who come in contact with such wastes. On the other hand, selection of appropriate treatment alternatives in infectious waste management has become a challenging task for public health authorities especially in developing countries. The objective of this paper is to select the best infectious waste treatment alternative by the modified Sustainability Assessment of Technologies (SAT) methodology, developed by the International Environmental Technology Center of the United Nations Environment Program (IETC-UNEP).

Methods: SAT methodology consists of three main components, including screening, scoping and detailed assessment. In screening, different infectious waste treatment alternatives undergo screening using the finalized environmental and technical criteria. Short-listed treatment options from the previous step, then go through the comprehensive scoping and detailed assessment (2nd and 3rd components) which is more qualitative and quantitative in nature. An empirical case in Tehran, the largest city in Iran, is provided to illustrate the potential of the proposed methodology.

Results: According to the final score, "Hydroclave", was the most suitable infectious treatment technology. The ranking order of the treatment alternatives were "Autoclave with a shredder", "Autoclave", "Central Incineration" and "chemical treatment" on the basis of technical, economical, social and environmental aspects and their related criteria.

Conclusions: According to the results it could be concluded that the top ranking technologies basically have higher scores in all the aspects. Hence it is easier to arrive at a decision for the final technology selection based on the principles of sustainability.

Keywords: Health-care waste, Infectious waste treatment, SAT methodology, Hospital, Tehran

* Correspondence: rnabizadeh@tums.ac.ir
[2]Department of Environmental Health Engineering, School of Public Health, Tehran University of Medical Sciences, Tehran, Iran
[4]Center for Air Pollution Research (CAPR), Institute for Environmental Research (IER), Tehran University of Medical Sciences, Tehran, Iran
Full list of author information is available at the end of the article

Background

Today health-care wastes (HCWs) have become a substantial public health and environmental concern all over the world, particularly in developing countries [1, 2]. According to the World Health Organization (WHO), the term HCWs includes all the waste generated within health-care institutions, research centers and laboratories related to medical practices. HCWs can be classified into two major categories: "non-hazardous" or "general HCW_S" which represents about 75–90 % of the total HCWs; and "hazardous" which represent 10–25 % of the total HCWs. Hazardous HCWs include, but are not limited to, infectious, chemical and radioactive wastes and may pose various environmental and health risks. Infectious waste refers to any waste type either known or suspected to contain pathogens (bacteria, viruses, parasites or fungi) in enough concentrations and/or quantities which lead to disease in susceptible hosts [3–5].

Although infectious waste is only a small part of the total HCWs, however, mismanagement in practices can cause this waste to be mixed with other non-hazardous waste [6, 7]. HCWs and infectious waste specifically may play an important role in the transmission and spread of many diseases such as human immunodeficiency virus (HIV), hepatitis B or C virus, and other agents associated with blood borne diseases [8–10]. A multi-language systematic review of HCW_S management in 40 low and middle-income countries worldwide declared that crucial problems in urban regions in Asia, Africa and the Middle East intensified by increasing quantities of HCWs and inappropriate treatment and disposal activities [11].

A survey conducted by WHO on HCWs management in 22 developing countries revealed that the proportion of health care facilities with improper waste treatment practices was between 18 and 64 % [12].

The goal of infectious waste treatment is to reduce the potential hazards of this type of wastes, and consequently protect public health and the environment [13]. To improve the HCWs management, implementation of appropriate methods is necessary [14–16]. However, selecting the best alternative for treating the HCWs and specially infectious waste is not always a simple task. To assess various HCWs management scenarios, Liu et al. [1] developed a hybrid multi-criteria decision method (MCDM) model by integrating the 2-tuple DEMATEL technique and fuzzy MULTIMOORA method for selecting the best HCWS treatment alternatives in Shanghai, China [1]. Liu et al. [16] introduced a MCDM model based on the fuzzy set theory and VIKOR method to identify the most suitable HCWs treatment alternative [16]. Dursun et al. [17] suggested two fuzzy MCDM techniques for assessing HCW_S treatment alternatives, which allow conducting an analysis based on a multi-level hierarchical structure and to incorporate uncertain data defined as linguistic variables into the analysis [17]. Karagiannidis et al. [18] assessed the thermal treatment processes of infectious wastes in Central Macedonia, Greece by analytic hierarchy process (AHP) [18]. Hsu et al. [19] used (AHP) method to objectively select medical waste disposal alternatives based on the results of interviews with experts in the field.

During the selection of treatment alternatives for HCWs, decision makers usually consider different criteria and sub-criteria for optimal decisions [19]. All the studies discussed above developed and applied different methods for selection of HCWs treatment alternatives. The main limitation of the existing decision analysis methods is that most of them are only mathematical models without focusing on important issues such as the sustainability concept. In response to the need for a technology assessment framework to identify and select the best possible environmental technology option, the International Environmental Technology Center of the United Nations Environment Program (IETC-UNEP) developed a new methodology known as Sustainable Assessment of Technologies (SAT). The focus of this methodology is both on the process and outcome, with an interest towards informed and participatory decision-making. The methodology employs a progressive assessment involving initial screening, scoping and detailed assessment. Importantly, the methodology takes a systems approach and stresses information, expertise and stakeholder participation [13]. In applying this methodology to developing countries, it seems necessary to make some changes on its criteria, based on local conditions. The aim of this study was to select the best treatment alternative for the infectious waste by modified Sustainability Assessment of Technologies (SAT) methodology.

Methods

Study area

The present study was performed in Tehran, the capital of Iran and one of the most crowded areas in Iran and in the Middle East, with eleven million inhabitants, in mid 2014 [20]. The average health-care waste generation in Tehran public hospitals is 65000 kg/day [6]. To illustrate the application of the suggested methodology for selecting the best alternative for infectious waste treatment, a case study conducted at the Imam Khomeini hospital complex. The complex, which is the largest and most advanced educational and medical center in Iran, is located in the center of Tehran in an area of 25 Hectares and a capacity of 1400 hospital beds out of which 1200 are considered active beds. The complex includes Imam Khomeini and Vali-e-Asr hospitals, cancer institute, radiology center, polyclinics and an emergency ward.

Application of SAT methodology

As stated above, SAT is a suitable methodology for integrating technical, environmental, social, and economic considerations with main focus on environmental issues and developmental aspects. This methodology consists of three main steps, including screening, scoping and detailed assessment. In order to adapt the methodology to national conditions, country specific parameters and constraints, we made some changes on its criteria and applied modified methodology to select the best alternative.

Screening

In this step, at first baseline data, including information on HCWs generation rate, number of beds, average occupancies and identifying stakeholders were collected from the studied hospital. Then, common thermal, chemical and radiation infectious waste treatment alternatives were screened by using screening criteria based on objective yes/no type answers. The total of participants in screening step were 25 individuals, that included doctors, nurses, environmental health experts, and hospital manager, 5, 5, 14, and 1 respectively. The technologies that didn't meet the basic criteria were directly excluded and the rest, were selected for further assessments. Autoclave, autoclave with a shredder, chemical treatment, hydroclave, demolizer, microwave, chem-Clav and central incineration were selected in this step. The criteria for this step described in SAT methodology included compliance with local environmental laws, compliance with national environmental laws, compliance with multilateral environmental agreements and consistency with WHO policies. Since Iran lacks local environmental laws, the criteria of "compliance with local environmental laws" weren't considered in this study. Instead, in order to increase the accuracy of the results of this step, some specific scoping criteria which were applicable to this step were added. Table 1 show the modified screening criteria in the screening component.

Scoping

After the screening step, technologies that did not qualify for the conditions were excluded and other technologies were assessed against specific criteria. Demolizer, Microwave and Chem-Clav technologies were eliminated in the earlier step and the shortlisted treatment alternatives (including autoclave, autoclave with a shredder, chemical treatment, central incineration and hydroclave) then underwent the comprehensive scoping assessment. The scoping step, which is a comprehensive and qualitative type (High/Medium/Low) assessment, uses selected technical, economic, social and environmental criteria (Fig. 1). This step lends an advantage in narrowing the decision range of scores, for a particular criteria in the detailed assessment level. For instance, if low/medium/Highscores are assigned on a basis of a scale of 0–9, then evaluation as 'medium' would scope the scores say between 4 and 6. This allows a narrowing of the range and therefore better compliance of opinions and thus reduced subjectivity. In order to select the most preferred infectious waste treatment technology, different groups of experts in HCWs field, were asked to fill the scoping questionnaire. The experts were divided into two groups. Group A, included 25 academic members of the Environmental science and Environmental Health Engineering departments across the country (associate and full

Table 1 Adjusted Screening Step Worksheet (UNEP, 2012)

Criteria	Autoclave	Autoclave with aShredder	Hydroclave	Chem-Clav	Microwave	Chemical treatment	Demolizer	Central incineration
Compliance with national environmental laws	Y/N	Y/N	Y/N	Y/N	Y/N	Y/N	Y/N	Y/N
Compliance with multilateral environmental agreements	Y/N	Y/N	Y/N	Y/N	Y/N	Y/N	Y/N	Y/N
Consistency with WHO policies	Y/N	Y/N	Y/N	Y/N	Y/N	Y/N	Y/N	Y/N
Added criteria to screening step of the basic SAT methodology								
Meets capacity requirement	Y/N	Y/N	Y/N	Y/N	Y/N	Y/N	Y/N	Y/N
Availability of spare parts	Y/N	Y/N	Y/N	Y/N	Y/N	Y/N	Y/N	Y/N
Safe to use	Y/N	Y/N	Y/N	Y/N	Y/N	Y/N	Y/N	Y/N
Volume reduction	Y/N	Y/N	Y/N	Y/N	Y/N	Y/N	Y/N	Y/N
Mass reduction	Y/N	Y/N	Y/N	Y/N	Y/N	Y/N	Y/N	Y/N
Air emissions	Y/N	Y/N	Y/N	Y/N	Y/N	Y/N	Y/N	Y/N
Technology Economically Viable	Y/N	Y/N	Y/N	Y/N	Y/N	Y/N	Y/N	Y/N

Y yes, *N* no

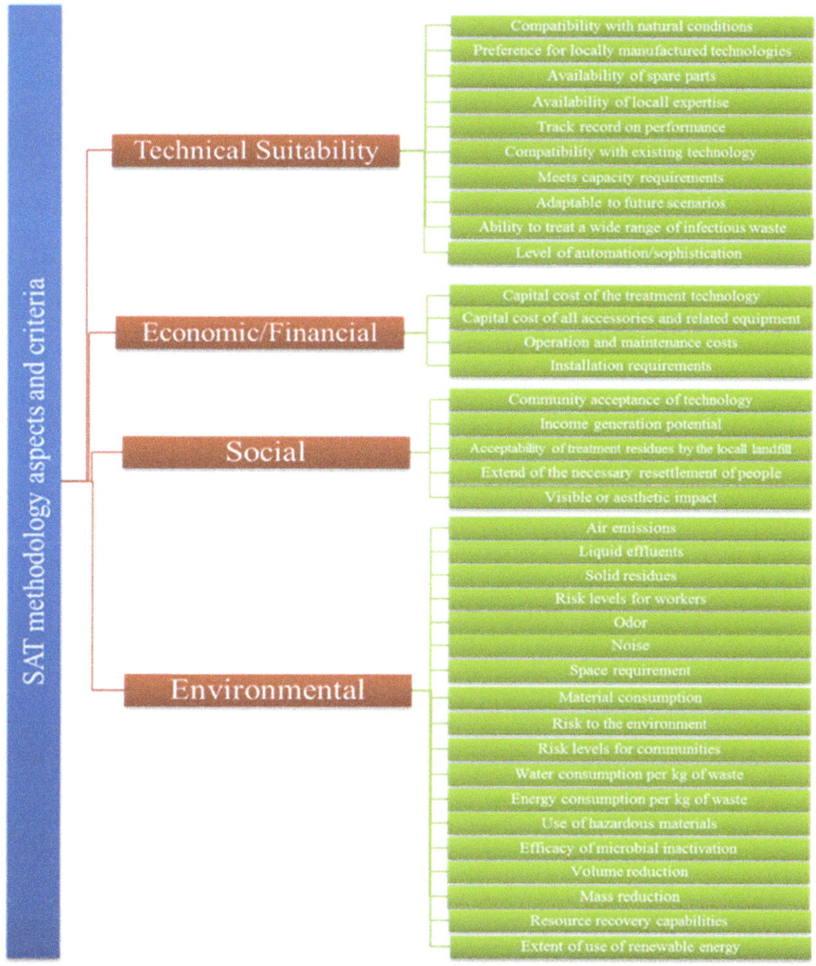

Fig. 1 SAT methodology aspects and their related criteria

professors), 5 experts from infectious waste disposal companies and 5 experts from the Ministry of Health and Medical Education. Group B included 35 graduate students (20 PhD and 15 masters students) in environmental health engineering. At first, the experts were requested to rank the relative importance of each four topics (technical suitability, economic/financial, social/cultural and environmental) by scoring from 0 to 100 so that the sum of all the ranking scores becomes 100. Each four topics were ranked environmental (45), economic/financial (25), technical suitability (20), and social/cultural (10). Then, experts asked to establish weighting factors (0 to 9) for each criteria (1 to 3 for low, 4 to 6 for medium, 7 to 9 for high). Besides, in order to determine the most important criteria in each aspects, the experts were asked to score the each criterion. The importance of each criteria assigned by the experts divided into five groups: very low (1), low (2), medium (3), high (4), essential (5).

Detailed assessment

The technologies with best overall ratings from the scoping step were selected for further assessment in this step. Different multi-criteria decision methods

Table 2 Imam Khomeini hospital complex average healthcare waste generation

Names of hospitals	Quantity of wastes (kg d^{-1})		
	General waste	Infectious waste	Sharps waste
Imam Khomeini	857.32	795.72	115.15
Vali-Asr	418.68	349.07	116.95
Cancer Institute	264	235.21	117.9
Total	1540	1380	350

Table 3 Screening step results

Technology	Positive score	Negative score	Net score
Hydroclave	75	24	51
Autoclave + Shreeder	67	31	36
Central incineration	63	32	31
Autoclave	55	33	22
	Excluded alternatives		
Chemical treatment	51	36	15
Microwave	34	43	-9
Demolizer	23	45	-15

(MCDMs) can be used for quantitative assessment of treatment alternatives in this step. In this study and in order to keep the integrity of the methodology, a weighted sum matrix method was used. The weight assigned to each criterion within a category was based on the importance given by the expert's judgment. The number or rating assigned to each technology based on the expert reflects how well the technology complies with each defined criteria. It should be noted that there were 10 technical, 4 financial, 5 social and 18 environmental criteria. For each criterion multiplying factors need to be calculated. For this at the first step, maximum scores for each topic were calculated as follows [13]:

Maximum score for Technical Suitability (MST):

$$\mathrm{MST} = 9 \times (\mathrm{W}_1 + \mathrm{W}_2 + \mathrm{W}_3 + \mathrm{W}_4 + \mathrm{W}_5 + \mathrm{W}_6 + \mathrm{W}_7 + \mathrm{W}_8 + \mathrm{W}_9 + \mathrm{W}_{10})$$

Maximum score for Economic/Financial (MSEn):

$$\mathrm{MSEc} = 9 \times (\mathrm{W}_{11} + \mathrm{W}_{12} + \mathrm{W}_{13} + \mathrm{W}_{14})$$

Maximum score for Social/Cultural (MSS):

$$\mathrm{MSS} = 9 \times (\mathrm{W}_{15} + \mathrm{W}_{16} + \mathrm{W}_{17} + \mathrm{W}_{18} + \mathrm{W}_{19})$$

Maximum score for Environment (MSEn):

$$\mathrm{MSEn} = 9 \times (\mathrm{W}_{20} + \mathrm{W}_{21} + \mathrm{W}_{22} + \mathrm{W}_{23} + \mathrm{W}_{24} + \mathrm{W}_{25} + \mathrm{W}_{26} + \mathrm{W}_{27} + \mathrm{W}_{28} + +\mathrm{W}_{29} + \mathrm{W}_{30} + \mathrm{W}_{31} + \mathrm{W}_{32} + \mathrm{W}_{33} + \mathrm{W}_{34} + \mathrm{W}_{35} + \mathrm{W}_{36} + \mathrm{W}_{37})$$

Where Wi is the weight of each criterion.

Then, the multiplying factors (MF) for each topic were calculated as follows:

Multiplying factors for Technical Suitability aspect:

Table 4 Qualitative assessment of Technical suitability, Economic/Financial and Social/Cultural aspects

Alternatives						
Criteria		Autoclave	Autoclave with a shredder	Chemical treatment	Central incineration	Hydroclave
Technical suitability	Compatibility with natural conditions	Medium	High	Medium	Medium	High
	Preference for locally manufactured technologies	Medium	Medium	Medium	Low	Medium
	Availability of spare parts	Medium	Medium	High	Medium	Medium
	Availability of local expertise	Medium	Medium	Medium	Medium	Medium
	Track record on performance	Medium	High	Medium	High	High
	Compatibility with existing technology	Medium	Medium	Medium	Medium	High
	Meets capacity requirement	Medium	Medium	Medium	High	High
	Adaptable to future situations	Medium	Medium	Medium	High	High
	Ability to treat a wide range of infectious wastes	Medium	High	Medium	High	High
	Level of automation/sophistication	Medium	Medium	High	Medium	Medium
Economic/ Financial	Capital cost of the treatment Technology	High	Medium	High	Low	Medium
	Capital costs of all accessories and related equipment	Medium	Medium	High	Low	Medium
	Operation and maintenance costs	Medium	Medium	Medium	Low	Medium
	Installation requirements	Medium	Medium	High	Medium	Medium
Social/Cultural	Community acceptance of the technology	High	High	Medium	Low	High
	Income generation potential	Low	Low	Low	High	Low
	Acceptability of treatment residues by the local landfill	Medium	Medium	Medium	Medium	Medium
	Extent of necessary resettlement of people	High	High	Medium	Low	High
	Visible or aesthetic impact	Medium	Medium	Medium	Low	High

$$MF_1 = W_1 \times R_T / MST$$

.

.

.

$$MF_{10} = W_{10} \times R_T / MST$$

Multiplying factors for Economic/Financial aspect:

$$MF_{11} = W_{11} \times R_{Ec} / MSEc \quad MF_{13} = W_{13} \times R_{Ec} / MSEc$$

$$MF_{12} = W_{12} \times R_{Ec} / MSEc \quad MF_{14} = W_{14} \times R_{Ec} / MSEc$$

Multiplying factors for Social/Cultural aspect:

$$MF_{15} = W_{15} \times R_S / MSS \quad MF_{18} = W_{18} \times R_S / MSS$$

$$MF_{16} = W_{16} \times R_S / MSS \quad MF_{19} = W_{19} \times R_S / MSS$$

$$MF_{17} = W_{17} \times R_S / MSS$$

Multiplying factors for Environmental aspect:

$$MF_{20} = W_{20} \times R_T / MST$$

.

.

.

$$MF_{37} = W_{37} \times R_T / MST$$

Results and discussion

Quantities and characteristics of wastes generated in studied hospital complex

The average HCWs generated by Imam Khomeini hospital complex during March to June 2014 was 3270 kilograms per day (Table 2). The percentage of general, infectious and sharps waste were 47.1, 42.2 and 10.7 %, respectively. WHO reported that 75- 90 % of total HCWs are general waste and 10- 25 % are infectious and hazardous wastes [3]. Results showed that the infectious and hazardous wastes measured in this study were higher than those reported by WHO. This indicates that segregation of different types of wastes wasn't properly implemented in the studied hospitals. According to the results, the mean generation rate for total, general, infectious and sharp wastes were 2.72,1.28, 1.15, and 0.29 kg occupied bed^{-1} day^{-1},respectively. HCWs generation rate previously reported in different studies in Iran which conducted in other cities including Mashhad, Tabriz, Isfahan, and Shiraz have been reported in the range of 2.6 to 4.45 kg occupied bed^{-1} day^{-1} for total HCWs,1.5 to 2.44 kg occupied bed^{-1} day^{-1} of general for non-infectious waste, and 1.039 to 1.59 kg occupied bed^{-1} day^{-1} for infectious waste [21–24]. Furthermore, Farzadkia et al 2008, reported a mean medical waste generation rate of 2.75 kg occupied bed^{-1} day^{-1} which was similar to the results of this study [25]. Among the different wards of the studied hospitals, operation rooms had the highest infectious waste generation rate. This can be caused by the types of services provided in this ward which comprises of various surgical procedures. A significant difference was observed based on weighed infectious wastes, which showed a statistically higher

Table 5 Qualitative assessment of **Environmental** aspect

Alternatives					
Criteria	Autoclave	Autoclave with a shredder	Chemical Treatment	Central incineration	Hydroclave
Air emissions	Medium	Medium	Low	Low	Medium
Liquid effluents	Medium	Medium	Low	Medium	High
Solid residues	Medium	Medium	Low	High	Medium
Risk levels for workers	Medium	Medium	Low	Medium	Medium
Odor	Medium	Medium	Low	Medium	Medium
Noise	Medium	High	High	Medium	Medium
Space requirement	Medium	Medium	High	Low	Medium
Material consumption	Medium	High	Low	Medium	High
Risk to the environment	Medium	High	Low	Low	High
Risk levels for communities	Medium	High	Medium	Low	High
Water consumption per kg of waste	Low	Medium	Medium	High	High
Energy consumption per kg of waste	Medium	Medium	High	Medium	Medium
Use of hazardous materials	High	High	Low	High	High
Efficacy of microbial inactivation	Medium	High	Medium	High	High
Volume reduction	Low	Medium	Low	High	High
Mass reduction	Low	Low	Low	High	High
Resource recovery capabilities	Medium	Medium	Low	Low	Medium
Extent of use of renewable energy	Medium	Medium	Low	Medium	High

Table 6 Scores obtained for different Technical Suitability, Economic/Financial and Social/Cultural criteria

Criteria		Alternatives Autoclave		Autoclave with a shredder		Chemical Treatment		Central incineration		Hydroclave	
		Score	Score × MF	Score	Score × MF	Score	Score × MF	Score	Score × MF	Score	Score × MF
Technical suitability	Compatibility with natural conditions	6	1.45	7	1.81	6	1.33	5	0.93	7	1.68
	Preference for locally manufactured technologies	6	1.45	6	1.33	5	0.93	3	0.33	6	1.23
	Availability of spare parts	6	1.45	5	0.93	7	1.81	5	0.93	5	0.85
	Availability of local expertise	5	1.01	5	0.93	6	1.33	5	0.93	5	0.85
	Track record on performance	5	1.01	7	1.81	5	0.93	7	1.81	7	1.68
	Compatibility with existing technology	5	1.01	6	1.33	5	0.93	4	0.59	8	2.19
	Meets capacity requirement	5	1.01	6	1.33	5	0.93	9	3.00	7	1.68
	Adaptable to future situations	5	1.01	6	1.33	4	0.59	8	2.37	7	1.68
	Ability to treat a wide range of infectious wastes	6	1.45	7	1.81	6	1.33	9	3.00	8	2.19
	Level of automation/sophistication	6	1.45	5	0.93	8	2.37	4	0.59	5	0.85
Economic/ Finanial	Capital cost of the treatment technology	7	6.19	6	4.75	8	8.47	2	0.53	5	3.31
	Capital costs of all accessories and related equipment	5	3.16	5	3.31	7	6.48	3	1.19	5	3.31
	Operation and maintenance costs	5	3.16	5	3.31	5	3.31	3	1.19	5	3.31
	Installation requirements	5	3.16	5	3.31	7	2.02	4	2.12	6	4.75
Social/Cultural	Community acceptance of the technology	7	2.27	8	2.63	5	1.03	3	0.37	7	2.02
	Income generation potential	1	0.05	2	0.16	2	0.16	7	2.02	2	0.16
	Acceptability of treatment residues by the local landfill	4	0.74	5	1.03	5	1.03	6	1.48	6	1.48
	Extent of necessary resettlement of people	7	2.27	7	2.02	6	1.48	3	0.37	7	2.02
	Visible or aesthetic impact	5	1.16	5	1.03	5	1.03	3	0.37	7	2.02

($p < 0.001$) quantity of HCWs in summer than that of winter.

Screening step

After gathering the stakeholders comments and choices, treatment alternatives that didn't meet the basic criteria, were excluded. The results of the screening step are presented in Table 3. As shown in Table 3, demolizer, Chem-cloth and microwave were excluded at this step, which may be due to the inability of these technologies to reduce the volume and mass of infectious waste, inadequate capacity of them or lack of stakeholders familiarity with these technologies.

Scoping step

Qualitative assessment based on the expert's opinion was performed during this step. The results of the scoping step for each aspect provided in Tables 4 and 5.

As the results show, autoclave obtained a medium score for all technical suitability aspects criteria. A similar result was observed for autoclave with a shredder, chemical treatment and central incineration. Also for most technical suitability criteria, the hydroclve obtained high scores.

Regarding the economic/financial aspect criteria, as shown in Table 4, high and low scores were obtained for chemical treatment and central incineration, respectively. Regarding this aspect, chemical treatment was the preferable choices of experts. Moreover, hydroclave and autoclave with a shredder obtained the medium scores for all economical aspects criteria. The similar result was observed for autoclave.

As shown in Table 4, regarding the social aspect, the high, medium and low scores for almost criteria were obtained for hydroclave, chemical treatment, and central incineration, respectively. Also, results were similar for autoclave and autoclave with a shredder regarding social aspect.

As shown in Table 5, based on qualitative assessment, hydroclave and chemical treatment obtained high and low scores for almost environmental aspect criteria, respectively. Autoclave, autoclave with a shredder and central incineration obtained medium scores for the most environmental aspect criteria.

Table 7 Scores obtained for different Environmental criteria

Criteria	Alternatives									
	Autoclave		Autoclave with a shredder		Chemical Treatment		Central incineration		Hydroclave	
	Score	Score × MF	Score	Score × MF	Score	Score × MF	Score	Score × MF	Score	Score × MF
Air emissions	6	2.07	6	1.75	3	0.44	2	0.20	6	1.75
Effluents	4	0.92	4	0.78	2	0.20	6	1.75	7	2.40
Solid residues	4	0.92	5	1.23	3	0.44	7	2.40	5	1.23
Risk levels for workers	5	1.44	5	1.23	2	0.20	4	0.78	6	1.75
Odor	4	0.92	4	0.78	3	0.44	4	0.78	4	0.78
Noise	6	2.07	6	1.8	7	2.40	4	0.78	6	1.75
Space requirement	6	2.07	6	1.75	7	2.40	3	0.44	6	1.75
Material consumption	6	2.07	7	2.40	3	0.44	6	1.75	8	3.14
Risk to the environment	6	2.07	7	2.40	3	0.44	2	0.20	7	2.40
Risk levels for communities	6	2.07	7	2.40	5	1.23	3	0.44	7	2.40
Water consumption per kg of waste	3	0.52	5	1.25	4	0.8	7	2.40	7	2.40
Energy consumption per kg of waste	5	1.44	6	1.75	7	2.40	6	1.75	6	1.75
Use of hazardous materials	7	2.82	7	2.40	2	0.20	8	3.2	7	2.40
Efficiencyof microbial inactivation	6	2.07	7	2.40	6	1.75	9	3.97	8	3.14
Volume reduction	2	0.23	6	1.75	2	0.20	9	3.97	8	3.14
Mass reduction	1	0.06	3	0.44	1	0.05	8	3.12	8	3.14
Resource recovery capabilities	6	2.04	5	1.23	3	0.44	2	0.20	5	1.23
Extent of use of renewable Energy	7	2.38	7	2.73	2	0.20	5	1.23	7	2.40
Final Score		28.18		30.51		14.68		29.39		39

Detailed assessment

Different MCDMs can be used to perform a detailed assessment step. In this study, to maintain the integrity of the methodology, the weighted sum matrix method was used. The results of this step for each aspect are presented in Tables 6 and 7. The distribution of technical, economic, social and environmental aspects considered by the experts is shown in Fig. 2. The final scores obtained by different treatment alternatives for the technical suitability, economical, social and environmental aspects related criteria, are shown as a radar diagram provided in Figs. 3, 4, 5 and 6. Also, the distribution of

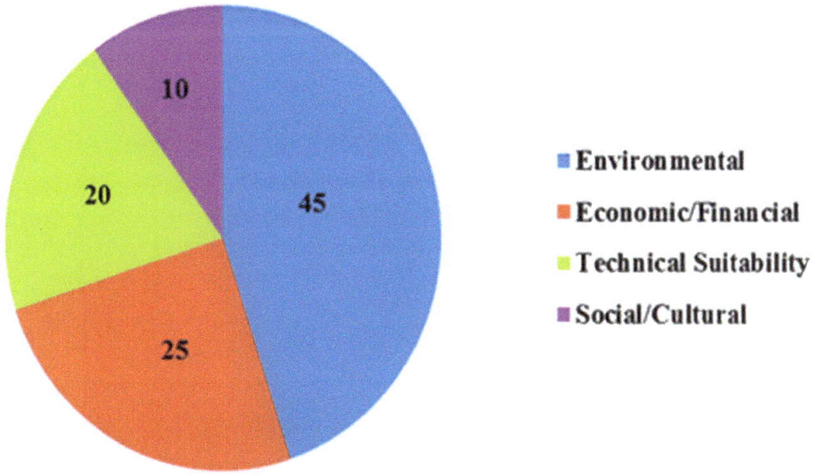

Fig. 2 The distribution of scores for technical,economic, social and environmental aspects

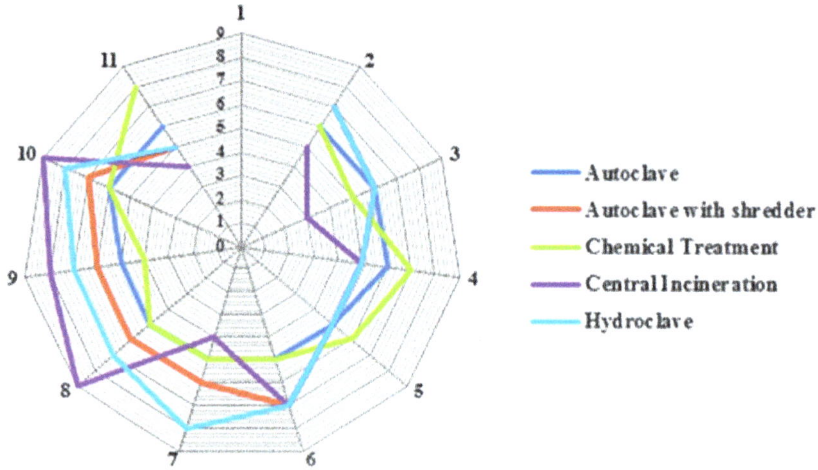

Fig. 3 Star diagram for detailed assessment: Technical suitability

the final weights of criteria for alternatives is presented in Fig. 7.

As the results show, environmental aspect was the most important aspect of the SAT methodology based on the expert's opinion. Among the different criteria in technical suitability aspect, the most important criteria considered by experts were ability to treat a wide range of infectious wastes, ideal capacity, track record on performance and availability of spare parts and usage of local materials, respectively. Regarding the economic/financial aspect, experts considered the capital cost of the treatment technology, operation and maintenance costs and installation requirements as the most important criteria, respectively. The most important criteria in the social aspect were community acceptance of the technology, acceptability of treatment residues by the local landfill and extent of necessary resettlement of people, respectively. In the environmental aspect, experts considered the criteria of efficiency of microbial inactivation, volume and mass reduction, emissions, risk levels for communities and the environment to be the most important criteria, respectively.

As the results show, regarding the technical suitability aspects, the highest scores were obtained for hydroclave and central incineration technologies. These results indicate that there is no significant difference between hydroclave and central incineration in terms of technical suitability ($p < 0.001$) that indicates the suitability of incineration for treatment of infectious waste as well as hydroclave. Moreover, among various technical suitability criteria, the highest scores were obtained for two criteria, including ideal capacity, and

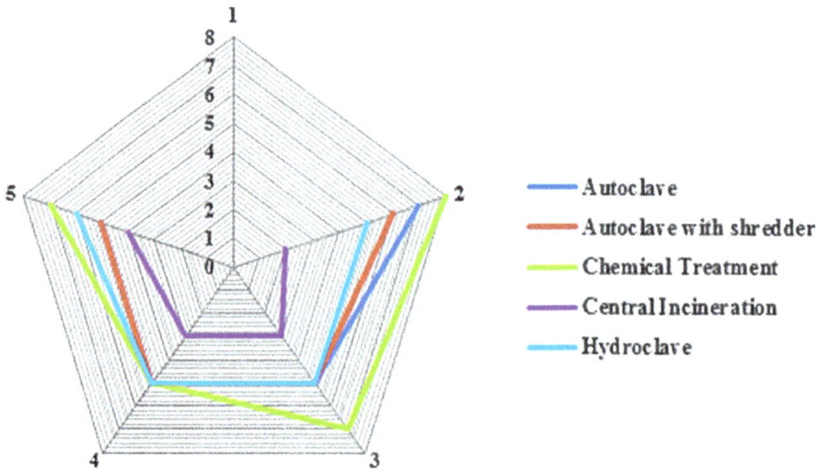

Fig. 4 Star diagram for detailed assessment: **Economic/Financial**

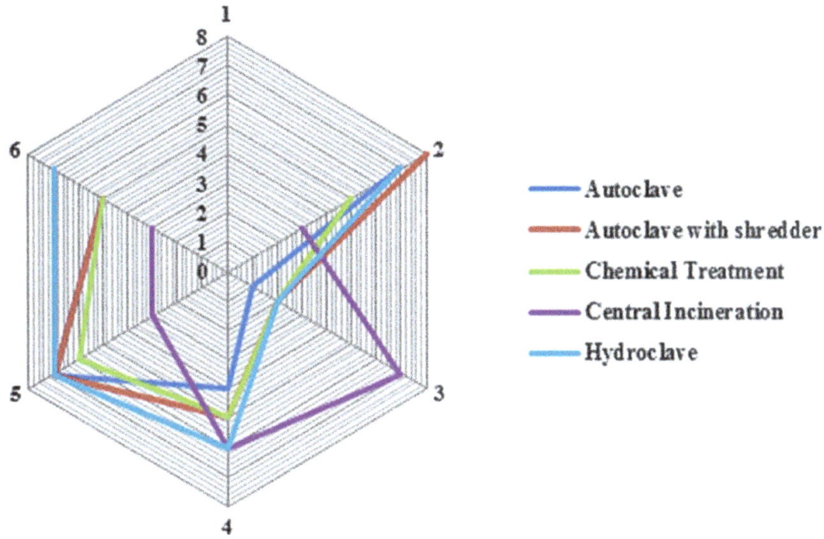

Fig. 5 Star diagram for detailed assessment: **Social/Cultural**

ability of treating a wide range of infectious waste. These high scores were obtained for incineration technology. These results are consistent with results reported by Pudussery who studied different medical waste management options in the Norfolk and Norwich university hospital and in which the incineration obtained the highest scores for type of waste treated, and volume and mass reduction of HCWs [26].

Regarding the economic/financial aspect, as shown in Table 6 and Fig. 4, the highest and lowest scores were obtained for chemical treatment and central incineration, respectively. The capital cost of implementation for chemical treatment is lower than those for other alternatives which is the main advantage of this treatment technology in terms of economic and financial aspect. On the other hand, although incineration acquired ahigh score regarding the technical suitability, however the higher capital and also operational and maintenance costs for incineration compared with other treatment alternatives are one of the disadvantages of this treatment technology regarding the financial aspect. These results are consistent with results reported by Pudussery, indicating that incinerators have higher capital and maintenance costs than other treatment alternatives [26].

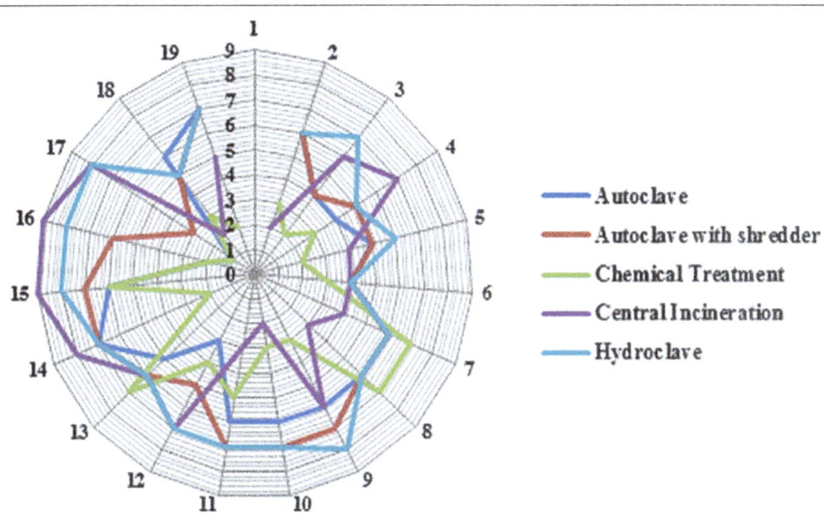

Fig. 6 Star diagram for detailed assessment: **Environmental**

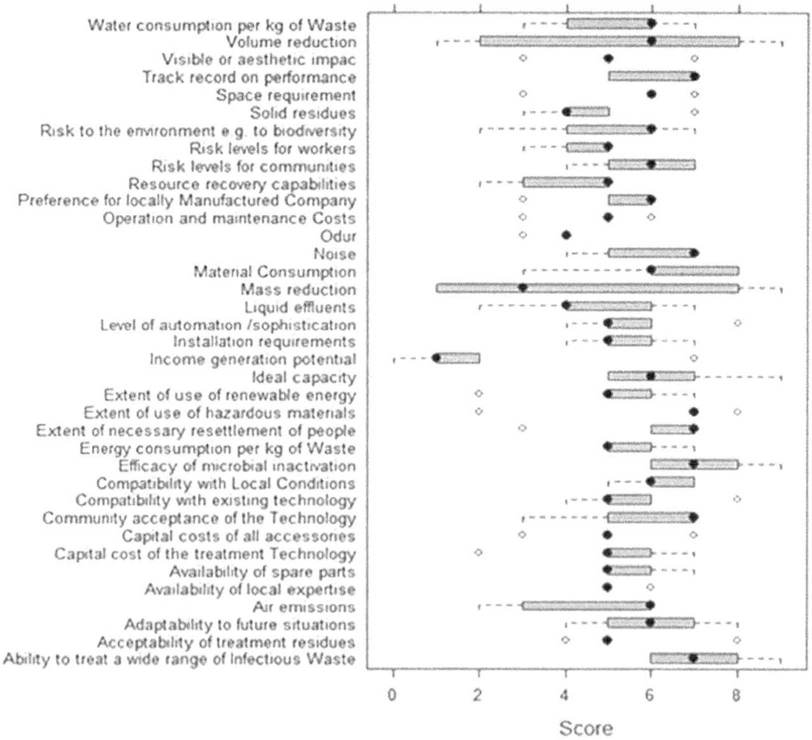

Fig. 7 The box and whisker of scores for each criteria acquired by treatment alternatives

As shown in Table 6, regarding the social aspect the highest score was obtained for hydroclave. The similar result was observed for autoclave and autoclave with a shredder. Among various criteria in social/cultural aspect, the highest score was obtained for the community acceptance of the technology which was acquired for autoclave with a shredder. On the other hand, the lowest score was obtained for the criterion of income generation potential.

One of the most important aspects of SAT methodology is the environmental aspect which has 18 specific criteria. According to the results that presented in Table 7 and Fig. 6, hydroclave and chemical treatment got highest and lowest scores for the environmental aspect, respectively. The highest score among environmental criteria is associated with central incineration for efficiency of microbial inactivation and volume reduction that are the main advantages of it. Also, the lowest scores in environmental criteria are associated with the autoclave and chemical treatment for mass reduction criteria.

As shown in Table 8, regarding all aspects of SAT methodology, the highest score was obtained for hydroclave. However, it may so happen that the selected best technology may be found to be inadequate or inappropriate in the future. This may happen due to changes in the situation, local requirements, legislations, or even the new developments in technology. Similar studies have been conducted in other countries. For instance, in a comparative study, Karagiannidis et al [18] assessed the thermal treatment processes of infectious hospital

Table 8 Final score of infectious waste treatment alternatives

Alternatives					
Criteria	Autoclave	Autoclave with a shredder	Chemical Treatment	Central incineration	Hydroclave
Technical Suitability	12.3	13.54	12.48	14.48	14.88
Economical	15.67	14.69	20.28	5.03	14.69
Social	6.49	6.87	4.73	4.61	7.7
Environmental	28.18	30.51	14.68	29.39	39
Total	62.64	65.61	52.17	53.51	76.27

wastes in Central Macedonia, Greece via the analytic hierarchy process (AHP). The results demonstrated that a centralized hydroclave or autoclave plant is the best alternative, which was similar to our findings [18]. A study was conducted in china that proposed a hybrid multi-criteria decision making (MCDM) model by integrating the 2-tuple DEMATEL technique and fuzzy MULTI-MOORA method for selection of HCWs treatment alternatives. Results showed that steam sterilization was found to be the most suitable HCWs treatment technology [1]. Puddussery utilized MCDA matrix method to find out the best technology for the on-site HCWs treatment in at the NORFOLK and NORWICH university hospital, in England. According the results, incineration was the optimum technology for the hospital [26]. Dursun et al proposed two fuzzy MCDM techniques which were based on fusion of fuzzy information, 2-tuple linguistic representation model, and TOPSIS for the evaluation of HCWs treatment alternatives for Istanbul. According to the results of the study, steam sterilization was determined as the most suitable treatment technology [17].

The box and whisker of scores for each criterion, are shown in Fig. 7. As the results show, for volume reduction 50 % of scores, were between 2 to 8. For mass reduction 50 % of scores were between 1 to 8. This result indicated the wide range of scores for these criteria. In addition, the distribution of final weights for treatment

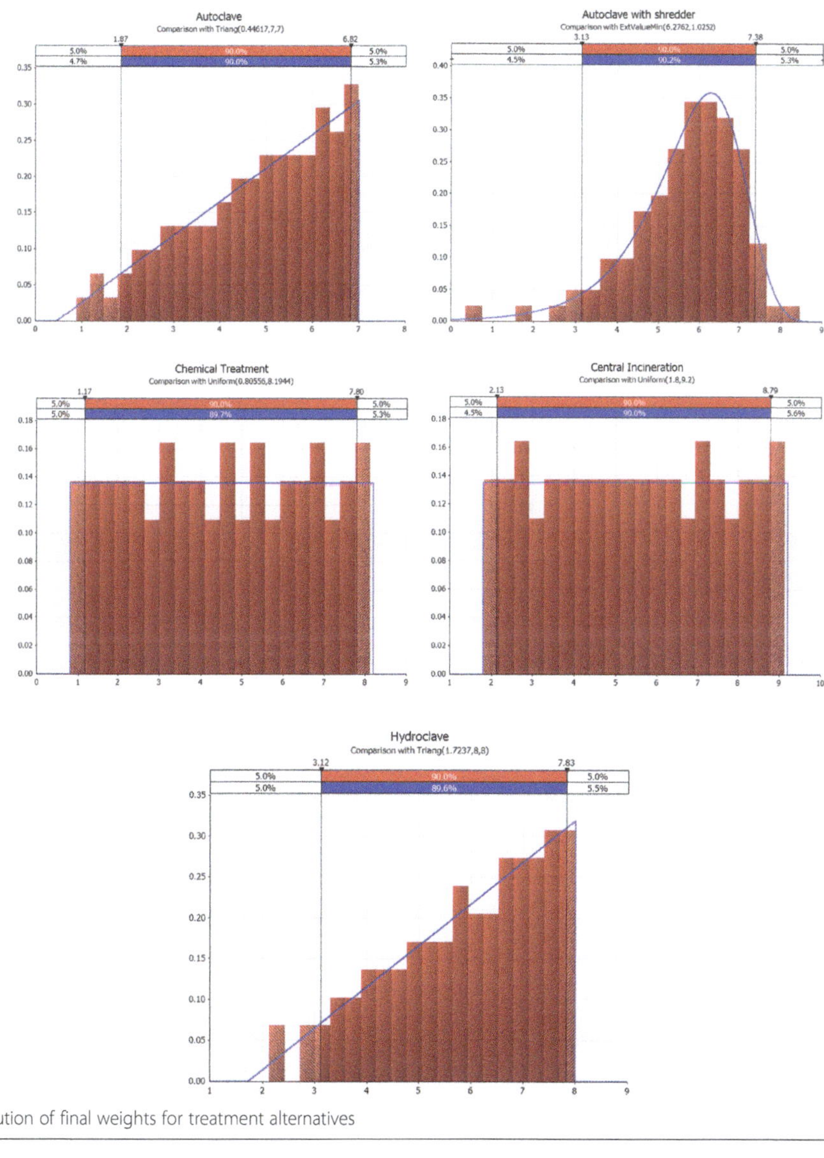

Fig. 8 The distribution of final weights for treatment alternatives

alternatives is given in Fig. 8. For chemical treatment and central incineration, the type of the distribution was uniform. Distribution types for autoclave and hydroclave were the triangle type. For autoclave with a shredder, extreme value min distribution was observed.

Conclusion

The most appropriate infectious waste treatment technology was selected based on the highest score. According to obtained final score, hydroclve, was the most suitable infectious waste treatment technology. The ranking order of the alternative treatments were Autoclave with a shredder, Autoclave, Central Incineration and Chemical treatment on the basis of the technical, economic, social and environmental aspects and their related criteria. So, as mentioned in SAT methodology, it could be concluded that the top ranking technologies basically have higher scores in all the aspects. Hence it is easier to arrive at a decision for the final technology selection based on the principles of sustainability. One limitation of the present study is that the results are subjected to the reliability on the response of experts on the questions in the survey. Also, the questionnaire surveys were time consuming and only 70 out of 150 questionnaires send were replied. Although to the best of our knowledge, this study is the first comprehensive study in which SAT methodology have been used to select the best treatment alternative for infectious waste in developing countries; however, there are a number of areas in which further research could be conducted. First, since the objective weights of the criteria were not considered and also the subjective weights were dependent on the experts' personal judgments, which may result in some errors or mistakes, there is a need to develop a new approach accounting subjective and objective weights of criteria simultaneously. Second, the fuzzy MCDMs for SAT methodology can be performed based on the most important criteria in each aspect determined in this study. Finally, the present study was conducted in a developing country. So it would be useful to conduct similar studies in developed countries and comparing the results with the results of this study.

Abbreviations

AHP: analytic hierarchy process; CSWR: Center for Solid Waste research; HCWs: health-care wastes; HIV: human immunodeficiency virus; IER: Institute for Environmental Research; IETC-UNEP: International Environmental Technology Center of the United Nations Environment Program; MCDM: multi-criteria decision method; SAT: Sustainable Assessment of Technologies methodology; WHO: World Health Organization.

Acknowledgments

The authors would like to acknowledge all of the experts and stakeholders that participated in the study.

Funding

This paper was part of a Master thesis of the first author and has been funded by the Center for Solid Waste research (CSWR), Institute for Environmental Research (IER) of Tehran University of Medical Sciences under grant no. 94-01-46-28616.

Availability of data and materials section

The authors do not wish to share their data. All the necessary data have been mentioned in the paper. If other researchers need our data for their studies, they can contact with first Autor via email.

Authors' contributions

AR has participated in all stages of the study (design of the study, collecting and analyzing of data and manuscript preparation). RN and KY were supervised the study. AHM and MY were advisors of the study. MH participated in manuscript preparation. MKH participated in the intellectual helping in different stages of the study. SP performed data collection. All authors read and approved the final manuscript.

Competing interests

The authors declare that they have no competing interests.

Consent for publication

Not applicable.

Ethics approval and consent to participate

Not applicable.

Author details

[1]Center for Solid Waste Research (CSWR), Institute for Environmental Research (IER), Tehran University of Medical Sciences, Tehran, Iran. [2]Department of Environmental Health Engineering, School of Public Health, Tehran University of Medical Sciences, Tehran, Iran. [3]Department of Environmental Health Engineering, School of Public Health, Shiraz University of Medical Sciences, Shiraz, Iran. [4]Center for Air Pollution Research (CAPR), Institute for Environmental Research (IER), Tehran University of Medical Sciences, Tehran, Iran. [5]Environmental and occupational health center, Ministry of health medical education, Tehran, Iran.

References

1. Liu H-C, You J-X, Lu C, Chen Y-Z. Evaluating health-care waste treatment technologies using a hybrid multi-criteria decision making model. Renew Sustain Energy Rev. 2015;41:932–42.
2. Hossain MS, Santhanam A, Norulaini NN, Omar AM. Clinical solid waste management practices and its impact on human health and environment–A review. Waste Manag. 2011;31(4):754–66.
3. Prüss A, Emmanuel J, Stringer R, Pieper U, Townend W, Wilburn S, et al. Safe management of wastes from health-care activities. 2014.
4. Graikos A, Voudrias E, Papazachariou A, Iosifidis N, Kalpakidou M. Composition and production rate of medical waste from a small producer in Greece. Waste Manag. 2010;30(8):1683–9.
5. Jaafari J, Dehghani MH, Hoseini M, Safari GH. Investigation of hospital solid waste management in Iran. World Review of Science, Technology and Sustainable Development. 2015;12(2):111–25.
6. Malekahmadi F, Yunesian M. Analysis of the healthcare waste management status in Tehran hospitals. Journal of Environmental Health Science and Engineering. 2014;12(1):1–5.
7. Sawalem M, Selic E, Herbell J-D. Hospital waste management in Libya: A case study. Waste Manag. 2009;29(4):1370–5.
8. El-Salam MMA. Hospital waste management in El-Beheira Governorate, Egypt. J Environ Manage. 2010;91(3):618–29.
9. Tsakona M, Anagnostopoulou E, Gidarakos E. Hospital waste management and toxicity evaluation: a case study. Waste Manag. 2007;27(7):912–20.
10. Chaerul M, Tanaka M, Shekdar AV. A system dynamics approach for hospital waste management. Waste Manag. 2008;28(2):442–9.
11. Harhay MO, Halpern SD, Harhay JS, Olliaro PL. Health care waste management: a neglected and growing public health problem worldwide. Trop Med Int Health. 2009;14(11):1414–7.

12. Water S, Organization WH. Safe health-care waste management: policy paper. 2004.
13. Compendium of Technologies for Treatment/Destruction of Healthcare Waste,. United Nations Environment Programme, Division of Technology, Industry and Economics International Environmental Technology Centre; 2012.
14. Diaz L, Savage G, Eggerth L. Alternatives for the treatment and disposal of healthcare wastes in developing countries. Waste Manag. 2005;25(6):626–37.
15. Rogers DE, Brent AC. Small-scale medical waste incinerators–experiences and trials in South Africa. Waste Manag. 2006;26(11):1229–36.
16. Liu H-C, Wu J, Li P. Assessment of health-care waste disposal methods using a VIKOR-based fuzzy multi-criteria decision making method. Waste Manag. 2013;33(12):2744–51.
17. Dursun M, Karsak EE, Karadayi MA. Assessment of health-care waste treatment alternatives using fuzzy multi-criteria decision making approaches. Resour Conserv Recycl. 2011;57:98–107.
18. Karagiannidis A, Papageorgiou A, Perkoulidis G, Sanida G, Samaras P. A multi-criteria assessment of scenarios on thermal processing of infectious hospital wastes: a case study for Central Macedonia. Waste Manag. 2010; 30(2):251–62.
19. Hsu P-F, Wu C-R, Li Y-T. Selection of infectious medical waste disposal firms by using the analytic hierarchy process and sensitivity analysis. Waste Manag. 2008;28(8):1386–94.
20. Hoseini M, Yunesian M, Nabizadeh R, Yaghmaeian K, Ahmadkhaniha R, Rastkari N, et al. Characterization and risk assessment of polycyclic aromatic hydrocarbons (PAHs) in urban atmospheric Particulate of Tehran, Iran. Environ Sci Pollut Res. 2016;23(2):1820–32.
21. Davoodi R, Eslami Hasan Abadi S, Sabouri G, Salehi M, Ghooshkhanei H, Rahmani S, et al. Medical Waste Management in the second largest City of Iran (Mashhad) with Three-Million Inhabitants. Journal of Patient Safety & Quality Improvement. 2014;2(4):160–4.
22. Taghipour H, Mosaferi M. Characterization of medical waste from hospitals in Tabriz, Iran. Sci Total Environ. 2009;407(5):1527–35.
23. Ferdowsi A, Ferdosi M, Mehrani Z, Narenjkar P. Certain hospital waste management practices in Isfahan, Iran. International journal of preventive medicine. 2012;3(Suppl1):S176.
24. Askarian M, Vakili M, Kabir G. Results of a hospital waste survey in private hospitals in Fars province, Iran. Waste Manag. 2004;24(4):347–52.
25. Farzadkia M, Moradi A, Mohammadi MS, Jorfi S. Hospital waste management status in Iran: a case study in the teaching hospitals of Iran University of Medical Sciences. Waste Manag Res. 2009;27(4):384–9.
26. Pudussery KP. Study On the Medical Waste Management in the Norfolk AND Norwich University Hospital, MS Thesis. School of Environmental Sciences: University of East Anglia; 2010.

Detection of parasitic particles in domestic and urban wastewaters and assessment of removal efficiency of treatment plants in Tehran, Iran

Kareem Hatam-Nahavandi[1], Amir Hossein Mahvi[2], Mehdi Mohebali[1,3], Hossein Keshavarz[1], Iraj Mobedi[1] and Mostafa Rezaeian[1*]

Abstract

Background: In recent years, decreasing annual rainfalls in some countries and population growth have led to a shortage of freshwater resources. Thus, recycled wastewaters has been suggested for agricultural activities. Contamination of wastewaters with pathogens is a major concern for the use of these waters. This study aimed to (i) investigate the occurrence of helminth eggs and protozoan (oo)cysts in human and livestock wastewaters, and (ii) evaluate the parasite removal efficiencies of urban and slaughterhouse treatment plants in Tehran province, Iran. One hundred and eight samples were collected from five urban and domestic wastewater treatment plants in Iran. Wastewater samples were concentrated by centrifugal-concentration and filtration methods.

Results: The quantity of helminths egg and protozoa (oo)cyst per liter of urban raw wastewater ranged from 1.2×10^1 to 2.9×10^1 and from 9.6×10^2 to 1.9×10^3, respectively. The number of eggs and (oo)cysts per liter of animal raw wastewater ranged from 1.6×10^3 to 4.9×10^3 and 3.1×10^4 to 6.0×10^4, respectively. The helminths and protozoa identified in urban treatment plants included hookworms, *Hymenolepis* and *Rhabditis* (or probably *Strongyloides*), *Entamoeba*, *Isospora*, *Giardia*, *Chilomastix* and *Cryptosporidium*, while in slaughterhouses *Trichuris*, *Trichostrongylus*, *Moniezia*, *Dicrocoelium*, *Fasciola*, *Entamoeba*, *Cryptosporidium*, *Eimeria* and *Giardia* were isolated. The overall removal efficiency of eggs and (oo)cysts in the treatment plants ranged from 94.8 to 95.7% and from 79.3 to 85.8%, respectively.

Conclusion: The study results revealed that the efficacy of removal of nematode eggs, and not protozoan (oo)cysts, in urban wastewater treatment plants, is in compliance with the WHO parasitological guideline (<1 nematode per liter) required for unrestricted irrigation.

Keywords: Protozoan (oo)cyst, Helminth egg, Wastewater treatment plant, Slaughterhouse, Iran

Background

Water is life. In 2025, water shortages will be more prevalent among poorer regions such as Africa and parts of Asia, where resources are limited, anuall rainfall is low, population growth is rapid, and water concumption is high [1]. Under these circumstances, treated wastewaters can be used for irrigation of parks, playgrounds and agricultural farmlands [2]. Contamination of wastewaters with pathogens and chemical pollutants is a major concern for the use of these waters. Parasitic particles, including the helminth ova and protozoan (oo)cyst, are detected more frequently in wastewater than in other surface waters and are resistant to chlorination or ozonation used commonly in the water and wastewater treatment systems [3,4]. Pathogenic protozoa are major causes of human gastroenteritis transmitted by water and significant challenges of public health worldwide [5]. Several water-borne giardiasis, amoebiasis, cryptosporidiosis, balantidiosis, cyclosporidiosis and microsporidiosis outbreaks have been reported throughout the world [6]. The first outbreak of plant-borne fascioliasis, the biggest in the world, occurred in Iran (Bandar Anzali) in

* Correspondence: rezaiian@sina.tums.ac.ir
[1]Department of Medical Parasitology and Mycology, School of Public Health, Tehran University of Medical Sciences, Tehran, Iran
Full list of author information is available at the end of the article

February 1988. Total number of infected inhabitants estimated to be 10,000 [7]. All of trematodes have an indirect life cycle, unlike nematodes, and humans can't be infected by eating the eggs of these flukes, therefore, the efficiency of wastewater treatment plants in removing eggs can lead to interruption of transmission cycle. Of all the helminth eggs likely to be present in wastewaters, *Ascaris*, *Trichuris* and hookworm are of particular public health concern because of severe socioeconomic consequences of an estimated 39 million DALYs (disability adjusted life year) lost to these infections [8]. Generally, parasite removal in wastewater has been synonymous with the removal of intestinal nematode ova, particularly those of *Ascaris*, *Trichuris* and the hookworms, because they occur commonly and simple purification and microscopic identification methods were available to determine their present. Many of these parasites are zoonotic, thus, can be realized to the importance of various studies based on the removal efficiency of domestic and municipal wastewater treatment plants. Many studies have been conducted to determine the prevalence of these pathogens in surface waters and vegetables in Iran [9-12]. The objectives of the present study were to investigate the occurrence of helminth eggs, protozoan (oo)cysts and pseudoparasitic structures in human and livestock wastewaters, and to evaluate the egg and (oo)cyst removal efficiencies of urban and slaughterhouse wastewater treatment plants by egg and (oo)cyst recoveries in both influent- and final effluent wastewaters.

Methods

Study sites and samples

Wastewater samples were collected from three municipal treatment plants and two slaughterhouse treatment plants.

Municipal wastewater treatment plants were located at the west and southwest of Tehran: Shahrak-e Ekbatan (WWTP1), Shahrak-e Gharb (WWTP2) and south Tehran wastewater treatment plant (WWTP3), and recycled water discharged into creek of firoozabad, Sheikh-Fazlollah highway surface water channel and Varamin agricultural lands, respectively.

Domestic wastewater treatment plants were located in one suburb area of Tehran: Meisam-robat-dam (SWWTP4) and Dam-pak (SWWTP5).

The animals slaughtered in these two slaughterhouses were included cattle, sheep and goat, and the plants treated only domestic wastewater and reclaimed water was reused for the irrigation of Shahriār agricultural farm lands.

The main features in each of the five treatment plants are described in Table 1.

Grab samples of untreated (5 L each) and treated (10 L each) wastewater were collected at the inlet and outlet points of treatment plants monthly once, from December 2013 to November 2014.

The determination of samples volume was conducted in compliance with Analysis of Wastewater for Use in Agriculture - A Laboratory Manual of Parasitological and Bacteriological Techniques [2].

Water samples were collected in carboys and transported to the intestinal protozoan laboratory of the faculty of public health at the Tehran University of Medical Sciences (TUMS) where they were stored at 4°C until used for the analyses. The samples analyses were completed within 7 days. To reduce the potential for cross-contamination between samples, all sampling carboys used for raw and treated effluent were kept separate.

Recovery efficiency of *Giardia* cyst concentration procedures

The cyst recovery efficiency of four concentration methods was evaluated and compared to demonstrate acceptable method performance and included (i) modified Bailenger method (MB), as recommended by WHO in "Analysis of wastewater for agricultural use" [2] (ii) scraping and rinsing of membrane method (RM), (iii) acetone-dissolution method (ADM) [13], and (iv) centrifugal-(water-ether) concentration method (CC method) [14].

For each concentration method, six aliquots of 5 litres (untreated and treated) samples were collected. For each concentration procedure, two aliquots of raw and two aliquots of treated samples were used as matrix spikes and were seeded with estimated numbers of *Giardia* cysts.

The cysts used in assays were a gift from Dr. Meamar, School of Medicine, Iran University of Medical Sciences, Tehran, Iran, and were isolated and purified from feces of diarrheal patients by sucrose flotation (specific gravity of 1.18). The number of cysts ($\sim 4 \times 10^3$) was determined by microscopic examination and the pellet was suspended in one milliliter deionized water.

All of seeded and unseeded samples were sieved through a sries of stainless steel and polyester meshes of 40 (pore size 400-μm), 50 (pore size 297-μm), 200 (pore size 74-μm) and 400 (pore size 37-μm) before filtration to avoid filter blockage by large particles.

The first set of raw (2 seeded and 1 unseeded) and treated (2 seeded and 1 unseeded) samples were transferred to 5000 ml separatory funnel (decanter) (which was designed for this purpose, with two valves built in the bottom of the funnel) and allowed to settle for 24 hours, separately during the consecutive days. The sediments were transferred to 50 ml conical centrifuge tubes through the valves in the bottom of the funnel and centrifuged at 1000 × g for 15 minutes and further processed by modified Bailenger method as described by Mahvi and Kia [10].

Table 1 The main characteristics of the five wastewater treatment plants

Wastewater treatment plants	Population served	Primary treatment	Secondary treatment	Tertiary treatment and disinfection	Biochemical parameter			Water turbidity*		Use of treated water
					Flow rate (m^3/s)	BOD*** (mg/L)	TSS**** (mg/L)	influent	effluent	
WWTP1	100000	Screening and grit removal	Activated sludge and A2/O*****	Sand filtration followed by chlorination	0.46	<6	<30	High	Moderate	Discharged into creek
WWTP2	85000	Screening and grit removal	Conventional activated sludge	Chlorination	0.27	<30	<30	High	Moderate	Discharged to the highway surface water channel
WWTP3	2100000	Screening, grit removal and sedimentation	Trickling filter followed by activated sludge	Chlorination and UV radiation	5.2	28	28	High	Moderate	Agriculture irrigation
SWWTP4	ND**	Sedimentation	Activated sludge and oxidation with O_2	Chlorination	ND	ND	ND	High	Moderate	Agriculture irrigation
SWWTP5	ND	Sedimentation	Activated sludge and oxidation with O_2	Chlorination	ND	ND	ND	High	Moderate	Agriculture irrigation

*Low = <1 NTU; moderate = 1–10 NTU; high = >10 NTU; **ND = Not data; ***BOD = Biochemical oxygen demand; ****TSS = Total suspended solids; *****A2/O = Anaerobic/anoxic/oxic.

The second set of test samples (2 raw seeded, 1 raw unseeded, 2 treated seeded and 1 treated unseeded) were filtered by membrane filters (pore size 0.8-μm, 50-mm diameter; Sartorius, Germany), entrapped particles were achieved by scraping the membrane with a smooth-edged plasticine molder and rinsing with PBS elution fluid (pH 7.4) (containing 0.1% Tween-80 and antifoam agent B) and centrifugation (2100 × *g*, 10 min, 4°C) (RM method).

The third set of test samples (3 raw and 3 untreated) were concentrated by filtration on cellulose-acetate membrane filters (pore size 0.8-μm, 50-mm diameter; Sartorius, Germany) by vacuum pump (model XX 5522050, Millipore). The membrane filters with entrapped particles transferred to a 50 ml conical centrifuge tube, dissolved in acetone and centrifuged (3000 × *g*, 10 min, 4°C). The supernatant fluid was discarded by pipette Pasteur, and the pellet was successively resuspended and centrifuged in 95% ethanol, 70% ethanol, and eluting solution (pH 7.4). The eluting solution consisted of 0.1% (vol/vol) Tween-80 detergent, 0.1% (w/v) sodium dodecyl sulfate, NaCl, KH_2PO_4, $Na_2HPO_4 \cdot 12H_2O$ and 0.001% (vol/vol) antifoam agent B (Sigma-Aldrich) (ADM method).

Fourth set of test samples (3 raw and 3 untreated) were centrifuged (2100 × *g*, 15 min, 4°C), and the sediment was concentrated by water-ether concentration procedure following the steps described below.

Microscopic enumeration of cysts was performed in a Thoma counting cell at a magnification of × 400.

The matrix spike recovery was determined from the simple formula as described by Skotarczak [15].

Parasite particles concentration

The wastewater samples were sieved through a polyester mesh of 40 (400 μm) to remove large particles.

Raw wastewater samples were centrifuged (2100 × *g*, 15 min, 4°C) in a 4 × 500 ml-capacity-swinging-bucket rotor of a refrigerated centrifuge (Beckman, GS-6R Centrifuge).

The supernatant fluids were carefully aspirated by vacuum pump, without disturbing the sediment and about 100 ml of supernatant was left on top of the sediment at the bottom of the canisters (Beckman Aerosolve® Cannisters).

The residues were transferred to 50 ml conical centrifuge tubes and centrifuged as before.

A water-ether concentration procedure was performed with 30 ml deionized water and 9 ml diethyl ether (CC method) [16]. This concentration method was followed by flotation with zinc sulfate ($ZnSo_4 \cdot 7H_2O$) (w/v) (specific gravity 1.364) [17].

The upper layer of the flotation solution was decanted into a container, and this solution was diluted with water to lower the specific gravity of the solution to below that of the protozoan (oo)cysts and helminth eggs, and then the (oo)cysts and eggs were collected in the sediment after centrifugation.

The other hand, treated samples were filtered by cellulose-acetate membrane filter (pore size 0.8-μm, 50-mm diameter; Sartorius, Germany) to retain the particles. Sample elution was achieved by scraping the membranes with a smooth-edged plasticine molder and rinsing with PBS elution fluid (containing 0.1% Tween 80 and 0.001% antifoam agent B). The eluate was collected in a clean glass petri-dish and transferred to a 50-ml centrifuge tube and centrifuged at 2100 × *g* for 10 min.

Microscopic examination and enumeration of (oo) cysts and eggs was performed in a Thoma counting cell at 400× magnification for *Giardia* cysts and other protozoan (oo)cysts and in a McMaster counting cell (weber England) at 100× magnification for helminthic eggs [18].

Protozoan (oo)cysts and helminth eggs were identified by morphometric parasitological criteria including the size, which was measured by a calibrated microscope, and shape of eggs and (oo)cysts at 100×, 400× and 1000× magnifications.

Data analysis

Results of egg and (oo)cyst quantitation were analyzed with Microsoft Excel (version 2010) and Statistical Package for Social Science version 22 (IBM SPSS Inc., Chicago, IL, USA). Kolmogorov-Smirnov test (test of normality) was realized prior to Student's *t*-test (Paired *T*-test). Geometric and arithmetic means were also calculated. To evaluate the (oo)cyst and egg removal efficiency of treatment plants, the logarithm of egg and (oo) cyst concentrations were calculated and the difference between the number of eggs and (oo)cysts present in the influent and in the effluent samples was considered. A p-value < 0.05 was considered statistically significant.

Results

Recovery efficiency of *Giardia* cysts in test samples

Figure 1 shows the results as the mean percentage recovery and ± SD, and co-efficient of variance.

The microscopic assessment and cyst enumeration results show that CC method has the highest cyst recovery at 96.1% (±0.7) and 95 (±1.4) for raw and treated samples, respectively (Figure 1).

Recoveries of cysts were higher when using RM method than when using ADM method.

The acetone-dissolution method, due to the formation of a hardened pellet (solid robbery pellet) in the bottom of the tube after the centrifugation step that has interfered with the detection of cysts, exhibited cyst recovery of less than expected.

Background solids from the raw test samples contributed to filter blockage for both the scraping and rinsing

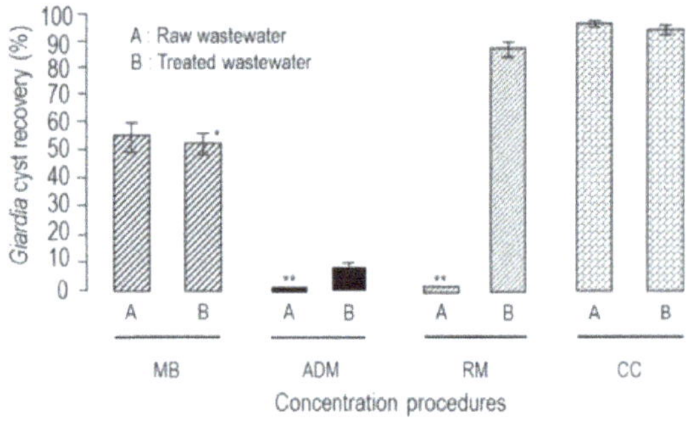

Figure 1 Comparison of the cyst concentration in raw and treated samples measured by different methods. Overall mean recoveries are expressed as a percentage. Co-efficient of variance (CV %) was 12, 2.5, lost, 11.8, lost, 1.9, 0.7 and 1.4 in raw and treated samples for MB method, ADM method, RM method and CC method, respectively. *Bars denote SD. **Lost raw samples.

of membrane method and the acetone-dissolution method, and their results were excluded.

The RM method produced the second highest recovery with 88% (±1.6) cysts isolated for treated samples. The MB method produced the third highest cysts recovery with 55% (±7.0) and 56.4 (±1.4) for raw and treated test samples.

The ADM method exhibited cyst recovery of 10.7% (±1.2) for treated test samples.

Interestingly, a large number of trophozoite forms of protozoa including amoeba, flagellate and cilliate, and a few protozoan cysts, such as *Bodo* spp., *Entamoeba* spp. and *Giardia duodenalis* were found in the supernatant remaining from the modified Bailenger method.

Frequency and distribution of parasitic particles in raw wastewaters

Eggs, (oo)cysts and pseudoparasitic structures detected in raw and treated wastewaters are shown in Figures 2, 3 and 4.

(Oo)cysts and eggs were detected in wastewater influents of all plants throughout the year.

In all plants, the highest and the lowest number of (oo)cysts and eggs were found in autumn and summer, respectively.

The estimated number of eggs and (oo)cysts per liter of raw wastewaters from urban treatment plants ranged

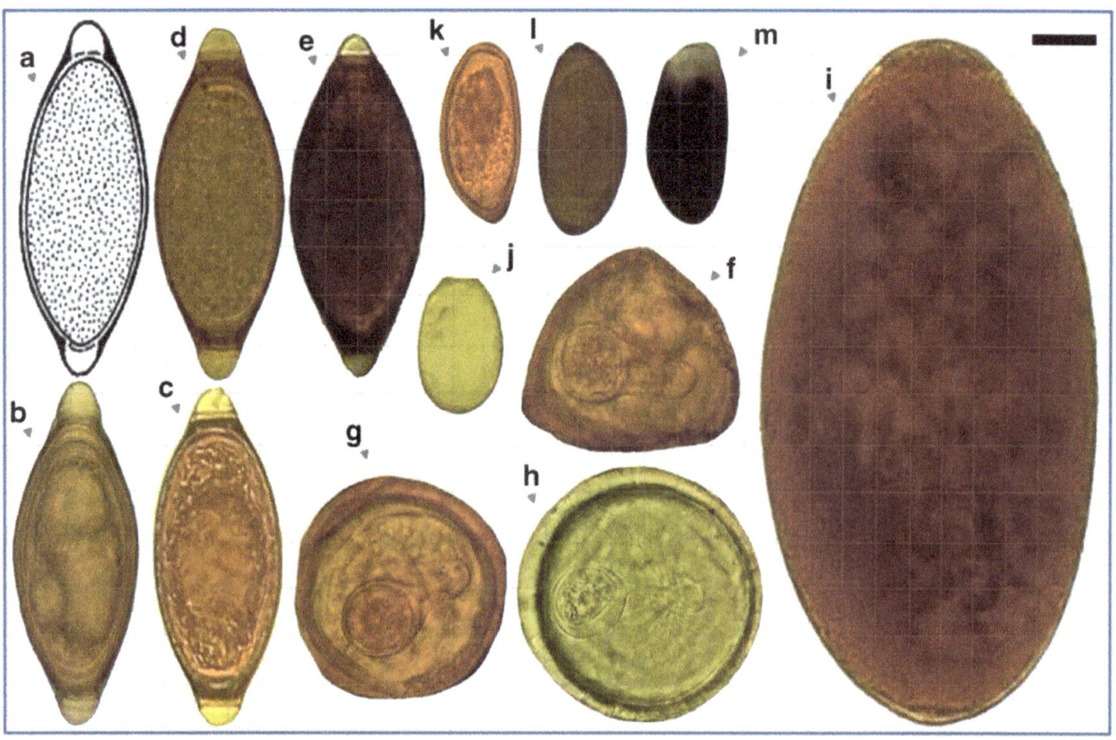

Figure 2 Relative sizes of some of the parasitic (anthropo-zoonotic) particles found in domestic wastewater treatment plants. (a), **(b)**, **(c)** ,**(d)**, **(e)** *Trichuris* spp.; **(f)** *Moniezia expansa* (triangular shape with pyriform apparatus); **(g)**, **(h)** *Moniezia* spp.; **(i)** *Fasciola hepatica*; **(j)** *Eimeria* spp. (damaged oocyst); **(k)**, **(l)** *Dicrocoelium dendriticum*; **(m)** *Dicrocoelium dendriticum* (damaged due to the aeration process) (Photographed under the light microscope at 1000x magnification using by Samsung Mobile, GT-B5512) (Bar showing 20 μm).

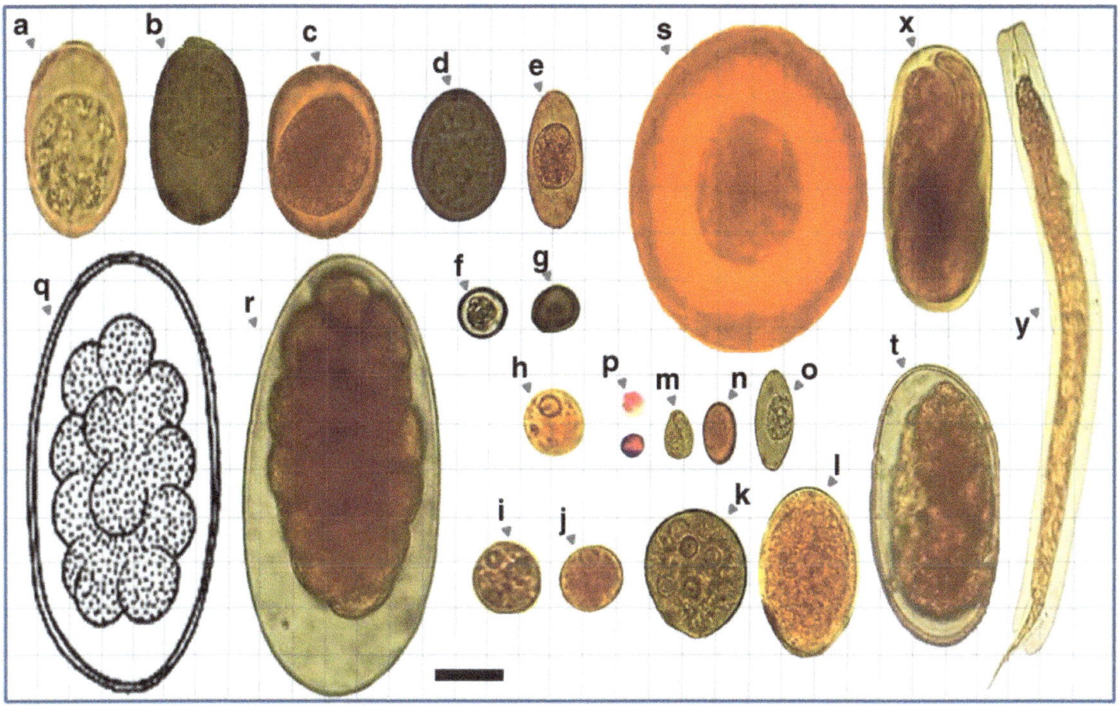

Figure 3 Relative sizes of some of the parasitic (anthropo-zoonotic) particles found in WWTPs and SWWTPs. a) *Eimeria* spp.; **(b)** *Eimeria* spp.; **(c)**, **(d)**, **(e)**, **(f)**, **(g)** coccidian spp. (This oocyst is typical of *Eimeria* spp. found in ruminant feces. The micropyle cap would indicate that this specimen came from sheep or goats. Cattle coccidia usually don't have micropyle caps) (h) *Entamoeba* spp. (*E. ovis/debliecki/dilimani/bovis*); **(i)** *Entamoeba wenyoni*; **(j)**, **(k)**, **(l)** *Entamoeba coli*; **(m)** *Chilomastix mesnili*; **(n)** *Giardia duodenalis*; **o)** *Isospora* spp; **(p)** *Cryptosporidium* spp. (probably *C. andersoni* or *parvum*); **(q)**, **(r)** *Trichostrongylus* spp.; **(s)** *Hymenolepis diminuta*; **(t)** hookworms; **(x)** *Rhabditis* spp. (or probably *Strongyloides*); **(y)** Free living larvae (probably *Rhabditidae*) (Bar showing 20 μm).

from 1.2×10^1 to 2.9×10^1 and from 9.6×10^2 to 1.9×10^3, respectively (Figure 5).

In the slaughterhouse treatment plants, the estimated number of eggs and (oo)cysts per liter of wastewater influents ranged from 1.6×10^3 to 4.9×10^3 and 31×10^3 to 60×10^3, respectively (Figure 5). Parasite quantification is necessary to evaluate the impact of the wastewater treatment processes on the prevalence of helminth eggs and protozoan (oo)cysts. The geometric mean concentrations of (oo)cysts and eggs per liter of wastewaters are shown in Figure 6.

In livestock wastewaters, eggs belonging to 3 groups of parasitic helminths were identified: the nematodes *Trichuris* spp., *Trichostrongylus* spp., the cestodes *Moniezia expansa* and the trematodes *Fasciola hepatica* and *Dicrocoelum dendriticum*. In urban wastewaters, eggs of 4 groups of helminths were observed: hookworms (*Ancylostoma duodenale* and *Necator americanus*), *Hymenolepis* spp. and *Rhabditis* spp. In these plants, (oo)cysts of 6 groups of parasitic protozoa were found: *Giardia* spp., *Entamoeba* spp., *Cryptosporidium* spp., *Eimeria* spp., *Isospora* spp. and *Chilomastix mesnili* (Figures 2, 3 and 4).

Entamoeba spp., the most commonly encountered cysts, were frequently found (60.9%) in urban raw wastewaters (Figure 7).

Sporolated and unsporolated oocysts of *Eimeria* spp. were frequently observed (56.1%) in slaughterhouse wastewater influents (Figure 7).

The highest number of egg in urban and livestock wastewaters was attributed to the nematodes *Rhabditis* (or probably *Strongyloides*) (47%) and *Trichostrongylus* (36%), respectively (Figure 7).

There were a large number of the cystic form particles, with a size of about 40–45 μ, and many pseudo-parasitic structures including protozoan (oo)cyst like particles and helminth egg like particles that we were unable to identify most of them (Figure 4).

We found many type of the small flagellates and amoebas in the raw and treated wastewaters that were rarely encountered.

The types of free-living protozoa and microorganisms in treated wasewater samples including rotifers, water bears, testate amoebas (*Arcella* spp. and *Euglypha* spp.), peritrichs (*Epistylis* spp, *Vorticella* spp.), Carnivorous

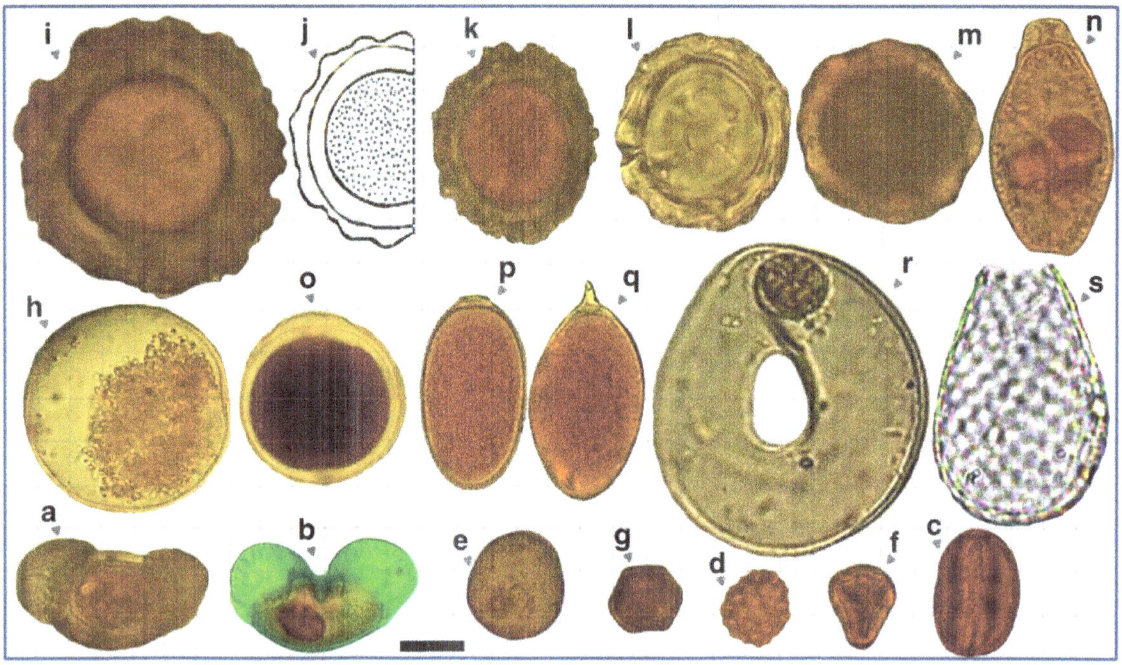

Figure 4 Relative sizes of some of the pseudo-parasitic particles including pollens, free living protozoa and their fossils found in WWTPs and SWWTPs. **(a)**, **(b)** Pollen grain (*Pinus contorta*, Family *Pinaceae*); **(b)** Pollen grain stained with trichrome; **(c)** pollen grain (*Eriogonum crocatum*, Grain Type: Tricolporate); **(d)** *pollen grain* (*Atriplex patula*, Grain Type: Periporate); **(e)** pollen grain; (f) pollen grain (*Eucaliptus globulus*, Myrtaceae Family); **(g)** pollen grain; **(h)** pecan pollen grain; **(i)**, **(k)**, **(l)**, **(m)** *Ascaris* egg-like particles in raw domestic wastewaters; **(j)** *Ascaris lumbricoides*; **(n)** *Epistylis* spp.; **(o)** parasite egg- or oocyst-like particle in municipal raw wastewaters; **(p)**, **(q)** Trematodes egg like particles in raw domestic wastewaters; **(r)** *Arcella discoides*; **(s)** *Euglypha* spp. (Bar showing 20 μm).

ciliates (*Acineria uncinata* and *Plagiocampa* rouxi), *Bodo* spp. and *Amoeba* spp. (cysts and trophozoites of unshelled amoebas) were also observed (Figure 4).

Removal efficiency of treatment plants

The overall average reduction in protozoan (oo)cysts (80.7%) was significant ($P < 0.05$) in all plants (Table 2). A similar reduction was observed in helminth eggs by municipal WWTPs and livestock SWWTPs ($P < 0.05$); however, the difference in reduction was not significant ($P > 0.110$) in WWTP 3 (Table 3).

The rate of egg overall removal in plants 1, 2, 3, 4 and 5 was 94.8, 95, 95.5, 95.5 and 95.7%, respectively (Table 4).

Overall removal efficiencies of protozoa (oo)cysts were also 81, 83.6, 85.8, 79.3 and 80.9% for plansts 1, 2, 3, 4 and 5, respectively (Table 4).

Discussion

The role played by animal and human wastewaters as sources of parasitic pathogens infecting human is very significant [19].

Many of these intestinal parasites of domestic animals are zoonotic and can be transmitted to humans through ingestion of eggs or (oo)cysts in contamintated water and food (vegetables) and those that do not cause human disease cause severe disease in livestock and have the potential to cause substantial economic losses.

The infected hosts, whether human or animal, shed large numbers of (oo)cysts and eggs via the faeces into the environment, and these parasites are very resistant and may survive in the environment for over a year [20,21].

Moreover, disinfection processes cannot destroy protozoa (oo)cyst and helminths egg, and they have been found in the final effluents of treatment plants [22].

In this study 108 samples were analysed in order to compare the presence of parasitic fauna in untreated and treated wastewaters contaminated by human and livestock feces.

In urban wastewater samples, *Entamoeba coli*, *Entamoeba histolytica*/*dispar*/*moshkovskii*, *Giardia* spp., *Isospora* spp., *Cryptosporidium* spp. and *Chilomastix mesnili* were found.

Our investigation of the municipal treatment plants revealed that *Entamoeba* spp. and *Giardia* spp. were ubiquitous, whereas *Cryptosporidium* spp. were quite rare. Results reported in our study correspond with those from

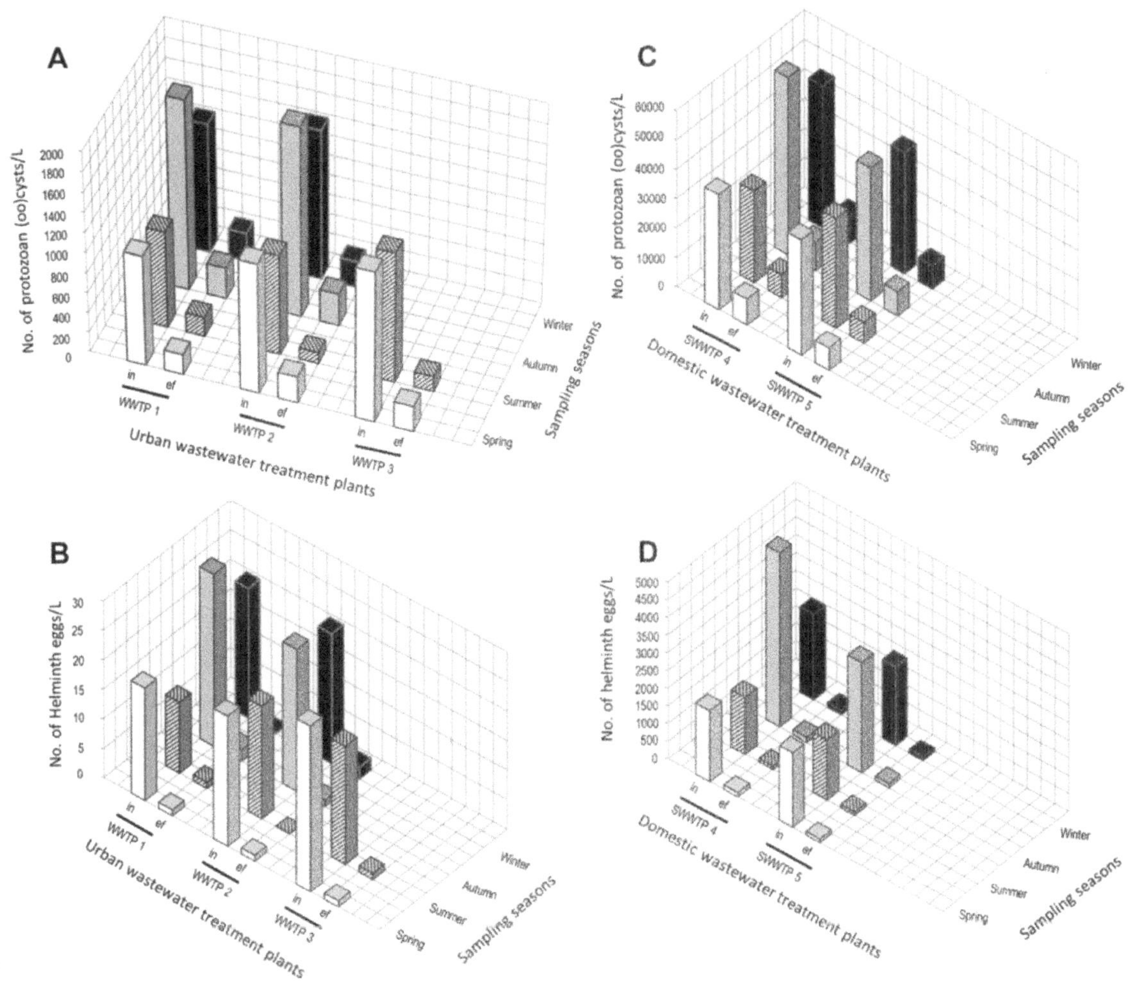

Figure 5 Number of protozoan (oo)cysts and helminth eggs in wastewater influent samples. (A) Protozoan (oo)cysts/L of urban wastewaters; **(B)** helminth eggs/L of urban wastewaters; **(C)** protozoan (oo)cysts/L of slaughterhouse wastewaters; **(D)** helminth eggs/L of slaughterhouse wastewaters (in = influent samples; ef = effluent samples).

studies published in several countries. Studies carried out in Italia [13,23], China [24], France [25], Malaysia [26], Tunisia [27,28] reported a prominence of *Giardia duodenalis* and *Entamoeba* spp. in municipal raw wastewaters. In a recent study conducted by Kitajima and colleagues [29] in the USA, 24 raw wastewater samples from 2 municipal treatment plants were analyzed for the presence of *Giardia* and *Cryptosporidium*, that the mean concentration of cysts in the influent has been higher than that of oocysts (4800–6400 versus 74–100 (oo)cysts per liter).

In domestic wastewater samples, *Eimeria* spp., *Entamoeba* spp. and *Giardia duodenalis* were frequently descried.

Similar prevalence rates were reported in raw wastewater collected at a slaughterhouse treatment plant in Tabriz, a city in the northwest of Iran, where the species of *E. ahsata*, *E. ovina*, *E. Faurei*, *E. parva*, *E. pallida* and *E. intricata* were identified [30].

In our study, some of the uni-, tetra-, and octanucleated cyst-forming *Entamoeba* species were detected. *Entamoeba wenyoni* in goats is a species of amoebas that has octanucleated cysts. The taxonomic status of these uninucleated *Entamoeba* species over the years has been confusing. They have been identified in cattle, sheep and goats, and have been given separate names, such as *E. bovis* in cattle, *E. ovis* in sheep and *E. debliecki* in goats. However, the various species cannot be distinguished from each other morphologically, and whether they occur in humans or are even genetically distinct remains to be established [31].

The types of helminths ova were observed in this study included gastrointestinal nematodes, cestodes and trematodes.

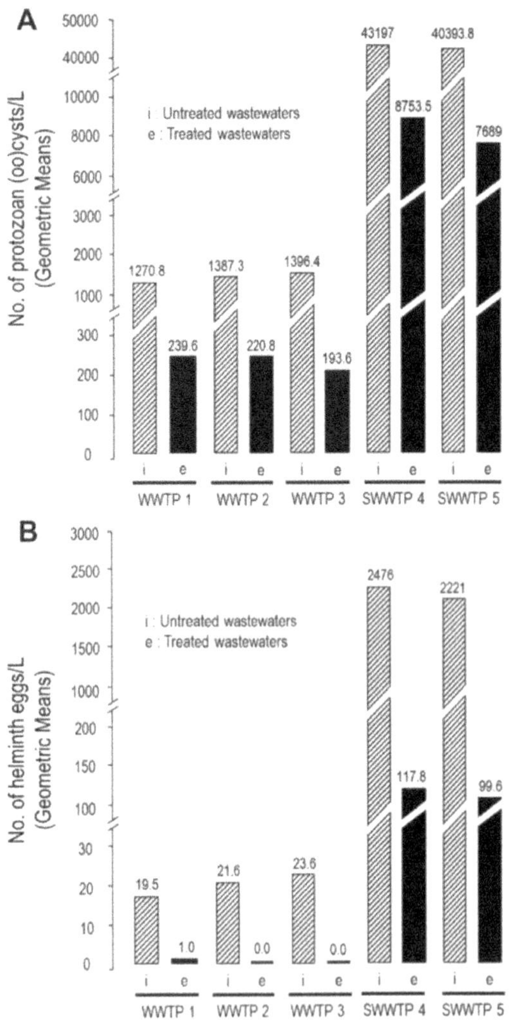

Figure 6 Geometric mean concentrations of protozoan (oo)cysts (A), and helminth eggs (B) per liter of raw and treated wastewater samples from urban (WWTPs) and domestic wastewater tratment plants (SWWTPs).

In the current study, eggs of 5 genus of parasitic helminths were detected in livestock wastewaters: *Trichostrongylus* spp., *Moniezia spp.*, *Fasciola hepatica*, *Trichuris* spp. and *Dicrocoelum dendriticum.*

We also found eggs of 4 genus of parasitic helminths in municipal wastewaters: hookworms (*Ancylostoma duodenale* and *Necator americanus*), *Hymenolepis diminuta* and *Rhabditis* spp. (thin-shell eggs and rhabditoid larvae). These eggs and larvae may be related to the free living forms of *Strongyloides stercoralis.*

It was difficult to distinguish individual species of some parasitic helminths whose eggs and larvae were observed (*Strongyloides* spp, *Rhabditis* spp., *Trichostrongylus* spp. and hookworms), and due to the other objectives pursued in our research project and financial constraints, we did not incubate the above mentioned nematode eggs in order to test their viability.

Results reported in our study correspond with those from studies published in Tehran, Isfahan and Shahrekord cities by our colleagues [10,32].

In our study, helminth ova content in municipal raw wastewater was lower than that reported by Sharafi et al. [33].

Raw wastewater helminth ova contamination found in our study is higher than those of reported for developed countries such as the United State America (1–8 egg per liter) and France (9 egg per liter) and is lower than those of reported for developing countries such as Brazil (166–202 egg per liter), Morocco (840 egg per liter), Jordan (300 egg per liter) [34].

We never found eggs of *Ascaris, Taenia saginata, Enterobius vermicularis* and *Hymenolepis nana* in untreated human wastewater samples. Most of the eggs were related to aquatic and soil nematodes that are nonpathogenic and the causative agent of spurious infection in humans. In most other studies, these nematode eggs have been reported as Strongyles.

It could stem from the fact that the prevalence of these entric parasites is low in Tehran in the recent years and the fact that eggs of *Enterobius vermicularis* and *Hymenolepis nana* cannot survive in wastewater and are quickly destroyed [35]. *E. vermicularis* and *H. nana* have a direct life cycle and this probably is the secret of their survival.

However, we found some intact eggs of *Hymenolepis diminuta* in urban raw wastewater. This cestode is a common parasite of rats living in sewage drains.

This has led to the suggestion that the enumeration of enteric parasites in wastewaters can be used as an indicator of infection level within a community [36].

Results of parasite removal efficiencies of treatment plants from each of these studies are not strictly comparable since treatment processes were done on different ways. In addition, because of differences in analyses methodologies, the timeframes in which studies were undertaken and how and where samples were collected.

The overall removal efficiency ranged from 79.3 to 85.8% for (oo)cysts and from 94.8 to 95.7% for eggs at the different plants, which is consistent with estimates from other treatment plants that use similar processes [10,33]. Helminth eggs were generally removed more effectively than protozoan (oo)cysts.

Performance for secondary treatment systems for egg removal range from 88 to 97%, whereas removal of (oo) cyst is more variable ranging from 80 to 97% [37].

The highest egg removal efficiency was at SWWTP5 (95.7%) and the highest (oo)cysts removal efficiency was

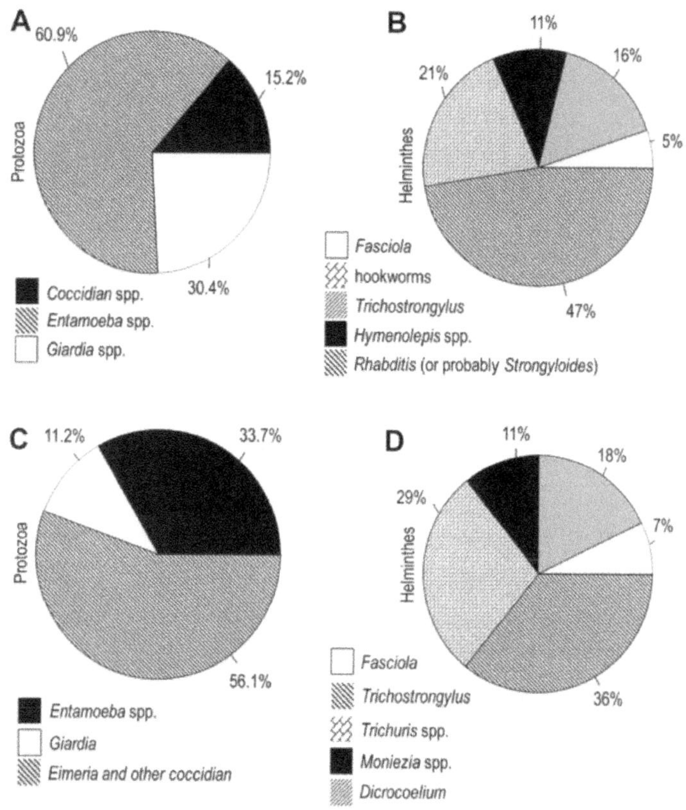

Figure 7 Cumulative percentages of protozoa (oo)cysts and helminth eggs in raw wastewaters. (A) and **(B)** municipal wastewaters; **(C)** and **(D)** slaughterhouse wastewaters.

at WWTP3, perhaps as a consequence of employing the trickling filter followed by activated sludge as secondary treatment system.

In the UK Robertson and colleagues reported more variable protozoan removal of 15–99% in activated sludge compared to 5–85% removal in trickling filters but no significant difference in efficacy of protozoan removal was found between the two processes [38].

Table 2 The mean concentrations of protozoan (oo)cyst in raw and treated wastewaters

Wastewater treatment plants	†No. of protozoan (oo)cysts/L samples		Mean difference	P-value
	Influent	Effluent		
WWTP1	1315.0 ± 414.2	245.0 ± 59.2	1070.0	0.010
WWTP2	1425.0 ± 377.5	237.5 ± 89.6	1187.5	0.004
WWTP3	1400.0 ± 141.4	200.0 ± 70.7	1200.0	0.027
SWWTP4	44500.0 ± 12449.0	8775.0 ± 694.6	35725.0	0.009
SWWTP5	40500.0 ± 3415.7	7700.0 ± 469.0	32800.0	<0.001

†Mean ± SD.

The overall mean reduction in protozoan (oo)cysts (80.7%) was significant ($P < 0.05$) in municipal WWTPs. A similar reduction was also observed in helminth eggs by municipal WWTPs ($P < 0.05$). The difference in reduction was not significant ($P > 0.110$) in WWTP 3; however, the number of egg in wastewater effluents of the three urban plants was in compliance with the WHO parasitological guideline (<1 nematode per liter) required for irrigation purposes.

The activated sludge process was employed in both SWWTP 1 and SWWTP 2, and their overall mean removal efficiencies were 79.3 ± 4.1 and 80.9 ± 0.5 for (oo) cysts and, 95 ± 1.5 and 95.5 ± 0.7 for eggs. In these plants, the overall mean reduction of (oo)cysts and eggs was significant ($P < 0.05$); however, the number of egg in treated wastewater was not in compliance with the WHO parasitological guidelines.

However, it should be noted that the two slaughterhouse plants were too old and there was no one to give us enough information about the plants.

In these abattoirs, we observed that the rumen contents of slaughtered animals were shipped separately and

Table 3 The mean concentrations of helminth egg in raw and treated wastewaters

Wastewater treatment plants	†No. helminth eggs/L samples		Mean difference	P-value
	Influent	Effluent		
WWTP1	20.5 ± 7.0	1.0 ± 0.8	19.5	0.010
WWTP2	21.8 ± 2.1	1.0 ± 0.8	20.8	<0.001
WWTP3	24.0 ± 5.7	1.0 ± 0.0	23.0	0.110
SWWTP4	2725.0 ± 1486.3	118.0 ± 16.7	2607.0	0.038
SWWTP5	2275.0 ± 76.8	100.0 ± 9.5	2175.0	0.005

†Mean ± SD.

used for agricultural-land fertilization and hence, it is thought that the use of slaughterhouse wastewater treatment plant is symbolic.

In the present study, in relation to the raw wastewater samples which were analysed by centrifugal-(water-ether) concentration procedure, primary sedimentation resulted in deposition of all particles and secondary sedimentation (the water-ether concentration) resulted in less turbid samples which could be more easily analysed with microscopic method. The use of this procedure significantly improves parasite (oo)cyst and egg purification, particularly for very turbid samples, and is recommended for use in epidemiological studies in which not only (oo) cyst and ova enumeration but also viability assessment are required.

Disadvantage of the membrane filter acetone-dissolution method is the hardening of the pellet containing particles after the centrifugation step and contributes to the overall ≥30 loss of parasitic particles. In addition, the study conducted by Carreno et al. found that the exposure of *Cryptosporidium* oocysts to solutions used for cellulose acetate membrane dissolution filtration reduce their infectivity in HCT-8 cells [39].

The RM method could potentially be used for monitoring parasitic particles in treated wastewater samples and not raw wastewaters in which contain high concentrations of suspended solids.

In the Bailenger method, background solids from the raw wastewater that are immersed in supernatant, not settled solids and particles with a density > 1.05, may have interfered with the precipitation of coccidian oocysts and other protozoan cysts, hence contributing to the overall 30-50% loss.

Dead (oo)cysts are lighter than live (oo)cysts and their settlement is not coincide with the deposition of live (oo)cysts. Therefore, the modified Bailenger method selectively concentrate viable (oo)cysts and more time may be required for settling parasite particles.

We found some of parasite particles consisting of helminth ova and protozoan (oo)cyst (along with trophozoite forms) in municipal and domestic treated wasewater samples.

Also, we found some of free-living protozoa in treated wasewater samples. A complete list of 228 species of protozoa has been reported by [40]. These microorganisms are commonly found in activated sludge and may be mistaken with human parasites.

Disinfection processes in the domestic and municipal wastewater treatment plants cannot destroy protozoa cyst and helminths egg, and they have been found in the final effluents of treatment plants [3,4,41].

Our data provide the first information about the distribution of the zoonotic parasitic particles in wastewater samples from treatment plants and slaughterhouses in Iran. A few studies described the presence of anthroponotic parasites in comparison with zoonotic parasites in faecal samples [25,42,43].

Conclusions

According to the results the efficiency of removal of nematode eggs and protozoan (oo)cysts in domestic wastewater treatment plants not only is not in compliance with the guidelines for the microbiological quality

Table 4 Overall mean removal efficiency of treatment plants for (oo)cysts and eggs

Sampling seasons	WWTP1		WWTP 2		WWTP 3		SWWTP 4		SWWTP 5	
	Removal efficiency*		Removal efficiency		Removal efficiency		Removal efficiency		Removal efficiency	
	Cysts and oocysts	Eggs	Cysts and oocysts	Eggs	Cysts and oocysts	Eggs	Cysts and oocysts	Eggs	Cysts and oocysts	Eggs
Spring	81.8	94.7	80	95.4	83.3	92.9	77.4	94	80.5	95.3
Summer	80.2	91.7	89	94.7	88.4	95	74.8	94	80.8	94.7
Autumn	83.6	93.1	83.1	91.6	ND**	ND	84.3	97.2	81.7	96.3
Winter	78.4	95.4	82.6	90.9	ND	ND	81	94.8	80.7	95.4
Overall mean ± SD†	81 ± 2	93.7 ± 1.6	83.6 ± 3.8	95.5 ± 3.7	85.8 ± 3.6	95.7 ± 0.9	79.3 ± 4.1	95 ± 1.5	80.9 ± 0.5	95.5 ± 0.7

*Removal efficiency calculated as a persentage (%).
**ND, no data.
†Mean removal efficiency (%) ± SD.
Results are expressed as the mean percentage removal efficiency and ± SD.

of treated wastewater used in agriculture but it also is at an alarming rate.

The release of contaminated outflows into surface waters and the use of these contaminated effluents for irrigation activities could increase the risk of human infection with these zoonotic parasites through the consumption of raw fruits and vegetables.

The study results revealed that the efficacy of removal of nematode ova in urban wastewater treatment plants, and not protozoan (oo)cysts, is in compliance with the WHO parasitological guideline (<1 nematode per liter) required for irrigation purposes.

This emphasizes the importance of the protozological control of effluents from urban wastewater treatment plants and the need for regulations that establish the acceptable concentrations of protozoan (oo)cysts based on the use of effluents, i.e., if they should be recycled in the cities for public, for industry, or for irrigation of corps.

However, in many areas, urban wastwater is directly used for the irrigation of corps and animal waste is used for agricultural-land fertilization and hence, these corps are contaminated with some of the zoonotic enteric parasites. Therefore, this is a way for these pathogens to travel further up the food chain, and this could be potential health risk associated with the agriculture application of sludges, manures and raw wastewaters for agricultural irrigation.

Abbreviations
WWTPs: Wastewater treatment plants; SWWTPs: Slaughterhouse wastewater treatment plants; BOD: Biochemical oxygen demand; TSS: Total suspended solids; A2/O: Anaerobic/anoxic/oxic; NTU: Nephelometric turbidity unit; MB: Modified Bailenger method; RM: Scraping and rinsing of membrane method; ADM: Acetone-dissolution method; CC: Centrifugal-(water-ether) concentration method.

Competing interests
The authors declare that they have no competing interests.

Authors' contributions
The overall implementation of this study was the results of efforts of all authors. All authors read and approved the final manuscript.

Acknowledgement
We thank Dr. Hamidreza Tashayoi and Mr. Rouhi at the Iran Water and Wastewater Treatment Company for their administrative cooperation. We are also grateful to Dr. Ahmadreza Meamar for providing *Giardia* cysts and to Dr. Khadijeh Khanaliha, Fatemeh Tarighi, Shohreh Farnia, Tahereh Rezaeian, Sorour Charehdar and Dr. Mohhamadbagher Molaei-Rad for their assistance in examination of wastewater. This result is a part of Ph.D. thesis for receiving Ph.D. degree in medical parasitology from the school of Public Health Tehran University of Medical Sciences. This study received financial support from research grant 92-02-160-23616, entitled "Assessment of phenotypic and genotypic of *Giardia* and *Cryptosporidium* in the influent and in the effluent of human and domestic animal wastewater treatment plants of Tehran" of the Institute for Environmental Research (IER), Tehran University of Medical Sciences, and Center for Research of Endemic Parasites of Iran (CREPI), Tehran University of Medical Sciences.

Author details
[1]Department of Medical Parasitology and Mycology, School of Public Health, Tehran University of Medical Sciences, Tehran, Iran. [2]Department of Environmental Health Engineering, School of Public Health, and Center for Water Quality Research, Institute for Environmental Research, Tehran University of Medical Sciences, Tehran, Iran. [3]Center for Research of Endemic Parasites of Iran (CREPI), Tehran University of Medical Sciences, Tehran, Iran.

References

1. Moe CL, Rheingans RD. Global challenges in water, sanitation and health. J Water Health. 2006;4 Suppl 1:41–5.
2. Hussain I, Raschid L, Hanjra MA, Marikar F, van der Hoek W. Wastewater use in agriculture: review of impacts and methodological issues in valuing impacts. Colombo, Sri Lanka: International Water Management Institute; 2002.
3. Levine AD, Asano T. Recovering sustainable water from wastewater. Environ Sci Technol. 2004;38:201A–8A.
4. Cai L, Zhang T. Detecting human bacterial pathogens in wastewater treatment plants by a high-throughput shotgun sequencing technique. Environ Sci Technol. 2013;47:5433–41.
5. Huang DB, White AC. An updated review on *Cryptosporidium* and *Giardia*. Gastroenterol Clin North Am. 2006;35:291–314.
6. Karanis P, Kourenti C, Smith H. Waterborne transmission of protozoan parasites: a worldwide review of outbreaks and lessons learnt. J Water Health. 2007;5:1–38.
7. WHO reports and collaborative reports. Control of foodborne trematode infections, Technical Report Series 849. World Health Organ Tech Rep Ser. 1995;849:1–157. http://apps.who.int/iris/handle/10665/41544.
8. Guandalini S. Textbook of Pediatric Gastroenterology and Nutrition. Florida, United States: CRC Press; 2004.
9. Gharavi M, Jahani M, Rokni M. Parasitic contamination of vegetables from farms and markets in Tehran. Iranian J Pub Health. 2002;31:83–6.
10. Mahvi A, Kia E. Helminth eggs in raw and treated wastewater in the Islamic Republic of Iran. East Mediterr Health J. 2006;12:137–43.
11. Fallah E, Mahdavi Poor B, Jamali R, Hatam-Nahavandi K, Asgharzadeh M. Molecular characterization of *Cryptosporidium* isolates from cattle in a slaughterhouse in Tabriz, Northwestern Iran. J Biol Sci. 2008;8:639–43.
12. Mahmoudi M, Ashrafi K, Abedinzadeh H, Tahvildar-Bideruni F, Haghighi A, Bandehpour M, et al. Development of sensitive detection of *Cryptosporidium* and *Giardia* from surface water in Iran. Iranian J Parasitol. 2011;6:43–51.
13. Cacciò SM, De Giacomo M, Aulicino FA, Pozio E. *Giardia* cysts in wastewater treatment plants in Italy. Appl Environ Microbiol. 2003;69:3393–8.
14. Franco RMB, Rocha-Eberhardt R, Cantusio Neto R. Occurrence of *Cryptosporidium* oocysts and *Giardia* cysts in raw water from the Atibaia river, Campinas, Brazil. Rev Inst Med Trop São Paulo. 2001;43(2):109–11.
15. Skotarczak B. Methods for parasitic protozoans detection in the environmental samples. Parasite. 2009;16:183–90.
16. Bukhari Z, Smith H. Effect of three concentration techniques on viability of *Cryptosporidium parvum* oocysts recovered from bovine feces. J Clin Microbiol. 1995;33:2592–5.
17. Zajac AM, Conboy GA. Veterinary Clinical Parasitology. Hoboken, New Jersey: John Wiley & Sons; 2012.
18. Ayres RM, Mara DD. Analysis of Wastewater for use in Agriculture: a Laboratory Manual of Parasitological and Bacteriological Techniques. Geneva: World Health Organization; 1996.
19. Dufour AP, Dufour A. Animal Wastewater Quality and Human Health. United Kingdom: IWA Publishing; 2012.
20. Olson M. Human and animal pathogens in manure. In: Conference on Livestock Options for the Future: 25-27 June 2001. Winnepeg: Manitoba, Canada: Agriculture and Agri-Food Canada; 2001. http://www.gov.mb.ca/agriculture/livestock/livestockopt/papers/olson.pdf.
21. Wichuk KM, McCartney D. A review of the effectiveness of current time-temperature regulations on pathogen inactivation during composting. J Environ Engin Sci. 2007;6:573–86.
22. Plym-Forshell L. Survival of salmonellas and Ascaris suum eggs in a thermophilic biogas plant. Acta Vet Scand. 1994;36:79–85.
23. Brandonisio O, Portincasa F, Torchetti G, Lacarpia N, Rizzi A, Fumarola L, et al. *Giardia* and *Cryptosporidium* in water: evaluation of two concentration methods and occurrence in wastewater. Parassitologia. 2000;42:205–9.
24. Li N, Xiao L, Wang L, Zhao S, Zhao X, Duan L, et al. Molecular surveillance of Cryptosporidium spp., Giardia duodenalis, and Enterocytozoon bieneusi by genotyping and subtyping parasites in wastewater. PLoS Negl Trop Dis. 2012;6:e1809.

25. Bertrand I, Schwartzbrod J. Detection and genotyping of *Giardia duodenalis* in wastewater: RELATION between assemblages and faecal contamination origin. Water Res. 2007;41:3675–82.
26. Lim Y, Wan Hafiz W, Nissapatom V. Reduction of *Cryptosporidium* and *Giardia* by sewage treatment processes. Tropical Biomed. 2007;24:95–104.
27. Khouja LBA, Cama V, Xiao L. Parasitic contamination in wastewater and sludge samples in Tunisia using three different detection techniques. Parasitol Res. 2010;107:109–16.
28. Layla BA, Yang W, Widmer G, Cama V, Ortega Y, Xiao L. Survey and genetic characterization of wastewater in Tunisia for *Cryptosporidium* spp., *Giardia duodenalis*, *Enterocytozoon bieneusi*, *Cyclospora cayetanensis* and *Eimeria* spp. J Water Health. 2012;10:431–44.
29. Kitajima M, Haramoto E, Iker BC, Gerba CP. Occurrence of *Cryptosporidium*, *Giardia*, and *Cyclospora* in influent and effluent water at wastewater treatment plants in Arizona. Sci Total Environ. 2014;484:129–36.
30. Yakhchali M, Zarei M. Prevalence of *Eimeria* infection in sheep of Tabriz suburb, Iran. Iran J Vet Res. 2008;9:277–80.
31. Verweij JJ, Polderman AM, Clark CG. Genetic variation among human isolates of uninucleated cyst-producing *Entamoeba* species. J Clin Microbiol. 2001;39:1644–6.
32. Miranzadeh M, Mahmodi S. Investigation into the removal of nematodes eggs in influent and effluent of shoosh wastewater treatment plant. J Water Wastewater. 2002;42:32–6 (In persian).
33. Sharafi K, Fazlzadehdavil M, Pirsaheb M, Derayat J, Hazrati S. The comparison of parasite eggs and protozoan cysts of urban raw wastewater and efficiency of various wastewater treatment systems to remove them. Ecol Eng. 2012;44:244–8.
34. Jimenez B. Helminth ova removal from wastewater for agriculture and aquaculture reuse. Water Sci Technol. 2007;55:485–93.
35. Horak P. Helminth eggs in the sludge from three sewage treatment plants in Czechoslovakia. Folia Parasitol . 1992;39:153–7.
36. Jakubowski W, Sykora JL, Sorber CA, Casson LW, Gavaghan PD. Determining giardiasis prevalence by examination of sewage. Water Sci Technol. 1991;24:173–8.
37. Mara D, Horan NJ. Handbook of water and wastewater microbiology. 2003. Academic press.
38. Robertson L, Paton CA, Campbell AT, Smith PG, Jackson MH, Gilmour RA, et al. *Giardia* cysts and *Cryptosporidium* oocysts at sewage treatment works in Scotland, UK. Water Res. 2000;34:2310–22.
39. Carreno RA, Pokorny NJ, Weir SC, Lee H, Trevors JT. Decrease in *Cryptosporidium parvum* oocyst infectivity in vitro by using the membrane filter dissolution method for recovering oocysts from water samples. Appl Environ Microbiol. 2001;67:3309–13.
40. Madoni P. Protozoa in wastewater treatment processes: a minireview. Ital J Zool. 2011;78:3–11.
41. Toze S. Microbial Pathogens in Wastewater: Literature Review for Urban Water Systems Multi-divisional Research Program. Australia: CSIRO Land and Water; 1997.
42. Bjorkman C, Svensson C, Christensson B, de Verdier K. *Cryptosporidium parvum* and *Giardia intestinalis* in calf diarrhoea in Sweden. Acta Vet Scand. 2003;44:145–52.
43. Hutchison M, Walters LD, Avery SM, Synge BA, Moore A. Levels of zoonotic agents in British livestock manures. Lett Appl Microbiol. 2004;39:207–14.

Liquid Phase adsorption kinetics and equilibrium of toluene by novel modified-diatomite

Reza Khalighi Sheshdeh[1*], Saeed Abbasizadeh[2], Mohammad Reza Khosravi Nikou[3], Khashayar Badii[4] and Mohammad Sadegh Sharafi[3]

Abstract

The adsorption equilibria of toluene from aqueous solutions on natural and modified diatomite were examined at different operation parameters such as pH, contact time, initial toluene concentration was evaluated and optimum experimental conditions were identified. The surface area and morphology of the nanoparticles were characterized by SEM, BET, XRD, FTIR and EDX analysis. It was found that in order to obtain the highest possible removal of toluene, the experiments can be carried out at pH *6*, temperature *25C* , an agitation speed of *200 rpm*, an initial toluene concentration of *150 mg/L*, a centrifugal rate of 4000 rpm, adsorbent dosage = *0.1 g* and a process time of *90 min*. The results of this work show that the maximum percentage removal of toluene from aqueous solution in the optimum conditions for NONMD was *96.91%* (*145.36 mg/g*). Furthermore, under same conditions, the maximum adsorption of natural diatomite was *71.45%* (*107.18 mg/g*). Both adsorption kinetic and isotherm experiments were carried out. The experimental data showed that the adsorption follows the Langmuir model and Freundlich model on natural and modified diatomite respectively. The kinetics results were found to conform well to pseudo-second order kinetics model with good correlation. Thus, this study demonstrated that the modified diatomite could be used as potential adsorbent for removal of toluene from aqueous solution.

Keywords: Diatomite, Adsorption, Toluene, Isotherm, Kinetics

Introduction

Wastewater pollutants discharged from pharmaceutical and chemical industries contain various types of aromatic compounds, such as toluene, pyridine, and nitrobenzene, which are very harmful to human health and the ecosystem [1]. In the past decades, extensive attention has been paid to develop efficient and cost-effective methods for removal of these pollutants. Various technologies were used for the treatment of organic pollutants, including adsorption, biodegradation, chemical oxidation, photo-degradation, solvent extraction, membrane separation, etc. [2,3]. Among these approaches, adsorption is still the most versatile and widely used method because of its high efficiency and simple operation conditions. Various adsorbents, such as active carbon, coal, fly ash, modified clays, polymeric resins, metal oxides, silicas, and zeolites, were applied to adsorb aromatic compounds in aqueous solutions [4-7]. For example, Roostaei and Tezel investigated toluene or benzene adsorption on silica gel, activated alumina, activated carbon, and zeolites, and found that the latter two materials provide a higher adsorption capacity for phenol [8-10]. Rodriguez and co-workers described activated carbons as good adsorbents for toluene and benzene [11-13]. Magnetic porous carbon microspheres have been reported with good adsorption properties for toluene and benzene [14-16]. Toluene and benzene and often coexist in wastewater because they are widely used in many industrial products and processes. Due to their biological toxicity to microorganisms, traditional biotreatment cannot be applied for an economical and effective degradation. Additionally, their coexistence will lead to the loss of degradation ability of bacteria to other pollutants [17-19]. Therefore, it is necessary to separate benzene and toluene from wastewater prior to their discharge into water bodies. Toluene is a typical indoor pollutant and its discharge may produce irritation of the eyes and the respiratory tract, nausea,

* Correspondence: rezakhalighi@yahoo.com
[1]School of Chemical Engineering, College of Engineering, University of Tehran, Tehran, Iran
Full list of author information is available at the end of the article

headache, fatigue, dullness and thirst, even at very low concentrations [4-8]. Toluene is well known for its neurotoxicity and exposure to it may decrease neuronal activities in vitro and cause mental depression and cognitive impairment in humans [1,6]. Toluene inhalation also results in various symptoms such as fatigue, headache, vertigo and ataxia. It is rapidly absorbed through respiratory and gastrointestinal tracts and, to a lesser extent, through the skin. American Conference of Governmental Industrial Hygienists (ACGIH) has recommended an *8-h* time-weighted average (TWA) of *50 ppm* (*189 mg/m*^{3}) for toluene to protect against effects on the central nervous system. These studies also confirmed that porosity and surface oxygen group content have major influences on low-concentration-*VOC* adsorption [18-20]. Natural diatomite ($SiO_2 nH_2O$) is made up from the skeletons of aquatic plants called diatom that usually is a pale-coloured, soft, lightweight siliceous sedimentary rock [21]. Diatomite contains a wide variety of shape and sized diatoms, typically *10-200 μm*, in a structure including up to *80-90%* pore spaces [19-21]. Diatomite s extremely porous structure, low density and high surface area make it suitable as an adsorbent for organic and inorganic chemicals [22,23]. In general, the literature includes few experimental data for modified natural adsorbent for removal of VOCs pollutants. In the present investigation, for the first time, the usage of Nickel Oxide Nanoparticles-Modified Diatomite (NONMD) for the adsorption of toluene has been studied, as a less expensive adsorbent for removal of toluene from an aqueous medium. The equilibrium and kinetic study are investigated to observe the effects of various process parameters such as pH, contact time, initial toluene concentration, calcinations and sorbent dosage on the adsorption process. Equilibrium data are attempted by various adsorption isotherms including Langmuir, Freundlich and Brunauer-Emmett-Teller (BET) isotherms in order to select an appropriate isotherm model. Moreover, a kinetics study of the adsorption process is also considered to describe the rate of sorption. Comparing natural and modified diatomite (NONMD) well shows that this process was successful and the removal percentage increased [24,25].

Experimental procedure

Preparation of adsorbent

Diatomite sample was obtained from Tabriz, Iran. The sample was washed several times with distilled water and *HCl* (*1 M*) to remove fines and other adhered impurities and to achieve neutralization. The sample was finally filtered, dried at 60C for 24 h, and stored in closed containers for further use.

The nanoparticles of *NiO* were synthesized by using following reaction (Equation 1):

$$Ni_2SO_4 \quad 2NaOH \rightarrow Ni\ OH_{\ 2} \quad Na_2SO_4 \qquad 1$$

The nanoparticles of *NiO* were synthesized by adding $NiSO_4$ and *NaOH* (*1 M*) to the solution. It means that *2.0 g* of previously dried diatomite was added to *25 ml* of Nickel hydroxide (*1 M*), Stirrer speed of *200 rpm*, for *1 h*. The new material, *Ni*-diatomite was sequentially separated by filtration. The calcination process was carried out by placing Modified diatomite sample in the furnace at *250C* for *4.5 h*. The sample was then allowed to cool in a desiccator. The modified sample was used to examine the effect of nickel oxide nanoparticles, silanol groups and the role of pore size distribution on the adsorption process. FT-IR spectra and EDX analysis illustrate that the raise of metal oxide content at the modified diatomite can be the main reason for increasing the adsorption capacity. In industries, there are many heavy metals contaminated materials. Recovery of materials and clean up these contaminations is very difficult and expensive [26-34]. This investigation can be a useful method to change a poisonous industrial waste to a valuable by product.

Materials and solutions

Toluene (AR grade min. *99.6%* Merck) was supplied by Quick Lab Sdn. Bhd., Ipoh, Perak. Distilled water was throughout employed as solvent. For adsorption experiments, various concentrations of toluene solutions (*100, 150, 200, 250* and *300 mg/L*) were prepared. The pH measurements were made using Hach pH meter. These chemicals were purchased from Merck, Germany.

Adsorption procedure

The adsorption experiments were performed by mixing various amounts of diatomite (*0.03 0.12 g*) in *100 mL* of toluene solutions with varying concentrations (ranging from *100-300 mg/L*) at natural pH (*pH* = *6*). The natural pH to determine the maximum toluene removal could be achieved with diatomite, because this pH was more suitable for industrial purposes. Adsorption experiments were conducted at optimum amount of diatomite (*0.1 g*) at pH*6*, an agitation speed of *200 rpm* and temperature *25 1C* for *1 h* to attain equilibrium conditions. The changes of absorbance were determined at certain time intervals (*5, 10, 30, 60* and *90 min*) during the adsorption process. After adsorption experiments, the toluene solutions were centrifuged for 10 min in a Hettich EBA20 centrifuge at *4000 rpm* in order to separate the sorbent from the solution and toluene concentration was then determined. The amount of toluene adsorbed by the adsorbent at equilibrium, q_e *(mg/g)*, was calculated by using the following equation:

$$q_e \quad \frac{V\ C_0 - C_e}{W} \qquad 2$$

Where C_0 and C_e (mg/L) are the initial and equilibrium concentrations of toluene, respectively, V (L) is the volume of the toluene solution and W (g) is the adsorbent mass.

Analysis

The residual toluene concentrations in aqueous medium were determined using a Perkin-Elmer spectrophotometer corresponding to maximum wavelength (λ_{max}) of toluene. The XRD analysis was performed on natural and modified diatomite samples using a Philips Xpert x-ray diffractometer. Scanning electron microscopic (SEM) of both natural and modified diatomite were carried out using LEO 1455VP scanning electron microscope before and after modification process. The samples were coated with gold (Au) prior to the scanning in the electron microscope. By using nitrogen adsorption method the BET specific surface area adsorbents was measured, using Autosorb-*1MP* apparatus from Qantachrome at *77 K*. The analysis on compositions was determined by energy dispersive X-ray technique using EDX-System (Tescan Vega /2/ Instrument) which is fitted to the SEM instrument.

Results and discussion

Surface characterization

As the calcination process decreases the diatomite capacity for the removal of dye from aqueous solutions, therefore in this investigation, we decide to compare adsorption properties of modified diatomite with natural diatomite instead of modified diatomite. In order to explore the surface characteristics of diatomite, a Fourier Transformed Infra-Red (FTIR) analysis was performed in the range of *450* to $4000\ cm^{-1}$. Figure 1a and b show the FTIR spectra of natural and modified diatomite samples before the adsorption process, respectively. On the other hand, the FTIR spectra of both samples after the adsorption process are shown in Figure 2a and b. The FTIR spectral values and specific type of bonds are given in Table 1.

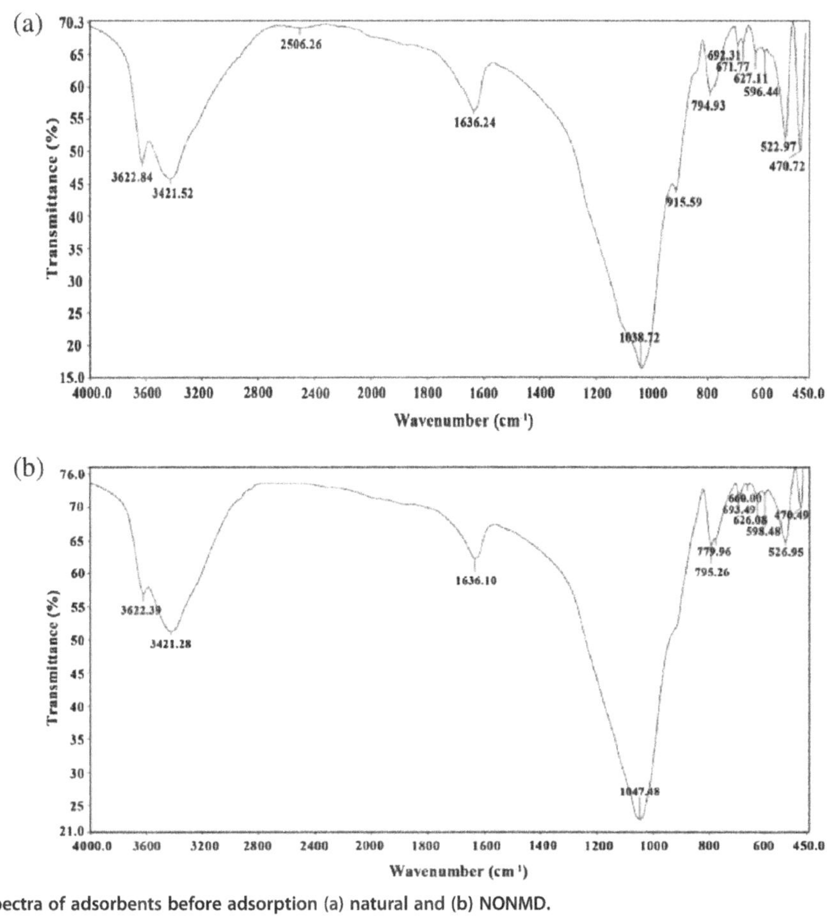

Figure 1 FT-IR spectra of adsorbents before adsorption (a) natural and (b) NONMD.

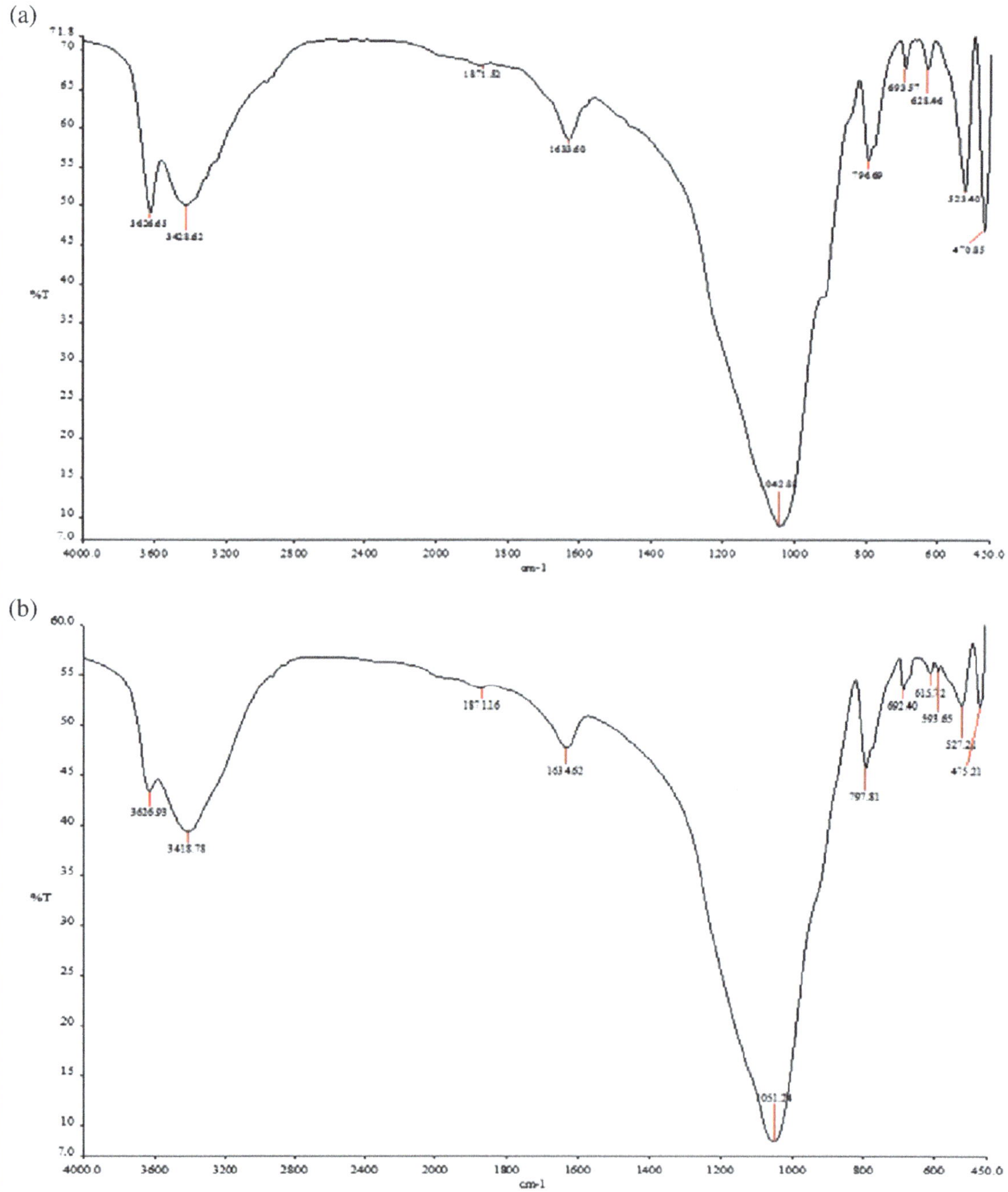

Figure 2 FT-IR spectra of adsorbents after adsorption (a) natural and (b) NONMD.

As can be seen in Figure 1b, the nickel content of NONMD is too low and there is a recognisable difference in this region regarding to nickel oxide nanoparticles on diatomite [35]. In addition, Figure 1a and b illustrate that the amount of silanol group has decreased slightly, and the metal oxide content has risen at the modified diatomite; however, the adsorption capacity has increased at NONMD. Comparison of Figures 1 and 2 show that there

Table 1 FTIR spectroscopy of spectra of natural and modified diatomite before and after the adsorption process

Steps	Adsorbents	Wavenumber (cm^{-1})	Specific type of bond
Before the adsorption process	Natural diatomite	470, 522, 596, 627, 671, 692	Si-O-Si bending vibration
		794, 915	SiO-H vibration
		1038	Siloxane group stretching (-Si-O-Si-)
		1636	Bending vibration of water (H-O-H)
		2506	Silanol group (Si-O-H)
		3421, 3622	Si-H
Before the adsorption process	Modified diatomite (NONMD)	470, 526, 598, 626, 660, 693	Si-O-Si bending vibration
		779, 795	SiO-H vibration
		1047	Siloxane group stretching (-Si-O-Si-)
		1636	Bending vibration of water (H-O-H)
		2506	Silanol group (Si-O-H)
		3421, 3622	Si-H
After the adsorption process	Natural diatomite	470, 523, 628, 693	Si-O-Si bending vibration
		796, 915	SiO-H vibration
		1042	Siloxane group stretching (-Si-O-Si-)
		1633	Bending vibration of water (H-O-H)
		1871	Combi group of aromatic rings
		2506	Silanol group (Si-O-H)
		3421, 3622	Si-H
After the adsorption process	Modified diatomite (NONMD)	475, 527, 593, 615, 692	Si-O-Si bending vibration
		797	SiO-H vibration
		1051	Siloxane group stretching (-Si-O-Si-)
		1634	Bending vibration of water (H-O-H)
		1871	Combi group of aromatic rings
		2506	Silanol group (Si-O-H)
		3418, 3626	Si-H

is a new peak at $1871\ cm^{-1}$ for the adsorption of dye (combi group of aromatic rings) on both samples after the adsorption process and peaks transmittance of silanol, siloxane, and metal oxide groups is slightly decreased in Figure 2.

Scanning electron micrographs (SEM) of natural and modified diatomite, before and after the adsorption process, are shown in Figure 3. These figures present that natural diatomite particles are amorphous, their pore spaces are lower than modified adsorbent, and particles of NONMD are more uniform and geometrical significantly. After modification and calcination process at *250C* , the structure of the adsorbent changed from amorphous sheets to semi-sphere shapes. Therefore, the volume of the pore spaces has increased, and the surface functional groups of modified diatomite have improved. Hence, the diffusion resistance of adsorption process has decreased, and the kinetics and capacity of dye adsorption process have risen. Moreover, adsorption of dye has caused a sticky phenomenon on structure of both adsorbents.

XRD analysis results of the natural and modified diatomite are shown in Figure 4. It can be seen from Figure 4 that the x-ray pattern of the natural diatomite is different from the pattern of the modified diatomite, suggesting that a phase transformation probably occurred during the modification and calcinations processes. The main composition of natural diatomite is quartz, anorthite and muscovite. It is evident that sanidine was appeared; while anorthite and muscovite were completely removed as the diatomite was calcined at *250C* .

In fact, some peaks in the diatomite disappeared and some peaks were created by modification process. It can be a trace of nickel oxide particles particles from modification process and ammonia ions because of calcination at high temperature and existence of nitrogen in air. Similar behaviour was previously investigated by other researchers [19,35].

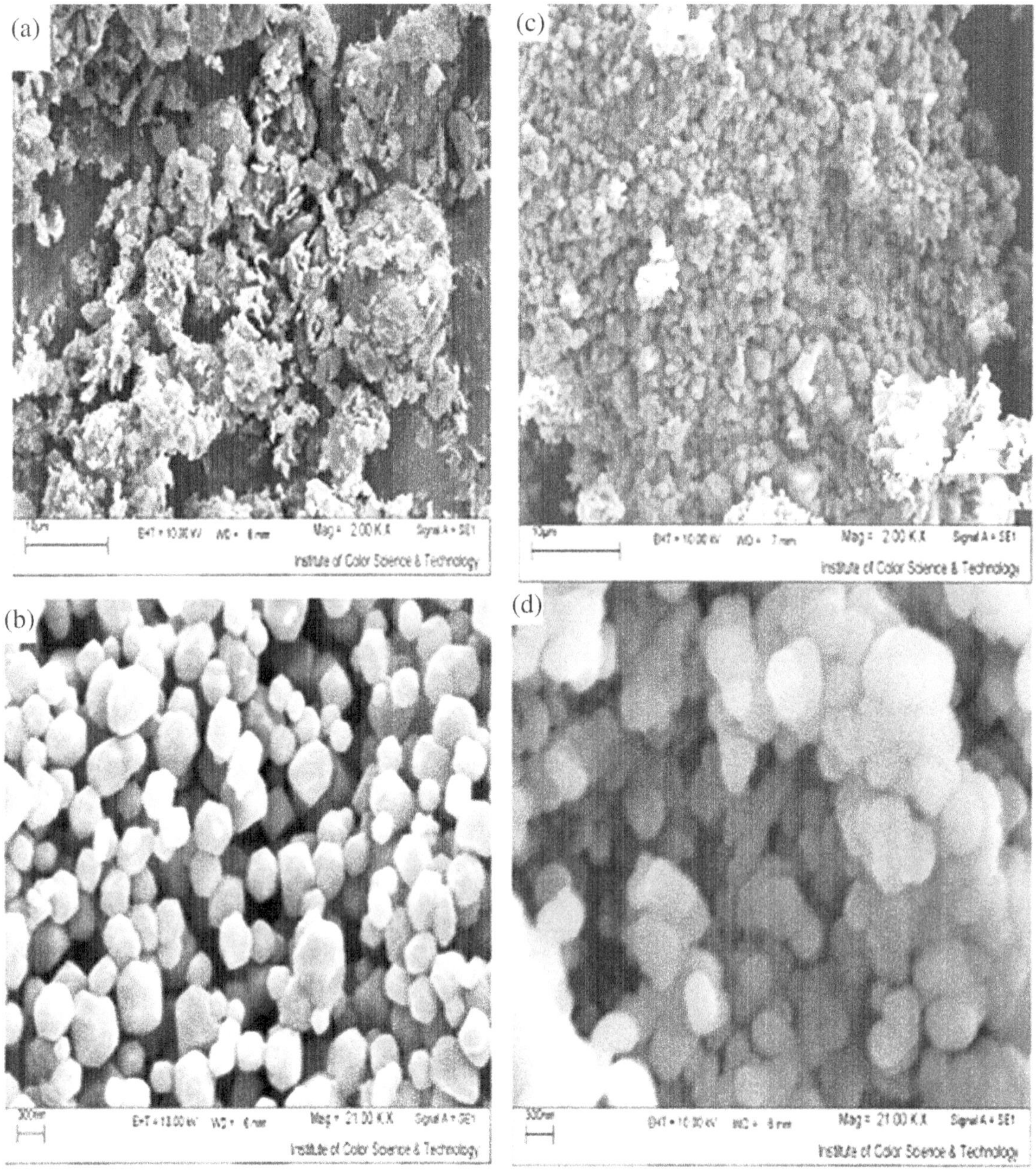

Figure 3 **Scanning electron micrographs before adsorption (a) natural and (b) NONMD, after adsorption (c) natural and (d) NONMD.**

As evident from EDX analyses (Figure 5), the natural diatomite did not have any Nickel but after modification process Ni was appeared (*3.96%W*). The surface area of the diatomite was determined by BET method (Figure 6). By using nitrogen adsorption method the BET specific surface area adsorbents was measured, using Autosorb-*1MP* apparatus from Qantachrome at *77 K*. In this investigation the values *7.5* (m^2/g) and *28.45* (m^2/g) for natural and modified diatomite were calculated respectively.

Effect of adsorbent dosage

The effect of natural and modified diatomite dosage on the adsorption of toluene was investigated at *25 1C* by varying the adsorbent amount from *0.03* to *0.12 g* while

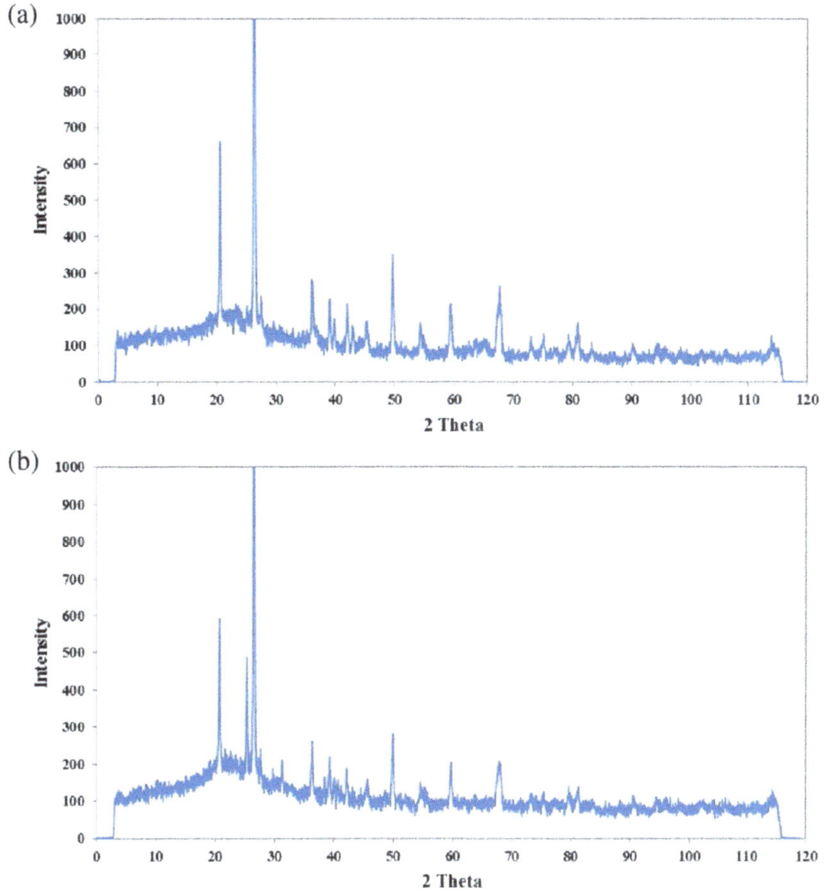

Figure 4 XRD patterns of (a) natural and (b) modified diatomite.

keeping the volume of toluene solution constant equal to *100 mL*, with an initial toluene concentration of *150 mg/L*. Figure 6 shows the percentage removal of toluene versus adsorbent amount. It is clear from the Figure 6, the removal percentage of toluene increased with an increase in the adsorbent amount. The main reason for this fact is due to the greater availability of the adsorption sites at higher concentrations of the adsorbent [19,35-37]. Based on the results shown in Figure 6, *0.1 g* of the natural and modified diatomite was used for further experiments.

Effect of initial toluene concentration

A change in the initial toluene concentration can considerably affect the adsorption process. Figure 7 depicts the effect of toluene concentration on the percentage removal of toluene by adsorbents. Evident from the Figure 7, when the toluene concentration increased from *100* to *300 mg/L* the percentage removal of toluene decreased from *97.68* to *88.09%* for modified and from *74.3* to *65.21* for natural diatomite.

As expected, when the concentration of toluene is increased, the limited capacity of the adsorbent checks any further adsorption of toluene and hence the overall removal percentage decreased.

Effect of contact time

The adsorption of toluene onto diatomite was evaluated as a function of contact time. Figure 8 shows the effect of contact time on the percentage removal of toluene in the aqueous phase by natural (Figure 8a) and modified diatomite (Figure 8b). The initial toluene concentration was varied from *100* to *300 mg/L*. At all initial toluene concentrations investigated, the adsorption occurs very fast initially. After *5 min* of adsorption process, the amount of adsorption by natural diatomite reaches to *66.99* and *64.09%* of the ultimate adsorption of toluene for initial

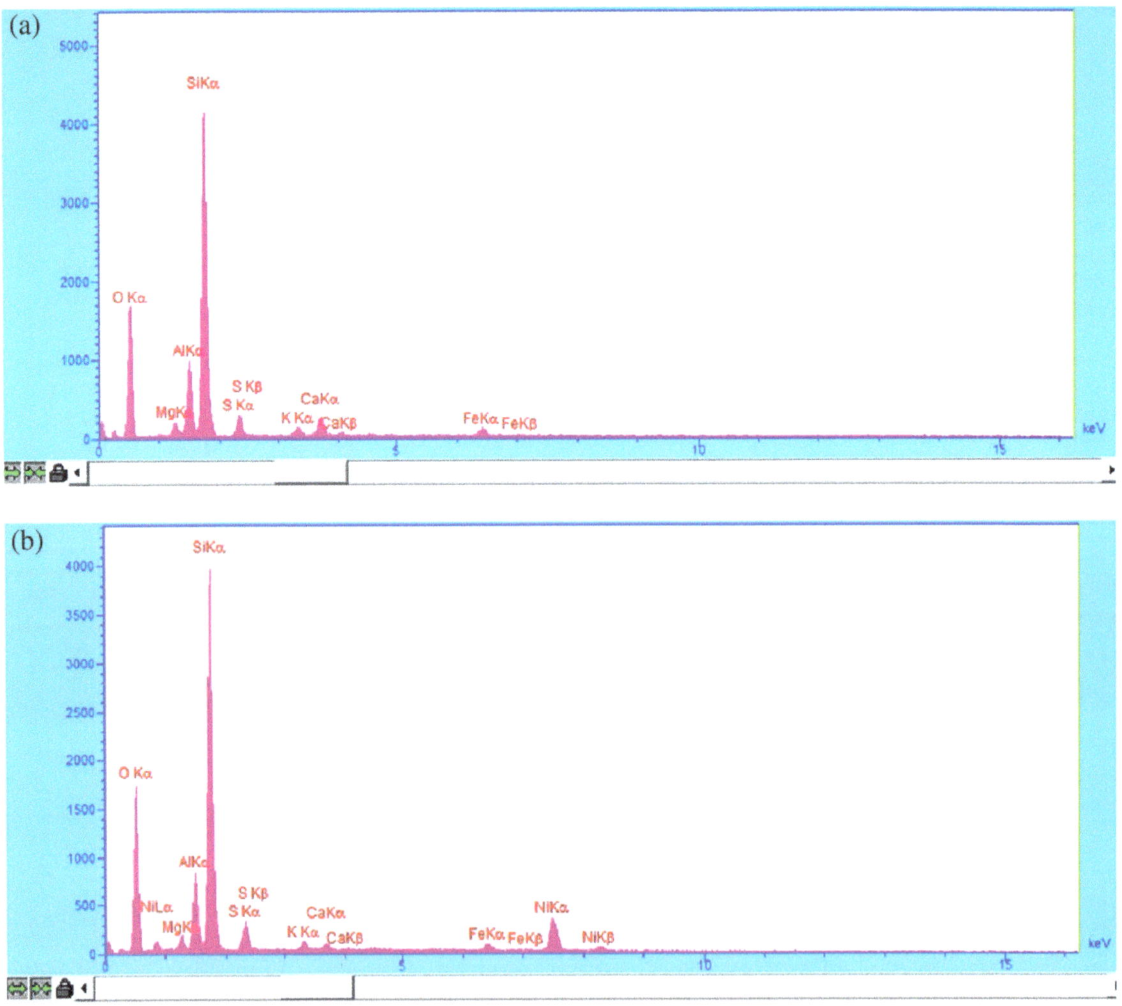

Figure 5 EDX patterns of (a) natural and (b) modified diatomite.

toluene concentrations of *100* and *150 mg/L* respectively. As illustrated in Figure 8b, the adsorption is also fast at early stage of the adsorption process for modified diatomite. Typically about *87.87%* of the ultimate adsorption of toluene with an initial concentration of *150 mg/L* takes place within the first *5 min* of contact and it almost remains constant thereafter. It means that the most of mass transfer resistance is in bulk of fluid and high rate agitation would decrease this resistant. In addition, these results show that the most of the toluene molecules are adsorbed on the external surface of the adsorbent, and transferred to the pores and internal surfaces layer. More experiments are necessary to be carried out to prove this investigation. As expected, when the concentration of toluene is increased, the limited capacity of the adsorbent checks any further adsorption of toluene and hence the overall removal percentage decreases.

Adsorption isotherms

The distribution of toluene between the adsorbent and the toluene solution at equilibrium is important in establishing the capacity of the adsorbent for toluene removal from aqueous systems. The adsorption isotherms of toluene on both natural and modified diatomite are shown in Figure 9. It is clearly seen from Figure 9 showed that the amount of adsorbed toluene on natural diatomite was much lower than that of modified diatomite.

The experimental data obtained were evaluated by various isotherm models incorporating Langmuir, Freundlich [37-39] and Brunauer-Emmett-Teller (BET) [39-41] isotherms.

Langmuir isotherm is applicable for monolayer adsorption on a surface containing a finite number of identical adsorption sites [42,43]. A linear expression for the Langmuir isotherm is as follows:

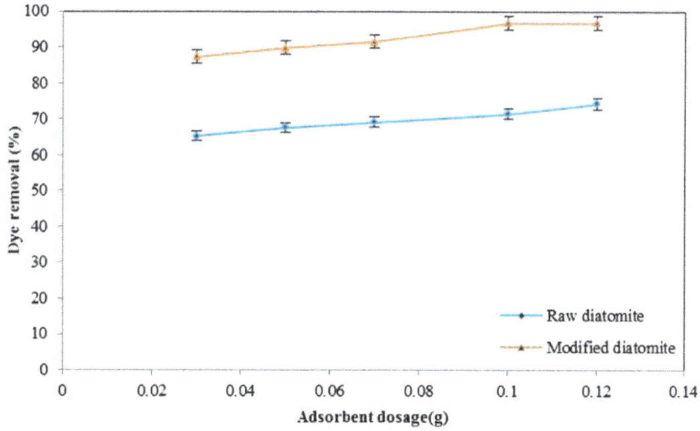

Figure 6 Effect of adsorbent dosage on the removal percentage of toluene by natural and modified diatomite, Temperature = *25 1C* , initial toluene concentration = *150 mg/L*, *pH = 6*, agitation speed = *200 rpm*.

$$1/q_e \quad \left(\frac{1}{K_L Q_0}\right) 1/C_e \quad 1/Q_0 \qquad 3$$

Where C_e is the concentration of toluene under equilibrium condition (*mg/L*), q_e denotes the amount of toluene adsorbed at equilibrium (*mg/g*), Q_0 indicates the maximum adsorption capacity and K_L is the Langmuir isotherm constant (*L/mg*). The values of K_L and Q_0 were calculated from the slope and intercept of the linear plot of $1/q_e$ versus $1/C_e$.

Freundlich equation was also applied for the adsorption of toluene on diatomite as given below:

$$q_e \quad K_F C_e^{\frac{1}{n}} \qquad 4$$

Where C_e is the equilibrium toluene concentration in aqueous system (*mg/L*), q_e is the amount of toluene adsorbed per weight of the adsorbent used (*mg/g*), K_F and n are Freundlich isotherm constants incorporating all factors affecting the adsorption process. Taking $\log_{10}$ from both sides of the Eq. (4) yields the following equation:

$$\log_{10} q_e \quad \log_{10} K_F \quad \frac{1}{n} \log_{10} C_e \qquad 5$$

Linear plot of $\log_{10} q_e$ versus $\log_{10} C_e$ gives the values of K_F and n.

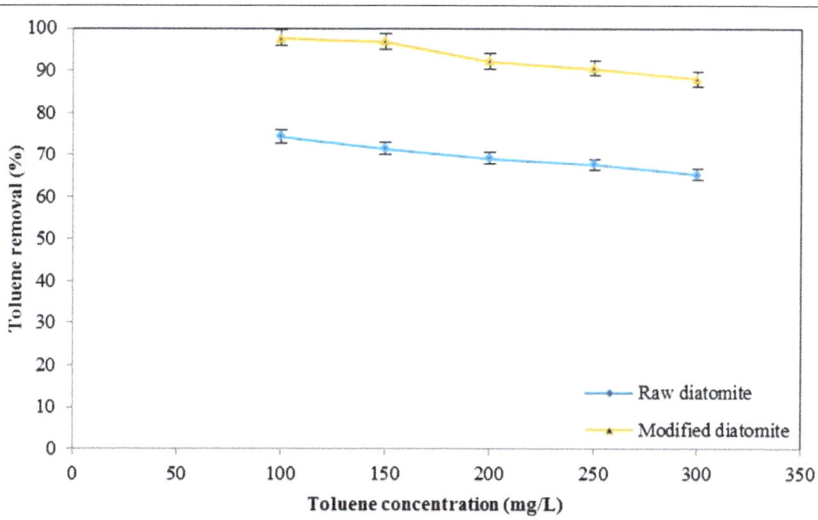

Figure 7 Effect of initial toluene concentration on adsorption of toluene by natural and modified diatomite, Contact time = *90 min*, Temperature = *25 1C* , *pH = 6*, agitation speed = *200 rpm*.

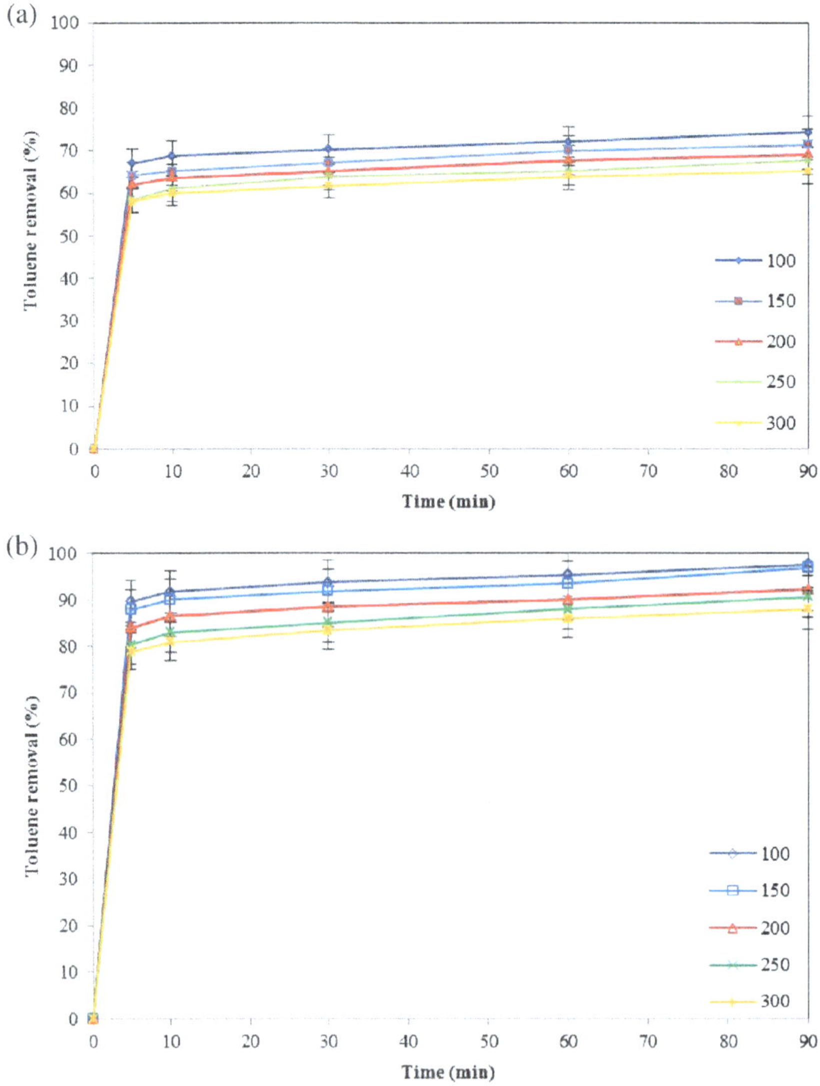

Figure 8 Effect of contact time on adsorption of toluene on (a) natural and (b) modified diatomite, Equilibrium time = *90 min*, *pH* = *6*, agitation speed = *200 rpm*, adsorbent dosage = *0.1 g*.

Brunauer-Emmett-Teller (BET) model was also used to fit the adsorption data according to the linear form of its rearranged adsorption isotherm model, which may be expressed as:

$$\frac{C_e}{C_s - C_e\ q_e} \qquad \frac{1}{K_b q_m} \qquad \left(\frac{K_b - 1}{K_b q_m}\right)\left(\frac{C_e}{C_s}\right) \qquad 6$$

where C_e is the concentration of toluene in solution (*mg/L*), C_s denotes the saturation concentration of toluene (*mg/L*), q_e is the amount of toluene adsorbed per weight of the diatomite used (*mg/g*), q_m is the amount of toluene adsorbed in forming a complete monolayer (*mg/g*), K_b indicates a constant explaining the energy of interaction with the surface. The values of K_b and q_m were calculated from the slope and intercept of the linear plot of $\left(\frac{C_e}{C_S - C_e}\right)\frac{1}{q_e}$ versus $\frac{C_e}{C_S}$.

The Q_0, K_L, r_1^2 (correlation coefficient for Langmuir isotherm), K_F, $1/n$, r_2^2 (correlation coefficient for Freundlich isotherm), K_b, q_m and r_3^2 (correlation coefficient for BET isotherm) are given in Table 2. The negative values of K_b related to the BET isotherm model describe that the adsorption process for natural diatomite did not follow the BET isotherm model, since this constant is indicative of the surface binding energy. In addition, standard statistics

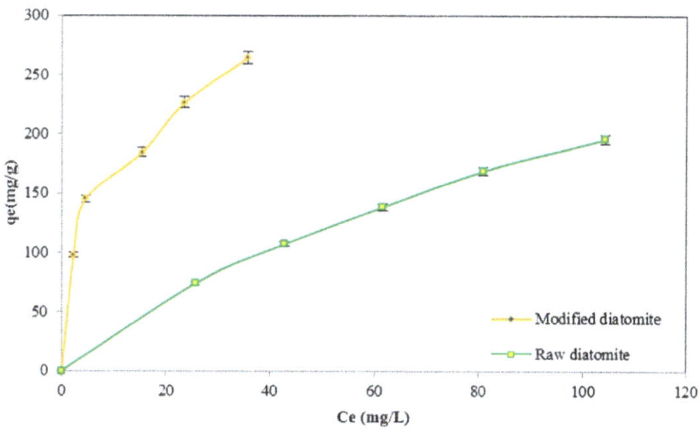

Figure 9 Adsorption isotherms of toluene onto natural and modified diatomite.

of root mean squared error (RMSE) was carried out to support the best fit adsorption model. RMSE can be expressed as:

$$RMSE \quad \left[\frac{1}{n}\sum\left(q_p - q_O\right)^2\right]^{\frac{1}{2}} \qquad 7$$

Where q_p is the predicted sorption capacity (mg/g), q_o is the observed sorption capacity (mg/g) and n is the number of samples. Thus, based on the high r^2 and low RMSE values, the results present that the adsorption of BR 46 on the natural diatomite and the NONMD follow the Langmuir model and the BET model, respectively [27]. It is evident from Table 2 that the isotherm data for the adsorption of toluene by natural diatomite were best-fitted using Langmuir model with a correlation coefficient of *0.997*. Furthermore, the Freundlich model is most appropriate for the adsorption of toluene on modified diatomite with a correlation coefficient of *0.998*.

Adsorption kinetics

The prediction of the adsorption kinetics of toluene from aqueous system is important in order to design a suitable treatment system. The kinetics of adsorption of toluene on diatomite may be described by the pseudo-first-order Lagergren rate equation [43-45] and the pseudo-second-order rate expression developed by Ho and McKay [46-49]. The Lagergren equation is:

$$\log\ q_e - q_t \qquad \log q_e - \frac{K_{1,ad}}{2.303}\, t \qquad 8$$

Where q_e and q_t are the amounts of toluene (mg/g) adsorbed at equilibrium and at time t (min) and $K_{1,ad}$ is the pseudo-first-order rate constant ($1/min$) [49].

The Ho and McKay equation is given below:

$$\frac{t}{q_t} \qquad \frac{1}{K_{2,ad}\, q_e^2} \qquad \frac{t}{q_c} \qquad 9$$

Where q_e and q_t are the amounts of toluene (mg/g) adsorbed at equilibrium and at time t (min) and $K_{2,ad}$ is the rate constant of the pseudo-second -order model ($g/mg.min$) [49].

Linear plot of $\log_{10}(q_e - q_t)$ against t gives the rate constant of $K_{1,ad}$ Moreover, the value of $K_{2,ad}$ is obtained from the intercept of the linear plot of t/q_t versus t. Adsorption kinetics constants of the pseudo-first-order and pseudo-second-order models at pH *6*, temperature *25 1C*, an agitation speed of 200 rpm, an initial concentration of 150 mg/L and for a time period of *90 min* are given in Table 3. From Table 3, the high values of correlation coefficients of the pseudo-second-order model for both natural and modified diatomite showed that the

Table 2 Parameters of various isotherms for adsorption of toluene onto natural diatomite and NONMD

	Langmuir				Freundlich				BET			
Adsorbent	Q_0	K_L	r_1^2	RMSE	K_F	1/n	r_2^2	RMSE	K_b	q_m	r_3^2	RMSE
Natural	263.150	0.008	0.997	0.250	7.760	0.697	0.970	0.410	0.873	1.922	0.819	0.490
NONMD	400.000	0.256	0.976	0.320	78.144	0.336	0.998	0.210	11.520	0.128	0.886	0.310

Table 3 Kinetics constants for toluene adsorption by natural diatomite and NONMD

	Pseudo-first-order				Pseudo-second-order			
Adsorbent	q_e (mg/g)	$K_{1,ad}$ (1/min)	R^2	RMSE	q_e (mg/g)	$K_{2,ad}$ (g/mg min)	R^2	RMSE
Natural	49.653	0.654	0.875	0.121	123.451	0.018	0.991	0.114
NONMD	73.345	0.873	0.888	0.117	193.431	0.053	0.993	0.111

adsorption data conformed well to the Ho and McKay kinetics model [Eq. (8)].

Conclusions

Diatomite has been studied for the removal of toluene from aqueous solution. Modification treatment of the adsorbent with nickel oxide nanoparticles was useful and its adsorption capacity increased. The adsorption process was not influenced by solution pH and used natural pH of the solutions. It was found that in order to obtain the highest possible removal of toluene, the experiments can be carried out at pH 6, temperature *25C* , an agitation speed of *200 rpm*, an initial toluene concentration of *150 mg/L*, a centrifugal rate of *4000 rpm*, adsorbent dosage = *0.1 g* and a process time of *90 min*. The results of this work show that the maximum percentage removal of toluene from aqueous solution in the optimum conditions for NONMD was *96.91%* (*145.36 mg/g*). Furthermore, under same conditions, the maximum adsorption of natural diatomite was *71.45%* (*107.18 mg/g*).

The most important thing to design and run an industrial adsorption plant is the knowledge of adsorption kinetics and isotherms. Hence, the experimental results were analyzed by using the Langmuir, Freundlich and BET equations. Equilibrium data for the adsorption of toluene by natural diatomite fit well to the Langmuir isotherm model. Furthermore, the Freundlich model is most appropriate for the adsorption of toluene on NONMD. In addition, the rate of adsorption process for both of them obeys the pseudo-second-order kinetics model.

Symbols used

C_0 $[mg\ L^{-1}]$ initial concentration of toluene
C_e $[mg\ L^{-1}]$ residual concentration at equilibrium
C_s $[mg\ L^{-1}]$ saturation concentration of toluene
$K_{1,ad}$ $[min^{-1}]$ rate constant of Pseudo-first-order
$K_{2,ad}$ $[min^{-1}]$ rate constant of Pseudo-second-order
k_F $[(mg\ g^{-1})(mg\ L^{-1})^{-1/n}]$ Freundlich constant
k_L $[L\ mg^{-1}]$ Langmuir constant
k_b [ ] BET constant
m $[g]$ mass of adsorbent used
n [ ] parameter indicating the intensity of adsorption
q_e $[mg\ g^{-1}]$ residual amount adsorbed at equilibrium
q_p $[mg\ g^{-1}]$ predicted sorption capacity
q_o $[mg\ g^{-1}]$ observed sorption capacity
Q_o $[mg\ g^{-1}]$ maximum sorption capacity
r^2 [ ] correlative coefficient for all models
V $[L]$ volume of toluene solution

Competing interests

The authors declare that they have no competing interests.

Authors contributions

The overall implementation of this study including design, experiments and data analysis, and manuscript preparation were the results of efforts by all of the authors. All authors have made extensive contribution into the review and finalization of this manuscript. All authors read and approved the final manuscript.

Acknowledgments

The authors are thankful to Petroleum University of Technology for providing the financial help and to Institute for Color Science and Technology (ICST), for supporting this research.

Author details

[1]School of Chemical Engineering, College of Engineering, University of Tehran, Tehran, Iran. [2]Department of Chemical Engineering, Tarbiat Modares University, Tehran, Iran. [3]Ahwaz Faculty of Petroleum, Petroleum University of Technology (PUT), Ahwaz, Iran. [4]Department of Environmental Researches, Institute for Color Science and Technology (ICST), Tehran, Iran.

References

1. Bouhamra WS, Baker CGJ, Elkilani AS, Alkandari AA, Al-Mansour AAA: **Adsorption of toluene and 1,1,1-trichloroethane on selected adsorbents under a range of ambient conditions.** *Adsorption* 2009, **15:**461 475.
2. Toh YC, Yen JJL, Jeffrey PO, Ting YP: **Decolourisation of azo dyes by whiterot fungi (WRF) isolated in Singapore.** *Enzyme Microb Technol* 2003, **35:**569 575.
3. Sivaraj R, Namasivayam C, Kadirvelu K: **Orange peel as an adsorbent in theremoval of acid violet 17 (acid dye) from aqueous solutions.** *Waste Manage* 2001, **21:**105 110.
4. Nacera Y, Aicha B: **Equilibrium and kinetic modelling of methylene blue sorption by pretreated dead Streptomyces rimosus: effect of temperature.** *Chem Eng J* 2006, **119:**121 125.
5. Zhang Y, Chen X, Bi HT S: **Application of wave propagation theory to adsorption breakthrough studies of toluene on activated carbon fiber beds.** *Carbon* 2010, **48:**2317 2326.
6. Khraisheh MAM, Al-Ghouti MA, Allen SJ, Ahmad MN: **Effect of OH and Silanol groups in the removal of dyes from aqueous solution using diatomite.** *Water Res* 2005, **39:**922 932.
7. Khalighi Sheshdeh R, Khosravi Nikou MR, Badii KH, Mohammadzadeh S: **Evaluation of Adsorption Kinetics and Equilibrium for the Removal of Benzene by Modified Diatomite.** *Chem Eng Technol* 2013, **36:**1713 1720.
8. Hachem C, Bocquillon F, Zahraa O, Bouchy M: **Decolourization of textile industry wastewater by the photocatalytic degradation process.** *Dyes Pigments* 2001, **49:**117 125.
9. Mahmoodi NM, Arami M, Yousefi Limaee N, Salman Tabrizi N: **Decolorization and aromatic ring degradation kinetics of Direct Red 80 by UV oxidation in the presence of hydrogen peroxide utilizing TiO_2 as a photocatalyst.** *Chem Eng J* 2005, **112:**191 196.
10. Pearce CL, Lloyd JR, Guthrie JT: **The removal of colour from textile wastewater using whole bacterial cells: a review.** *Dyes Pigments* 2003, **58:**179 196.

11. Vlyssides AG, Loizidou M, Karlis PK, Zorpas AA, Papaioannou D: **Electrochemical oxidation of a textile dye wastewater using a Pt/Ti electrode.** *J Hazard Mater* 1999, **70:**41 52.
12. Khattri SD, Singh MK: **Colour removal from synthetic dye wastewater using a bioadsorbent.** *Water Air Soil Pollut* 2000, **120:**283 294.
13. Benkli YE, Can MF, Turan M, elik MS: **Modification of organo-zeolite surface for the removal of reactive azo dyes in fixed-bed reactors.** *Water Res* 2005, **39:**487 493.
14. Shawabkeh RA, Tutunji MF: **Experimental study and modelling of basic dye sorption by diatomaceous clay.** *Applied Clay Sci* 2003, **24:**111 120.
15. Gong R, Ding Y, Li M, Yang C, Liu H, Sun Y: **Utilization of powdered peanut hull as biosorbent for removal of anionic dyes from aqueous solution.** *Dyes Pigments* 2005, **64:**187 192.
16. Fu Y, Viraraghavan T: **Removal of Congo Red from an aqueous solution by fungus Aspergillus niger.** *Adv Environ Res* 2002, **7:**239 247.
17. Gucek A, Sener S, Bilgen S, Mazmanci ML: **Adsorption and kinetic studies of cationic and anionic dyes on pyrophyllite from aqueous solutions.** *J Colloid Interf Sci* 2005, **286:**53 60.
18. Wang S, Boyjoo Y, Choueib A, Zhu ZH: **Removal of dyes from aqueous solution using fly ash and red mud.** *Water Res* 2005, **39:**129 138.
19. Netpradit S, Thiravetyan P, Towprayoon S: **Adsorption of three azo reactive dyes by metal hydroxide sludge: effect of temperature, pH, and electrolytes.** *J Colloid Interf Sci* 2004, **270:**255 261.
20. Pala A, Tokat E: **Color removal from cotton textile industry wastewater in an activated sludge system with various additives.** *Water Res* 2002, **36:**2920 2925.
21. Aksu Z: **Application of biosorption for the removal of organic pollutants: a review.** *Process Biochem* 2005, **40:**997 1026.
22. Shawabkeh R, Al-Harahsheh A, Al-Otoom A: **Copper and zinc sorption by treated oil shale ash.** *Sep Purif Technol* 2004, **40:**251 257.
23. Lin YH, Leu JY: **Kinetics of reactive azo-dye decolorization by Pseudomonas luteola in a biological activated carbon process.** *Biochem Eng J* 2008, **39:**457 467.
24. Annadurai G, Juang RS, Lee DJ: **Factorial design analysis for adsorption of dye on activated carbon beads incorporated with calcium alginate.** *Adv Environ Res* 2002, **6:**191 198.
25. Chakraborty S, De S, Das Gupta S, Basu JK: **Adsorption study for the removal of a basic dye: experimental and modeling.** *Chemosphere* 2005, **58:**1079 1086.
26. Deniz F, Karaman S: **Removal of Basic Red 46 dye from aqueous solution by pine tree leaves.** *Chem Eng J* 2011, **170.**67 74.
27. Deniz F, Saygideger SD: **Removal of a hazardous azo dye (Basic Red 46) from aqueous solution by princess tree leaf.** *Desalin* 2011, **268:**6 11.
28. Bennani Karim A, Mounir B, Hachkar M, Bakasse M, Yaacoubi A: **Removal of Basic Red 46 dye from aqueous solution by adsorption onto Moroccan clay.** *J Hazard Mater* 2009, **168:**304 309.
29. Olgun A, Atar N: **Equilibrium and kinetic adsorption study of Basic Yellow 28 and Basic Red 46 by a boron industry waste.** *J Hazard Mater* 2009, **161:**148 156.
30. Zaitana H, Korrir A, Chafik T, Bianchi D: **Evaluation of the potential of volatile organic compound (di-methylbenzene) removal using adsorption on natural minerals compared to commercial oxides.** *J Hazard Mater* 2013, **262:**365 376.
31. Aivalioti M, Vamvasakis I, Gidarakos E: **BTEX and MTBE adsorption onto natural and thermally modified diatomite.** *J Hazard Mater* 2010, **178:**136 143.
32. Aivalioti M, Papoulias P, Kousaiti A, Gidarakos E: **Adsorption of BTEX, MTBE and TAME on natural and modified diatomite.** *J Hazard Mater* 2012, **207 208:**117 127.
33. Senturk HB, Ozdes D, Duran C: **Biosorption of Rhodamine 6G from aqueous solutions onto almond shell (Prunus dulcis) as a low cost biosorbent.** *Desalin* 2010, **252:**81 87.
34. Senthil Kumar P, Ramalingam S, Senthamarai C, Niranjanaa M, Vijayalakshmi P, Sivanesan S: **Adsorption of dye from aqueous solution by cashew nut shell: studies on equilibrium isotherm kinetics and thermodynamics of interactions.** *Desalin* 2010, **261:**52 60.
35. Khraisheh MAM, Al-degs YS, Mcminn WAM: **A remediation of wastewater containing heavy metals using natural and modified diatomite.** *Chem Eng J* 2004, **99:**177 184.
36. Allen SJ, Gan Q, Matthews R, Johnson PA: **Comparison of optimised isotherm models for basic dye adsorption by kuzdu.** *Bioresour Technol* 2003, **88:**143 152.
37. Bhattacharyya KG, Sarma A: **Adsorption characteristics of the dye, Brilliant green, on Neem leaf powder.** *Dyes Pigments* 2003, **57:**211 222.
38. Demir H, Top A, Balkose D, Ulku S: **Dye adsorption behaviour of Luffa cylindrical fibers.** *J Hazard Mater* 2008, **153:**389 394.
39. Hameed BH: **Equilibrium and kinetic studies of methyl violet sorption by agricultural waste.** *J Hazard Mater* 2008, **154:**204 212.
40. Arami M, Limaee NY, Mahmoodi NM, Tabrizi NS: **Equilibrium and kinetics studies for the adsorption of direct and acid dyes from aqueous solution by soymeal hull.** *J Hazard Mater* 2006, **B135:**171 179.
41. Ferrero F: **Dye removal by low cost adsorbents: hazelnut shells in comparison with wood sawdust.** *J Hazard Mater* 2007, **142:**144 152.
42. Khalighi Sheshdeh R, Khosravi Nikou MR, Badii KH, Yousefi Limaee N: **Adsorption of Acid Blue 92 Dye on Modified Diatomite by Nickel Oxide Nanoparticles in Aqueous Solutions.** *Prog Color Colorants Coat* 2012, **5:**101 116.
43. Al-Degs Y, Khraisheh MAM, Tutunji MF: **Sorption of lead ions on diatomite and manganese oxides modified diatomite.** *Water Res* 2001, **35:**3724 3733.
44. Al-Ghouti M, Khraisheh MAM, Ahmad MNM, Allen S: **Thermodynamic behaviour and the effect of temperature on the removal of dyes from aqueous solution using modified diatomite. A kinetic study.** *J Colloid Interf Sci* 2005, **287:**6 13.
45. Colgecen G, Erdem E, Donat R: **The removal of Textile Dyes by Diatomite Earth.** *J Colloid interf Sci* 2005, **282:**314 319.
46. Hayat K, Gondal MA, Khaled MM, Ahmed S: **Effect of Operational Key Parameters on Photocatalytic Degradation of Phenol using Nano Nickel Oxide Synthesized by Sol Gel Method J.** *Mol Catal A- Chem* 2011, **336:**64 71.
47. Badii K, Doulati Ardejani F, Aziz Saberi M, Yousefi Limaee N, Shafaei SZ: **Adsorption of Acid blue 25 dye on diatomite in aqueous solutions.** *Indian J Chem Technol* 2010, **17:**7 11.
48. Mahmoodi NM: **Photocatalytic ozonation of dyes using copper ferrite nanoparticle prepared by co-precipitation method.** *Desalin* 2011, **279:**332 337.
49. Khalighi Sheshdeh R, Khosravi Nikou MR, Badii KH, Yousefi Limaee N, Golkarnarenji G: **Equilibrium and kinetics studies for the adsorption of Basic Red 46 on nickel oxide nanoparticles-modified diatomite in aqueous solutions.** *J Taiwan Ins Chem Eng* 2014, **45:**1792 1802.

Permissions

All chapters in this book were first published in JEHSE, by BioMed Central; hereby published with permission under the Creative Commons Attribution License or equivalent. Every chapter published in this book has been scrutinized by our experts. Their significance has been extensively debated. The topics covered herein carry significant findings which will fuel the growth of the discipline. They may even be implemented as practical applications or may be referred to as a beginning point for another development.

The contributors of this book come from diverse backgrounds, making this book a truly international effort. This book will bring forth new frontiers with its revolutionizing research information and detailed analysis of the nascent developments around the world.

We would like to thank all the contributing authors for lending their expertise to make the book truly unique. They have played a crucial role in the development of this book. Without their invaluable contributions this book wouldn't have been possible. They have made vital efforts to compile up to date information on the varied aspects of this subject to make this book a valuable addition to the collection of many professionals and students.

This book was conceptualized with the vision of imparting up-to-date information and advanced data in this field. To ensure the same, a matchless editorial board was set up. Every individual on the board went through rigorous rounds of assessment to prove their worth. After which they invested a large part of their time researching and compiling the most relevant data for our readers.

The editorial board has been involved in producing this book since its inception. They have spent rigorous hours researching and exploring the diverse topics which have resulted in the successful publishing of this book. They have passed on their knowledge of decades through this book. To expedite this challenging task, the publisher supported the team at every step. A small team of assistant editors was also appointed to further simplify the editing procedure and attain best results for the readers.

Apart from the editorial board, the designing team has also invested a significant amount of their time in understanding the subject and creating the most relevant covers. They scrutinized every image to scout for the most suitable representation of the subject and create an appropriate cover for the book.

The publishing team has been an ardent support to the editorial, designing and production team. Their endless efforts to recruit the best for this project, has resulted in the accomplishment of this book. They are a veteran in the field of academics and their pool of knowledge is as vast as their experience in printing. Their expertise and guidance has proved useful at every step. Their uncompromising quality standards have made this book an exceptional effort. Their encouragement from time to time has been an inspiration for everyone.

The publisher and the editorial board hope that this book will prove to be a valuable piece of knowledge for researchers, students, practitioners and scholars across the globe.

List of Contributors

Azadeh Tofighi and Shohreh Zare Karizi
Department of Biology, Varamin-Pishva Branch, Islamic Azad University, Pishva, Iran

Mahnaz Mazaheri Assadi
Departments of Biotechnology, Iranian Research Organization for Science and Technology, Tehran, Iran

Mohammad Hosein Arash Asadirad
Departments of Microbiology, Zanjan Branch, Islamic Azad University, Zanjan, Iran

Fariborz Omidi
Department of Occupational Health Engineering, School of Public Health, Shahroud University of Medical Sciences, Shahroud, Iran

Mohammad Behbahani and Hamid Sadeghi Abandansari
Department of Chemistry, Shahid Beheshti University, Tehran, Iran

Alireza Sedighi
Department of Occupational Health, School of Public Health, Tehran University of Medical Sciences, Tehran, Iran

Seyed Jamaleddin Shahtaheri
Department of Occupational Health Engineering, School of Public Health and Institute for Environmental Research, Tehran University of Medical Sciences, Tehran, Iran

Pranas Baltrėnas and Antonas Misevičius
Institute of Environmental Protection, Vilnius Gediminas Technical University, Vilnius, Lithuania

Afshin Maleki and Shiva Zandi
Kurdistan Environmental Health Research Center, Kurdistan University of Medical Sciences, Sanandaj, Iran

Hassan Amini
Department of Epidemiology and Public Health, Swiss Tropical and Public Health Institute (Swiss TPH), Socinstrasse 57, 4002 Basel, Switzerland
University of Basel, Petersplatz 1, 4003 Basel, Switzerland
Kurdistan Environmental Health Research Center, Kurdistan University of Medical Sciences, Sanandaj, Iran

Shahrokh Nazmara
Department of Environmental Health Engineering, School of Public Health, Tehran University of Medical Sciences, Tehran, Iran

Amir Hossein Mahvi
Department of Environmental Health Engineering, School of Public Health, Tehran University of Medical Sciences, Tehran, Iran
Center for Solid Waste Research (CSWR), Institute for Environmental Research (IER), Tehran University of Medical Sciences, Tehran, Iran

Marta Gmurek, Magdalena Olak-Kucharczyk and Stanisław Ledakowicz
Faculty of Process and Environmental Engineering, Department of Bioprocess Engineering, Lodz University of Technology, Wolczanska 213, 90-924 Lodz, Poland

Maryam Habibi and Mehry Esvand
Department of Environmental Health Engineering, School of Health, Arak University of Medical Sciences, Arak, Iran

Behrooz Karimi
Department of Environmental Health Engineering, School of Health, Arak University of Medical Sciences, Arak, Iran
Department of Environmental Health Engineering, School of Health, Tehran University of Medical Sciences, Tehran, Iran

Alireza Mesdaghinia, Simin Nasseri and Mahdi Hadi
Center for Water Quality Research (CWQR), Institute for Environmental Research (IER), Tehran University of Medical Sciences, Tehran, Iran

Amir Hossein Mahvi
Department of Environmental Health Engineering, Faculty of Health, Tehran University of Medical Sciences, Tehran, Iran
Center for Solid Waste Research (CSWR), Institute for Environmental Research (IER), Tehran University of Medical Sciences, Tehran, Iran

Hamid Reza Tashauoei
Department of Environmental Health Engineering, School of Public Health, Islamic Azad University-Tehran Medical Branch, Tehran, Iran

Samaneh Saber-Samandari and Jalil Heydaripour
Department of Chemistry, Eastern Mediterranean University, TRNC via Mersin 10, Gazimagusa, Turkey

Mahdi Farzadkia, Ali Esrafili and Mehdi Shirzad-Siboni
Department of Environmental Health Engineering, School of public Health, Iran University of Medical Sciences, Tehran, Iran

Edris Bazrafshan
Health Promotion Research Center, Zahedan University of Medical Sciences, Zahedan, Iran

Jae-Kyu Yang
Divisions of General Education, Kwangwoon University, Seoul 139-701, South Korea

Neda Molaee
Department of Microbiology and Immunology, Arak University of Medical sciences, Arak, Iran

Hamid Abtahi
Molecular and Medicine Research Center, Arak University of Medical Sciences, Arak, Iran

Mohammad Javad Ghannadzadeh
Department of Environmental Health, Faculty of Health, Arak University of Medical Sciences, Arak, Iran

Masoude Karimi
Department of Medical Microbiology and Immunology, Arak University of Medical sciences, Arak, Iran

Ehsanollah Ghaznavi-Rad
Molecular and Medicine Research Center, Arak University of Medical Sciences, Arak, Iran
Department of Medical Microbiology and Immunology, Faculty of Medicine, Arak University of Medical Sciences, Arak, Iran

Sara Taghizadeh, Hossein Najmabadi and Farkhondeh Behjati
Genetics Research Center, University of Social Welfare and Rehabilitation Sciences, Tehran, Iran

Koorosh Kamali
Department of Public Health, School of Public Health, Zanjan University of Medical Sciences, Zanjan, Iran

Reza Rezaee, Ramin Nabizadeh and Shahrokh Nazmara
Department of Environmental Health Engineering, School of Public Health, Tehran University of Medical Sciences, Tehran, Iran

Simin Nasseri
Center for Water Quality Research, Institute for Environmental Research, Tehran University of Medical Sciences, Tehran, Iran
Department of Environmental Health Engineering, School of Public Health, Tehran University of Medical Sciences, Tehran, Iran

Amir Hossein Mahvi
Department of Environmental Health Engineering, School of Public Health, Tehran University of Medical Sciences, Tehran, Iran
Center for Solid Waste Research, Institute for Environmental Research, Tehran University of Medical Sciences, Tehran, Iran

National Institute of Health Research, Tehran University of Medical Sciences, Tehran, Iran

Seyyed Abbas Mousavi
Department of Chemical and Petroleum Engineering, Sharif University of Technology, Tehran, Iran

Alimorad Rashidi
Nanotechnology Research Center, Research Institute of Petroleum Industry (RIPI), Tehran, Iran

Ali Jafari
Department of Environmental Health Engineering, School of Public Health, Lorestan University of Medical Sciences, Khorramabad, Iran

Ahed Zyoud, Amani Zu'bi and Hikmat S. Hilal
SSERL, Department of Chemistry, An-Najah National University, Nablus, Palestine

Muath H. S. Helal
College of Pharmacy and Nutrition, University of Saskatchewan, 116 Thorvaldson Building, Saskatoon S7N 5C9, Canada

DaeHoon Park
Dansuk Industrial Co, LTD. #1239-5, Jeongwang-Dong, Shiheung-Si, Kyonggi-Do 429-913, South Korea

Guy Campet
Institut de Chimie de la Matie're Condense'ıe de Bordeaux (ICMCB), 87 Avenue du Dr. A Schweitzer, Pessac 33608, France

Hai Yan
College of Landscape Architecture, Beijing Forestry University, Beijing 100083, China
School of Landscape Architecture, Zhejiang Agriculture and Forestry University, Lin'an, Zhejiang 311300, China

Li Dong
College of Landscape Architecture, Beijing Forestry University, Beijing 100083, China

Ali Jafari and Ramin Nabizadeh
Department of Environmental Health Engineering, School of Public Health, Tehran University of Medical Sciences, Tehran, Iran

Amir Hossein Mahvi
Center for Water Quality Research (CWQR), Institute for Environmental Research (IER), Tehran University of Medical Sciences, Tehran, Iran
Department of Environmental Health Engineering, School of Public Health, Tehran University of Medical Sciences, Tehran, Iran
Center for Solid Waste Research (CSWR), Institute for Environmental Research (IER), Tehran University of Medical Sciences, Tehran, Iran

Simin Nasseri
Center for Water Quality Research (CWQR), Institute for Environmental Research (IER), Tehran University of Medical Sciences, Tehran, Iran
Department of Environmental Health Engineering, School of Public Health, Tehran University of Medical Sciences, Tehran, Iran

Alimorad Rashidi
Nanotechnology Research Institute of Petroleum Industry (RIPI), West Blvd. Azadi Sport Complex, Tehran, Iran

Reza Rezaee
Kurdistan Environmental Health Research Center, Kurdistan University of Medical Sciences, Sanandaj, Iran

Shervin Jamshidi
Department of Environmental Engineering, Faculty of Environment, University of Tehran, Tehran, Iran

Abbas Akbarzadeh
Water Research Institute (WRI), Tehran, Iran

Kwang-Sung Woo and Alireza Valipour
Department of Civil Engineering, Yeungnam University, Gyungsan, South Korea

Stefan-Adrian Strungaru, Mircea Nicoara and Gabriel Plavan
Department of Biology, "Alexandru Ioan Cuza" University of Iasi, Faculty of Biology, 700505 Iasi, Romania

Oana Jitar
Department of Environmental Engineering and Management, "Gheorghe Asachi" Technical University of Iasi, 73, "Prof. Dr. D. Mangeron" Street, 700050 Iasi, Romania

Robert Pintaric, Joze Matela
Department of Radiology, University Medical Centre Maribor, Maribor, Slovenia

Stefan Pintaric
University of Ljubljana, Veterinary faculty, Ljubljana, Slovenia

Kanayochukwu C Ajah, Joel Ademiluyi and Chidozie C Nnaji
Department of Civil Engineering, University of Nigeria, Nsukka, Enugu StateNigeria

Zohreh Ghaemi, Faramarz Moattar, Amirhesam Hassani and Nematollah Khorasani
Department of Environmental Science, Graduate School of the Environment and Energy, Science and Research Branch, Islamic Azad University, Tehran, Iran

Abdolreza Karbassi
Graduate Faculty of Environment, University of Tehran, P.O. Box 14155-6135 Tehran, Iran

Ricardo A. Melo, Roberto L. Pimentel, Diego M. Lacerda and Wekisley M. Silva
Department of Civil and Environmental Engineering, Federal University of Paraíba, Campus I, Cidade Universitária, 58051-900 João Pessoa, Brazil

Ata Rafiee, Amirhosein Mahvi and Kamyar Yaghmaeian
Center for Solid Waste Research (CSWR), Institute for Environmental Research (IER), Tehran University of Medical Sciences, Tehran, Iran
Department of Environmental Health Engineering, School of Public Health, Tehran University of Medical Sciences, Tehran, Iran

Mohammad Hoseini
Department of Environmental Health Engineering, School of Public Health, Shiraz University of Medical Sciences, Shiraz, Iran

Saeid Parmy
Department of Environmental Health Engineering, School of Public Health, Tehran University of Medical Sciences, Tehran, Iran

Masud Yunesian and Ramin Nabizadeh
Department of Environmental Health Engineering, School of Public Health, Tehran University of Medical Sciences, Tehran, Iran
Center for Air Pollution Research (CAPR), Institute for Environmental Research (IER), Tehran University of Medical Sciences, Tehran, Iran

Mehran Khaefi
Environmental and occupational health center, Ministry of health medical education, Tehran, Iran

Kareem Hatam-Nahavandi, Hossein Keshavarz, Iraj Mobedi and Mostafa Rezaeian
Department of Medical Parasitology and Mycology, School of Public Health, Tehran University of Medical Sciences, Tehran, Iran

Amir Hossein Mahvi
Department of Environmental Health Engineering, School of Public Health, and Center for Water Quality Research, Institute for Environmental Research, Tehran University of Medical Sciences, Tehran, Iran

Mehdi Mohebali
Department of Medical Parasitology and Mycology, School of Public Health, Tehran University of Medical Sciences, Tehran, Iran
Center for Research of Endemic Parasites of Iran (CREPI), Tehran University of Medical Sciences, Tehran, Iran

Reza Khalighi Sheshdeh
School of Chemical Engineering, College of Engineering, University of Tehran, Tehran, Iran

Saeed Abbasizadeh
Department of Chemical Engineering, Tarbiat Modares University, Tehran, Iran

Mohammad Reza Khosravi Nikou and Mohammad Sadegh Sharafi
Ahwaz Faculty of Petroleum, Petroleum University of Technology (PUT), Ahwaz, Iran

Khashayar Badii
Department of Environmental Researches,Institute for Color Science and Technology (ICST), Tehran, Iran

Index

P

R

S

T

U

V

W